AIDS up to the year 2000

Research team:
Dr. F.M.L.G. van den Boom[1], project leader
Dr. J.C. Jager[2], project leader
D.P. Reinking[1]
M.J. Postma[2]
C.E.S. Albers[1]
[1] Netherlands Institute of Mental Health (NcGv)
[2] National Institute of Public Health and Environmental Protection (RIVM)

Scenario Committee on AIDS
Chairman: Prof. E.J. Ruitenberg

AIDS up to the year 2000

Epidemiological, Sociocultural and Economic Scenario Analysis for the Netherlands

Scenario report commissioned by the Steering Committee on Future Health Scenarios

Springer-Science+Business Media, B.V.

ISBN 978-0-7923-1895-8 ISBN 978-94-011-2848-3 (eBook)
DOI 10.1007/978-94-011-2848-3

Originally published by Kluwer Academic Publishers in 1992

Contents

Foreword

Three quarters of the total decline in mortality in the period 1850-1970 in the Western industrialized world may be attributed to a fall in mortality from infectious diseases. The success was so marked that in countries such as the Netherlands, infectious diseases constituted an ever-diminishing threat to public health. The totally unexpected epidemic of HIV infection and AIDS appears to represent a radical departure from this situation, as has indeed proved the case in the United States and Central Africa, where the mortality rate - especially among young adults - is once again rising rapidly (Chin, 1991).

In the Netherlands it appears that the effect of the epidemic on public health will remain containable. Here too, however, the advent of AIDS has been a shock, leading to a fundamental debate in health care and society in general, while there have also been considerable repercussions in the field of care and prevention and for patients' rights and scientific research. The scale and consequences are just beginning to become visible now, nearly ten years after the first Dutch AIDS case and five years after the introduction of a coherent AIDS policy.

AIDS is not just another infectious disease. In fact it is not even a disease, but a complex range of conditions which manifest themselves in combination, leading to death, by means of the steady decline and all but total elimination of the natural human immune system. This is brought about by the HIV virus, which often becomes discernible only after many years. In the early stages, the shock caused by AIDS is in large measure due to the shock at discovering that a potential fatal infection could have occurred unrecognised and remained so for such a long time. No defence was possible against such an invisible foe.

Defence has now become possible, though behaviour changes and measures to rule out exposure to the virus, but elimination of the virus or a cure for AIDS is not yet possible. AIDS is fatal and the prevailing view at present is that each HIV infection will ultimately lead to AIDS and, given enough time, death.

The socially disruptive nature of the infection is all the more pronounced because HIV is primarily transmitted by sexual contact and AIDS manifests itself particularly among young people: in Europe and the United States especially among homosexual males and injecting drug users, and in Africa among heterosexual men and women. Those confronted with the fatal disease form a young, vigorous and often well educated group of patients who will do all they can to stave off the inevitable.

The means of transmission and the inevitable consequences of HIV infection mean that the AIDS problem is more than just a social issue or a challenge for health care. AIDS touches on individial civil rights as well as the state's responsibility for protecting and promoting public health. In countries where AIDS is claiming many lives the economic, social and democratic consequences of the epidemic are becoming increasingly discernible (Mann, 1987; Turner et al., 1989). The risk of HIV infection means that reproduction, blood transfusions and medical interventions need extra safeguarding. AIDS creates difficulties for life insurance companies and their clients, imposes strains on gay emancipation and converts injecting drug users into a direct threat to public health. Now that AIDS is entering its second decade there is good reason to take stock of the situation and - in so far as possible - to look into the future. This is the essence of the AIDS scenario project. The retrospective analysis takes the form of baseline analyses. These analyses, which are divided into a socio-epidemiological, a sociocultural and an economic part, set out the results of literature studies and consultations with experts. Together these provide a single baseline analysis of ten years of AIDS in the Netherlands and the wide-ranging consequences for health care, prevention and society in general. At the same time this reconstruction of AIDS provides the basis for the projections in this report of the medium and long-term impact of AIDS.

Building on the methods of scenario research, this project has also developed its own methodology. This conceptual model specially devised for the AIDS scenario analysis describes the interrelationships between data drawn from epidemiological, economic and socio-scientific studies, which are then applied for the purposes of projections by applying a combination of mathematical simulations and data and insights from empirical research. This approach has enabled an overview to be provided of the epidemiological, economic and socio-cultural consequences, based where possible on recent insights and empirical data.

This methodological framework has been devised with a view to its continued usability in the future, in the sense that new research data can easily be integrated into the present or future mathematical models, thereby increasing the precision of the projections. Similarly developments in the field of medical technology can also be incorporated in such models.

The international nature of the project should also be emphasized. Among other things the Dutch scenario project on AIDS arises from a WHO initiative and the EC's Concerted Actions on AIDS. Dutch involvement has included participation in the "EC

Concerted Actions on Mathematical Modelling of AIDS" and the "Study on Economic Aspects of AIDS and HIV-infection", activities in the framework of the multinational study into the "Sociocultural and Economic Impact of AIDS on society" of the WHO in Copenhagen, and associated initiatives such as the EC-organized workshops on "Statistical Analysis and Mathematical Modelling of AIDS" and "AIDS-impact Assessment, Modelling and Scenario analysis" in Bilthoven in 1987 and 1989. The results of this project can be applied at both domestic and international level, thereby contributing towards greater knowledge and understanding of the consequences of AIDS and the further dissemination and refinement of the methodology for scenario analysis into the impact of AIDS.

This report is the fruit of two years' intensive study into the likely impact of AIDS in the medium and long term and, inextricably bound up with that, the necessary efforts to prevent the adverse implications of AIDS. On behalf of the Scenario Committee I hope that this report will make a contribution towards policy formulation in the field of AIDS, with the ultimate aim of banishing AIDS as a potential threat to public health.

Prof.dr. E.J. Ruitenberg
Chairman AIDS Scenario Committee

Summary

The scenario project "The Sociocultural and Economic Impact of AIDS" has been conducted under the aegis of the eponymous scenario committee by a research team drawn from the Netherlands Institute of Public Mental Health (NcGv) and the National Institute of Health and Environmental Protection (RIVM) on behalf of the Steering Committee on Future Health Scenarios (STG).

The project's terms of reference were four-fold:

1. *What is the likely incidence and prevalence of HIV/AIDS, if necessary subclassified into sub-epidemics, in the Netherlands in the short and medium term?*
2. *What impact will potential future trends in the epidemic have for health care and preventive policies?*
3. *What has been the sociocultural and economic impact of the AIDS epidemic and what consequences need to be anticipated in the future?*
4. *Which potential and realistic future situations may be formulated with respect to combating the AIDS epidemic and the treatment of HIV-infected persons, people with AIDS and groups heavily affected by AIDS?*

The research has been conducted by means of literature studies and the consultation of experts and with the aid of existing mathematical models. A conceptual model provided the framework for the research.

The research questions have been drawn up on the basis of a methodological framework for scenario analysis into the epidemiological, sociocultural and economic consequences of HIV/AIDS, building on the existing methodology of scenario research. The project focuses especially on the Dutch situation. In view of the complexity and wide-ranging nature of the AIDS problem - and given also the available research data - it was decided to develop ascenario analysis focused on risk behaviour, the effects of public information and education and promotion of behavioural changes, changes in the effects and organization of care and options for AIDS control. The scenario analysis has not been conducted with respect to such significant topics as changes in the size of the groups particularly at risk for HIV/AIDS, infectiousness of HIV, mobility aspects and the availability of a vaccine.

The reference point for analysing the consequences of AIDS is provided by the studies of the HIV/AIDS epidemic. The epidemiological trends are translated in terms of their economic impact and placed in the social context of the AIDS epidemic. The first scenario project, which is based around a disorder that can be transmitted by means of risk behaviour, is distinctly target-setting in nature. The exploratory scenarios provide an impression of possible consequences of AIDS that cannot be ruled out. In addition the exploratory scenarios have a target-setting component. Because AIDS control covers a number of undisputed goals such as combating the spread of HIV, the exploratory scenarios also indicate the extent to which AIDS control is achieving its goals. In doing so the exploratory scenarios indirectly provide an impression of present AIDS control strategies. By way of direct follow-up to the exploratory scenarios, alternative paths to the same goal are explored in the strategic scenarios.

The problem being addressed by the project has been tackled by means of a large number of scenarios: a reference scenario plus a separate subscenario, exploratory scenarios on behaviour, care and medical technology, and strategic scenarios on AIDS control and treatment. The reference scenario is based on the assumption that present trends will continue unchanged. One element of the reference scenario has been separated off to form a subscenario, which examines the consequences of the course taken by the HIV epidemic up to 1.1.1989. By analysing the subscenario in combination with the reference scenario an impression is obtained of the areas in which the consequences of AIDS can no longer be modified by interventions in the field of public information and education and promoting changes in behaviour.

The reference scenario and subscenario are worked out in terms of their economic consequences and linked to findings from the sociocultural baseline analysis. Alternative scenarios are devised by varying selected key parameters in the epidemiological, sociocultural and economic fields. The consequences of AIDS are then expressed both qualitatively and quantitatively in terms of indicators.

Mathematical simulations have been used in the scenario project for various purposes: describing and reconstructing the epidemiological pattern to date, estimating the number of HIV-infected persons, describing the distribution of the epidemic within and between groups and carrying out medium and long-term projections. The mathematical modelling has been separated into (1) statistical modelling of available data on the basis of empirical models and (2) dynamic population models.

The scenarios are based on three baseline analyses: (1) a baseline analysis of socio-epidemiological aspects; (2) a baseline analysis of sociocultural aspects; and (3) a baseline analysis of economic aspects. These baseline analyses provide a reconstruction of the consequences of and reaction towards AIDS to date and define the point of departure for the projections.

Baseline analysis of socio-epidemiological aspects
This analysis consists of a general section on influences on the course of the HIV/AIDS epidemic and a group-based reconstruction of the course of HIV/AIDS epidemic and the effects of HIV/AIDS prevention. On the reference date of 1.1.991, 1,531 people with AIDS have been recorded. Corrected for reporting delays this figure is expected to rise to 1,652. Some 50% of the cumulative number of people with AIDS are expected still to be alive. Only estimates are available on HIV incidence and prevalence in the Netherlands; as of 1.1.1989 the cumulative incidence was put at 6,000-8,000. The potential years of life lost (PYLL) per death due to AIDS is 33.7. This corresponds with the PYLL for road accidents and exceeds that for suicide, lung-cancer and infectious diseases other than AIDS.

Nearly 80% of people with AIDS consist of gay and bisexual men, while the remainder are primarily injecting drug users (IDU) and heterosexual contacts. The AIDS epidemic is beginning to spread less rapidly. The survival period of people with AIDS has been rising for a number of years and in 1989 had reached an average of 22 months.

The main risk factors for HIV infection are risky sexual contact - especially unprotected anal intercourse - and the shared use of injection equipment. The precise risk of HIV infection per contact or per partner cannot be established from the Dutch or international literature. A reasonable assumption for the speed of progression to AIDS would appear to be that 54% of HIV-infected persons develop AIDS 11 years after contamination with HIV.

With a view to scenario analysis and against the background of group-related differences in the spread of HIV/AIDS the following key data have been assembled: group size, the incidence of risky sexual contact and the number of sexual partners, the incidence of drug use and the shared use of injection equipment, the results of studies into developments in the HIV incidence and the effects of HIV/AIDS prevention. The baseline analysis also examines more specific points, varying from group to group, such as possible contacts with other risk groups and the possibilities of the national and international spread of HIV.

Among men who have sex with men a widespread change of behaviour occurred in a short space of time in response to HIV/-AIDS. Looking to the future it will obviously be important whether, and to what extent, the prevention effects will prove lasting. The most important preventive measure for IDUs consists of the new or accelerated needle-exchange programmes that have been set up on a large scale. While HIV/AIDS prevention activities may be said to have had an effect on IDUs, this does not amount to a large-scale and permanent change in behaviour. HIV does not appear to be spread wide scale among commercial sex workers; for the present the shared use of injection equipment among hard-drug using commercial sex workers is the most important risk factor. An independent epidemic of HIV infections among the heterosexual population is considered unlikely in the short term. In the longer term, however, a substantial spread of HIV among the heterosexual population cannot be ruled out. There is a brief examination of the special problems of people with haemophilia, health care workers, pregnant women and people from lower socio-economic categories.

Baseline analysis of sociocultural aspects
The baseline analysis examines the social context within which the AIDS epidemic has evolved and reconstructs the reaction to AIDS during the period 1982-1990.

It is noted that the advent of AIDS has not led to any radical break in patterns of sexuality and sexual behaviour, some of which was established decades ago. The age of first sexual contact has continued to decline, the number of sexual partners throughout life has remained reasonably constant and sexual contact remains closely linked to exclusive (in some cases short-lived) relationships. Instead of repression, AIDS appears if anything to have led to greater openness in the field of sexuality. With respect to the spread of HIV, socio-sexual research suggests that on the one hand a widespread dissemination of HIV is improbable in the short term, but that on the other there is a definite potential for it to spread more widely.

For gay men AIDS represented both an individual and a social threat, with potential consequences for their position in society and for gay emancipation of homosexuals. It is noted that AIDS has not had any negative impact for the (by international standards) liberal attitude towards homosexuality and the position of gay men as a group. Nor has AIDS led to any major increase in discrimination. The large part played by the organizations of and for gay men in drawing attention to the AIDS crisis and the launching of initiatives in the fields of AIDS prevention, care and support are also noted.

The AIDS and drug problem is described against the background of the rise in hard-drug use in the 1970s and the extensive system of outreach developed in response. Reference is made to the hierarchy of dependence relationships within the drugs world and the special problem of the large group of "heroin tourists". Recent developments in the 1980s include the increase in poly-drug use and the advent of hard-drug use among second-generation young people from ethnic minorities. The underlying principles of Dutch drug-dependence policy are also noted, under which the use of hard drugs is approached not from a criminal but from a health perspective. Reference is made to the fact that AIDS has not led to any change in the way in which the hard drug problem is being tackled and that AIDS and drugs policies are to a large extent coordinated.

The analysis notes evidence of growing commercialization, increases in scale and internationalization in prostitution. The policy of tolerance towards prostitution is briefly examined, together with the possible consequences of the proposed legalization of brothels.

The main points of Dutch AIDS policy are seen as: (1) preventing HIV infection; (2) the organization of care and support; (3) the formulation of a research programme; (4) countering undesirable social consequences of AIDS. The far-reaching cooperation between the various bodies concerned with AIDS control stands out internationally.

The rather conservative attitude towards HIV-testing in the Netherlands is described against the backdrop of the international trends towards greater emphasis on individual civil rights. A reconstruction is provided of the debate about the application of HIV-testing; in particular there were conflicting interests with respect to the use of HIV-testing for large-scale seroprevalence screening and in medical examinations. The application of HIV-testing for life insurance purposes was noted as a possible problem in the future.

The new strategy for HIV/AIDS prevention is discussed against the background of the control of classic infectious diseases and STDs. For the present, public information and the promotion of behavioural change remain the only available strategy. Attention is directed towards the undiminished importance of the underlying aims of AIDS control, namely that of preventing HIV infection and building up and sustaining public support for AIDS control. The systematic nature of HIV/AIDS prevention is presented in terms of a chart, in which group-oriented activities and universal campaigns both have a place.

Brief consideration is devoted to the special attention to care for people with AIDS, especially the setting up of regional hospital centres, the emphasis on psychosocial care and support (e.g. buddy help) and the impact of patients and patients' associations on the content of the care and clinical drug trials.

It is noted that in the Netherlands respect for privacy, self-determination, the personal responsibility of the individual and countering the social consequences of AIDS have played a *decisive* role in the reaction to AIDS.

Baseline analysis of economic aspects
The economic consequences of the AIDS epidemic are expressed in patient-related versus general programme costs. Direct patient-related costs are those costs directly related to the individual patient in the AIDS or pre-AIDS stage. These costs relate to treatment and care (both inpatient and outpatient). Indirect patient-related costs refer to the Potential Years of Life Lost (PYLL) and sickness absence. These have not been expressed in monetary terms in this project. General programme costs cover the costs of research, prevention, information and education and services provided for the population in general, such as facilities for HIV-testing.

Patient-related costs cover the costs of hospitalization or nursing-home admission, district nursing, home help and intensive home care, general practitioner care, psychosocial support by the Regional Institutes for Ambulant Mental Health Care (RIAGG), social work, the work of the Schorer Foundation and the consumption of medicines. Where possible the patient-related consequences are expressed in costs and in bed need, consultations and hours of care and support.

The hospitalization costs for CDC IV patients range from NLG 35,900 to NLG 47,400 per observation year, with an average period of hospitalization of over 50 days. The estimated costs for people with AIDS outside hospitals amount to over NLG 8,700 per person-year. This is a minimum estimate since the lack of data means that - as in the case of psychosocial care - a proportion of the costs is unknown. Wherever possible we have shown hours of help and care. The costs and scale of the care and support for HIV-infected persons are all but unknown.

The total patient-related costs for 1990 are estimated at at least NLG 51.2 million, of which NLG 44.1 million within hospitals. Expressed per person, from the point of infection to death, we estimate the patient-related costs at at least NLG 112,900-126,000.

The programme costs relate to the costs of research, prevention and testing. Excluding the costs of preventive measures for HIV infection control in the work place, these amounted in 1990 to NLG 47.3 million.

Reference scenario: the consequences of AIDS in 1995 and 2000
The reference scenario is the best possible approximation of the impact of AIDS up to the year 2000 given unchanged trends. The reference scenario is constructed on the basis of mathematical simulations, in which the present trend in the incidence of AIDS is projected forward to the year 2000. Substantively, this comes down to a projection showing a declining rate of growth of the AIDS epidemic.

One element of the reference scenario has been separated off, in which a survey has been conducted of the consequences of the trend of the HIV-epidemic up to 1.1.1989. This subscenario provides the best possible impression of the impact of AIDS that cannot be avoided anymore by public information, education and prevention. Since the subscenario underestimates the consequences of AIDS it must not be regarded as a best-case variant of the reference scenario.

Assuming that the growth of the AIDS epidemic tapers off, the AIDS incidence in the period 1991-2000 would amount to 6,366. The subscenario indicates that of this figure, 3,807 cases can no longer be avoided by means of prevention and the promotion of behavioural change. Because the subscenario is an underestimation the incidence of AIDS in the period 1991-2000 will certainly exceed 3,800 cases. This means that there are likely to be at least twice and perhaps five times as many people with AIDS in the second decade of the AIDS epidemic as there were in the first. The pre-AIDS prevalence amounts to 8,000 in 1995 and 9,000 in the year 2000. This means that the cumulative number of HIV-infected persons since 1979 will have risen from an estimated 6,700 at 1.1.1989 to 17,000 in the year 2000. By that year at least 5,000 and possibly in excess of 6,500 people will have died due to AIDS. The PYLL per 1,000 of population increases in the reference scenario from 1.27 in 1995 to 1.53 in 2000.

Under the reference scenario the patient-related costs of the care of HIV-infected persons and people with AIDS amount to NLG 77 million in 1995 and NLG 93 million in the year 2000. The subscenario indicates that a substantial proportion of the impact of AIDS could be averted by the prevention of new HIV infections. In the year 2000 the difference in patient-related costs between the reference scenario and the subscenario is nearly NLG 60 million.

The programme costs depend only in part on the epidemiological course. The figure of NLG 47 million per year from the baseline analysis has been retained in the reference scenario. It is further assumed that the social context of the reference scenario remains unchanged in relation to the sociocultural and socio-epidemiological baseline analysis.

The conclusion to emerge from the reference scenario is that the impact of AIDS will not become fully discernible until the second decade of the epidemic. Under the reference scenario the annual incidence of AIDS doubles between 1990 and 2000, while there is a three-fold increase in patient-related costs. A comparison of the reference scenario with the subscenario indicates that a highly effective HIV/AIDS-prevention strategy would not have a significant effect on the AIDS incidence until 1995-2000.

The analysis of the reference scenario includes an examination of the underlying assumption of unchanged trends. Consideration is also given to cross-cutting developments and the possibilities of averting as much of the impact of AIDS as possible by continued or intensified efforts at HIV/AIDS prevention.

Risk behaviour and the spread of HIV

The behaviour scenarios provide an impression of the (not always quantifiable, or pin-pointable in time) HIV incidence stemming from changes in risk behaviour that cannot be ruled out or effective prevention measures. The formulation and determination of the assumptions for scenario analysis are based on data from international literature, supplemented by individual consultation and a workshop. In total six behaviour scenarios have been drawn up examining some of the major HIV transmission routes within and between core groups. The lack of basic research data on such aspects as infectiousness, seroprevalence and trends in the HIV incidence, the prevalence of risk behaviour and the effects of prevention call for caution, especially when it comes to the quantitative interpretation of the results of scenario analysis.

For males with multiple male partners two scenarios have been developed: (I) HIV/AIDS according to the methodology of the reference scenario and subscenarios, and (II) temporary versus permanent relapse into risk behaviour. Scenario I puts the cumulative incidence of HIV among men who have sex with men at 7,500 in the period 1989-2000. As in scenario II it is evident that *a constant high level of safe behaviour* is necessary in order to control the spread of HIV infections. Against the background of the baseline analysis it is concluded that at the present time, a scenario assuming a permanent increase in risk behaviour seems unlikely.

The spread of HIV among IDUs has been explored in two scenarios: (III) an introduction and rapid spread versus a plateauingin HIV infection; (IV) spread of HIV via the shared use of injection equipment and/or sexual contact. The uncertainty about the course of the HIV epidemic among IDUs remains large, so that it is not possible to make any statements about the probability of the variants in scenario (III). With respect to the sexual transmission of HIV, simulations based on scenario (IV) have shown the particular importance for female IDUs of safe sexual behaviour and safe injection practices. In addition it would seem plausible that the spread of HIV to the heterosexual population will take place primarily through male IDUs. This group is three times as big as the female IDU group. Other factors include the differences in the assumed risk of male-female (and vice versa) transmission.

Scenario V explores the possibility of an independent epidemic among the heterosexual population in general. Simulations indicate that this is possible only *in special circumstances*. This scenario is consistent with the findings from the socio-epidemiological and the sociocultural baseline analyses.

Scenario VI relates to commercial sex workers and their clients. The simulations draw a distinction between HIV infections in these two categories. The conclusion to emerge is that in the absence of a high level of safer sexual behaviour hundreds of new HIV infections are possible within the world of prostitution in a period of five years. Commercial sex workers do not incur a substantial risk of acquisition until the seroprevalence among their clients reaches 10% or more. This does not eliminate the fact that both commercial sex workers and clients have a shared interest in safer sex.

The general analysis based on the behaviour scenarios underlines the importance of *a permanently high level of safe behaviour*. The scenarios indicate that this applies equally to men who have sex with men, IDUs and their sexual partners, commercial sex workers and clients. In the case of the heterosexual population the situation tends to be rather more complex, resulting in the conclusion that the information and education provided to the heterosexual population on AIDS should to a significant extent be integrated with public information on sexually transmitted diseases.

Care and medical technology

The three scenarios explore the impact of developments in medical technology and the care and treatment of HIV-infected persons and people with AIDS on the demand, delivery, coordination and organization of health care. Scenario I examines three variants that analyse the impact on care of an assumed extension in the survival period from diagnosis with AIDS to three years. The variants in scenario I are: (A) unchanged intensity of care (B) more intensive home-care and (C) substitution.

The conclusions to emerge from the care scenarios reinforce the findings from the reference scenario. The patient-related costs (amounting to at least NLG 93 million in the reference scenario) in scenario I amount to at least NLG 132 million in variant A in the year 2000 and at least NLG 137 million in variant B. Variant C results in a minor drop in the patient-related costs compared with the two other variants. The assumption here is that a day's intensive home-care corresponds with a substituted low-care day of hospitalization. Taken all in all, AIDS imposes a *substantial* but *manageable* burden on overall health care facilities and the costs of health care. Inpatient facilities appear sufficient to meet the need for beds. Given the anticipated intensification of home-care and the lengthier periods of hospitalization, particular attention needs to be devoted to the need for and organization of home care and the support provided by volunteers.

Scenario II examines early intervention. Under this scenario the progression to AIDS is deferred, with a reduced need for beds. On the other hand people with HIV come into contact with the health care system at an earlier stage. Under this scenario there is a large demand for psychosocial help. The costs of monitoring and early intervention are appreciable and could rise to NLG 27.5 million in the year 2000.

Scenario III examines AIDS as a chronic disorder. Developments in scenario I are set out more sharply in a description of the consequences for care in the long term. In this scenario problems are to be anticipated especially at the level where help is provided and in the organization and coordination of (out-of-hospital) care. The analysis based on the care scenarios examines the possibilities for the simultaneous occurrence of developments in scenarios I and II. It is also noted that AIDS remains a serious, complicated disease requiring intensive and specialized treatment and care. The consequences of AIDS for the health system after the year 2000 are briefly touched upon: the demand for help for people with AIDS is defered now, it could in due course lead to an increase in the burden of care.

Reaction to AIDS: strategies for AIDS control and care

The reaction to AIDS is explored on the basis of strategic scenarios relating to AIDS control and the care and support of people with AIDS and HIV-infected persons.

The strategies analysed in the field of AIDS control relate to two radically different ways of achieving the goal of "preventing HIV infection as far as possible". A "Self-determination strategy" builds on the present AIDS-control strategy, with the additional assumption that AIDS control is an example of the control of sexually transmitted diseases in general. A contrasting approach consists of the "Detection strategy", which is based on a reappraisal of the underlying principles of present AIDS control. Among other things the Detection strategy assumes that an active system of contact tracing and partner notification is required and that restrictive measures should if necessary be applied. In the analysis the scenarios are juxtaposed against the social context and the legal framework for AIDS control as derived from the sociocultural baseline analysis.

With respect to the organization of care, two strategies are described aimed at "the provision of high quality care to people with HIV and AIDS". Under a "Regular care strategy" the special arrangements for AIDS are dismantled and the care of people with AIDS is fully integrated into the existing system of health care facilities. This scenario is based on the principle that the care of people with AIDS and HIV-infected persons should as far as possible take place within the regular system of health care facilities. By contrast the "AIDS-specific care strategy" is based on the principle that the care of people with AIDS requires specially tailored facilities and care providers. In the analysis it is noted that it is still too early to come down in favour of either one of these strategies.

The general analysis contains a brief reflection based on the Policy Document on AIDS Control and the basic choice to be made between an AIDS-specific, a health-care facilities and a laissez-faire policy. It is noted that the seriousness of the AIDS problem does not permit a laissez-faire policy. It is possible that in certain sub-areas, a switch may take place from an AIDS-specific to a provision policy. In a societal sense special attention is drawn in this context to Dutch sociocultural traditions, the importance attached to individual civil rights and the basic principle of personal responsibility of the individual.

Concluding remarks

The final chapter contains a reflection on the findings from the scenario analysis.

Attention is drawn to the similar conclusions to emerge from the reference scenario, the subscenario and the care scenarios, namely that the consequences of AIDS will not emerge fully until the second decade of the epidemic. The possibility is examined that the efforts and initial successes of the 1980s will means that AIDS control in the 1990s will focus to a greater extent on efforts to control the consequences of the AIDS epidemic. Given the major potential for HIV/-AIDS to spread and the numerous transmission routes of the virus, it is concluded that watchfulness and a certain degree of caution are demanded. Reference is made to the lack of significant research data on seroprevalence, infectiousness, risk behaviour and its determinants, and the spread of HIV outside core groups. The potential consequences of the introduction of HIV-2 in the Netherlands or the rise in mobility are also uncertain. Further research on these aspects will permit more sharply focused long-range studies than at present.

It is noted that a common feature of the reference scenario, the subscenario and the care scenarios is that the financial consequences of AIDS will be considerable but not unmanageable. On the other hand AIDS is likely to remain an incurable disease up to the year 2000 requiring intensive and complex care. The next decade will at most see a deferment of suffering and death and the quality of life of people with AIDS will remain closely bound up with the quality of care for terminal diseases.

In a societal sense it is noted that AIDS has not led to radical sociocultural changes or panic reactions. This does not eliminate the fact that AIDS can still lead to undesirable social consequences. Nor can safe sexual behaviour be regarded as the social norm. It is noted that the preservation of public support for dealing with the epidemic and the need to prevent HIV infection requirs sustained efforts.

With respect to the medium term the impact of AIDS is expected to remain largely unchanged on the 1980s: until the year 2000 - and possibly for long thereafter - AIDS will remain an incurable, fatal disease constituting a threat to public health. Continuing efforts at AIDS control are required in the field of epidemiology, in HIV/AIDS prevention, within health care and in research and in the interests of maintaining public support for coping with the epidemic.

Introduction

At the initiative of the World Health Organization, the Steering Committee on Future Health Scenarios (STG) asked the Netherlands Institute of Mental Health (NcGv) and the National Institute of Public Health and Environmental Protection (RIVM) to conduct a pilot study into the feasibility of a scenario study into the sociocultural and economic impact of AIDS on society. The study, conducted by D.P. Reinking, researcher, and Dr. F.M.L.G. van den Boom, project leader, of the NcGv and M.J. Postma, researcher, and Dr. J.C. Jager, project leader, of the RIVM, got under way in November 1988. On the basis of the results it was decided in July 1989 to set up a full-scale project, and a scenario committee, chaired by Prof.Dr. E.J. Ruitenberg, was appointed. The aforementioned NcGv/RIVM research team was responsible for project implementation. In June 1990 the research group was expanded by the addition of Mrs. C.E.S. Albers from the NcGv.

The research group and the committee were asked to explore potential developments in the HIV/AIDS epidemic in the Netherlands in the medium and long term, together with the sociocultural and economic impact. The examination of potential situations in combating AIDS and the treatment of HIV-infected persons, people with AIDS and groups heavily affected by AIDS also formed part of the terms of reference.

The study was conducted by means of literature surveys, mathematical modelling, the consultation of experts and a workshop of experts. We should like to extend a special word of thanks to the members of the Scenario Committee for their productive cooperation, going beyond the meetings of the committee alone. Needless to say we are particularly grateful to M.J.J.C. Poos and Dr. J.A.M. van Druten for their support in the mathematical modelling carried out for this project, while we should also like to acknowledge our gratitude to the large number of experts whom we consulted for this project. Our special thanks go out to the Chief Medical Inspectorate of Public Health for allowing us consult the anonymous register of people with AIDS in the Netherlands. A list of the experts consulted during the main project is provided in Appendix IV.

The report consists of three parts.

Part I, consisting of Chapters 1 and 2, provides an elaboration of the terms of reference, the working method and the methodology developed for scenario analysis. Chapter 1 examines the design and implementation of the scenario project. Following a brief introduction of a number of central concepts it examines the methodology of scenario analysis and the conceptual model that provided the framework for tackling the project. The special nature of a scenario project into a transmittable disease is also examined. Chapter 2 discusses the working method adopted for the construction of the scenarios on the sociocultural and economic impact of AIDS and also introduces the models used and their potential applications.

Part II consists of Chapters 3, 4 and 5. Successively these examine the socio-epidemiological baseline analysis (Chapter 3), the baseline analysis of the sociocultural aspects of AIDS (Chapter 4) and the baseline analysis of the economic consequences of AIDS (Chapter 5). Together these chapters provide a retrospective review of the first decade of the AIDS epidemic and provide the point of departure for the projections.

Part III of the report, consisting of Chapters 6-10, contains the development of the scenarios. The reference scenario is described in Chapter 6. This sets out the impact of AIDS on the assumption that the trends in the baseline analysis continue unchanged. Chapters 7, 8 and 9 contain scenarios in which the consequences of alternative developments in specific areas of the reference scenario are explored. Chapter 7 examines the impact of behaviour and changes in behaviour on the course of the AIDS epidemic. The chapter examines the possibility of the distribution of HIV within and between various sub-epidemics. Chapter 8 describes the impact of developments in health care and medical technology on the delivery, demand, costs and organization of care for people with HIV and AIDS. Chapter 9 compares strategies in the field of AIDS control and care with one another and also with current control strategies and the organization of care. The final chapter consist of a summary of and reflection on the main findings from the scenarios.

In conducting the research choices had to be made as there were too many interesting aspects to be covered in a limited period. These choices were made by the scenario committee, often after lengthy and profound discussion.

One of the choices related to limiting the research to the Dutch situation. This choice was made in the first place because the scenario project forms part of an international project set up by the Regional Office for Europe of the World Health Organization. Together with other European countries the Netherlands was to develop a methodology with which the various data on the epidemic and its impact on society could be meaningfully compared with one another. As soon as a clear-cut methodology is available it will then be possible to identify more clearly the backgrounds to the differing epidemiological trends, policy differences and the consequences of transfrontier developments such as growing mobility. Now that the Dutch study has been completed it will certainly act as an example for other participating countries and for projections within the European Community and at global level.

Apart from this argument, it became increasingly clear as the research progressed how little research data there in fact was on the Dutch (let alone wider) situation with respect to mobility, regional distribution and the results of seroprevalance testing. In addition the available material is to some extent context-bound (e.g. for sociocultural reasons), which has made it more difficult to assess the value of foreign data for the Dutch situation.

A second important choice related to the exploration of the epidemiological aspects. This project has examined the impact of AIDS in a sociocultural and economic sense. Surveys of potential or not inconceivable epidemiological trends therefore occupy a central place in the scenario analysis. On the other hand a choice between the determinants of HIV infection was unavoidable. This report has opted in favour of scenarios in which risk behaviour and the effects of prevention are varied. An exploration of the effects of variations in infectiousness, group size and speed of progression of AIDS had to be left to one side.

A third significant choice consisted of the decision not to compare the costs associated with AIDS with those of other diseases. This was decided in the first place because the costs of AIDS have been calculated on the basis of an analytical framework that has yet to be developed for other diseases, so that a proper comparison was not possible. But even if this had been possible from a technical viewpoint, the question would remain as to which disease AIDS might then be compared with. Another consideration in the mind of the committee in deciding against such comparison was that it could otherwise provide a possible basis for making choices in health care. The committee considers it would be inappropriate to examine this highly complicated ethical problem indirectly in this report. A fundamental discussion is required before precise cost-benefit analyses can be conducted. This is also why the indicator for the potential years of life lost has not been translated into monetary terms or why no attempt has been made to convert the quality of life into economic terms. Furthermore, there are many statistical gaps in the field of costs: there are no figures available on the cost of lost output and the same applies to the costs of psychosocial and out-of-hospital care. Finally the committee took the view that if the costs incurred were to be calculated scrupulously and compared with other diseases, the "benefits" would also need to be calculated. The moral and ethical complications of such an exercise were, however, deemed excessive. Once again a fundamental discussion needs to take place first.

A fourth significant choice related to not taking the availability of a vaccine into account in the scenarios. The arguments against doing so were related to the unpredictability of the period in which such a vaccine might become available, uncertainty as to how effective such a vaccine would be and questions as to who would qualify for vaccination. In the final analysis the consequences of a vaccine for the HIV and AIDS epidemic are highly uncertain. The committee considers that justice would only be done to this complex subject by a separate study into the many variations that apply in this field and the large number of variables that need to be taken into account in the projections.

A fifth significant choice was the decision that the researchers would not develop new mathematical models for the project but instead build on existing ones. Doing so meant that frequent consultations were required with the relevant researchers concerning possible adaptations of their models on the basis of subsequent available information. This does not however mean that the results recorded in this report are meant as a validation of the model but should, instead, be seen as surveys of possible epidemiological developments.

Last but not least, choices had to be made as to which projections to carry out. In some cases these were determined by the lack of relevant data. There are for example no projections for ethnic minorities, as there is no information on sexual behaviour and HIV prevalence. This is not in any way to suggest that this was regarded as an unimportant subject. As in the case of mobility, the methodology that has been developed means that if new information becomes available in this field the consequences for developments in the HIV/AIDS epidemic can then be calculated. In other words, the methodology developed lends itself to on-going surveillance - something which both the committee and the research group considered exceptionally important.

Part I Scenarioproject AIDS

1 Scenario project "The sociocultural and economic impact of AIDS: design and working plan"

1.1 Introduction

"With the recent manifestation of the acquired immune deficiency syndrome, AIDS, society is being confronted for the first time since the polio epidemic of the 1950s with a serious infectious disease of epidemic proportions, to which medical science as yet has no answer ..... All the available information currently points ..... in the direction of a particularly serious development involving not just large-scale human suffering but also enormous costs" (Dutch Lower House, 1985). It was with these introductory remarks that State Secretary Van der Reijden submitted the first government memorandum on AIDS to the Lower House of Parliament on 20 September 1985. At that point a cumulative total of 66 people with AIDS had been notified to the Chief Medical Inspectorate for Public Health.

The Human Immuno Deficiency Virus (HIV) is transmitted by means of blood or semen. This until then virtually unknown virus ultimately causes AIDS[1]. With due caution it was estimated that the cumulative number of reported AIDS cases would rise to 150 at the end of 1985 and to perhaps 4,000 in 1990. It was further cautiously assumed that there would be at least 5-6,000 people infected with HIV in 1985. Without rapid and adequate preventive efforts this number would be considerably higher in 1990[2].

The concern about the impact of AIDS related not just to human suffering, the consequences for health care and the associated costs but also to the "social context" of the problem. It was feared that AIDS would lead to panic reactions among the population, risk groups and care providers. Among other things AIDS could lead to ostracism and discrimination. This fear was accentuated by the fact that in the Western world AIDS had until then primarily affected gay men and drug users. In this respect Mann (1989) referred to a third,

---

1 The virological and immunological aspects of HIV and AIDS fall outside the scope of this study and are not considered in further detail in this report.

2 As far as seroprevalence in the Netherlands is concerned estimates are still being used. In the first AIDS memorandum submitted to the Lower House the available methods for seroprevalence estimation in 1985 were still the subject of such caution that the authorities were unwilling to provide an estimate of the number of HIV-infected persons in 1990.

"sociocultural epidemic", in reaction to the epidemic of HIV infections and the subsequent AIDS epidemic.

1.2 Terms of reference of the project

A broad outline has been provided above of the major, wide-ranging consequences that need to be taken into account in the context of AIDS. Looking to the short term there is a need for effective AIDS control, high-quality care for people with AIDS and HIV and the containment of societally undesirable reactions. In addition there was, and remains, a need for insight into the possible impact of the epidemic in the medium and long term. Important questions include: How many people with AIDS and HIV may be expected in the coming years? What permanent effects may preventive strategies aimed at changing behaviour be expected to have? How fast, and by what means, should HIV be expected to spread and what countermeasures can be taken? What implications will the epidemiological trends have for health care? In what way can societally undesirable reactions to AIDS be prevented?

Among other things, the scenario project "The sociocultural and economic impact of AIDS on society" is concerned with the impact of AIDS in the medium and long term as seen in the light of these questions. The project is designed to provide insight into the impact of AIDS in the Netherlands in an epidemiological, sociocultural and economic sense with a view to the introduction of the most appropriate long-term policies to combat AIDS. A preliminary study carried out by the Netherlands Centre for Mental Health Care (NcGv) and the National Institute for Health and Environmental Protection (RIVM) during the period October 1988 - June 1989 resulted in the following terms of reference for the main project (Reinking et al., 1989):

1. What is the likely incidence and prevalence of HIV/AIDS, if necessary subclassified into sub-epidemics, in the Netherlands in the short and medium term?
2. What consequences will potential future trends in the epidemic have for health care and preventive policies?
3. What has been the sociocultural and economic impact of the AIDS epidemic and what consequences need to be anticipated in the future?
4. Which potential and realistic future situations may be formulated with respect to combating the AIDS epidemic and the treatment of people with HIV, AIDS and groups heavily affected by AIDS?

1.3 *Definitions and underlying principles*

Projections of the epidemic of HIV and AIDS occupy a central place in the project. A significant element of the projections of the consequences, e.g. with respect to the demand for health care and the need and effectiveness of prevention, are directly related to the epidemiological course taken by HIV and AIDS. A number of key concepts and underlying principles are introduced in section 1.2.1.

1.3.1 *HIV infection*

HIV shows up in blood, semen, vaginal fluid and breast milk. Documented HIV transmission routes are sexual intercourse, transfusions of blood or blood products, the shared use of injection equipment among injecting drug users and maternal-foetal transmission (Friedland and Klein, 1987; Houweling and Coutinho, 1989). The most common transmission route is sexual contact. Particularly risky is unprotected anal intercourse. The exact chance of HIV transmission by risk-laden activities is not readily determined (DeGruttola et al., 1989; Holmberg et al., 1989).

The transmission of HIV by means of blood transfusions and treatment with blood projects has been virtually ruled out in the Netherlands since early 1985: all blood donations are now screened by means of an HIV-antibody test, as are donor organs, while blood products also undergo heat treatment. These transmission routes are left out of account in the long-range studies and we shall instead be concentrating on the most prevalent transmission routes: sexual contact and the shared use of injection equipment in injecting drug use.

A distinction is drawn between two strains, HIV-1 and HIV-2. Infection in the Netherlands is chiefly due to the HIV-1 strain, although a few cases are also known of people with AIDS infected with HIV-2 (Van der Ende et al., 1990). HIV-2 is primarily encountered in West African countries and is probably transmitted in the same way as HIV-1. This report only examines HIV-1.

1.3.2 *Progression to AIDS*

Infection with HIV leads to an acute short-lived clinical syndrome, followed by a long period of asymptomatic infection. AIDS is diagnosed when the immune system is weakened to the point that resistance to a broad spectrum of disease symptoms is no longer possible. It is unknown whether every HIV-infected person also develops AIDS. Research in the US among gay men indicates that

54% of HIV-infected persons develop AIDS within 11 years (Lifson et al., 1990). There are as yet no data on the progression to AIDS for periods in excess of 11 years from infection, but it may be assumed that both the percentage of people with HIV who develop AIDS and the average incubation period will rise.

AIDS is a fatal disease that bears largely on people in the younger age groups, i.e. 20-50 years. The average life expectancy from diagnosis has risen from less than a year in the early 1980s to 16 months in 1988 and 22 months in 1989 (Bindels et al., 1990), and is thought to have risen further again since 1989. For epidemiological purposes the Netherlands uses the internationally standard "AIDS surveillance case definition" drawn up by the Centers for Disease Control (CDC, 1987ab; GHI, 1987). The surveillance case definition relates to both children and adults. Appendix A to this chapter contains a list of indicator diseases for the diagnosis of AIDS.

Apart from surveillance case definition there was also a need for a classification system for HIV infection based around clinical manifestations. The CDC classification distinguishes four mutually exclusive hierarchical classes:

CDC I:	acute infection
CDC II:	asymptomatic infections
CDC III:	generalized lymphadenopathy
CDC IV:	various clinical syndromes

Compared with the surveillance case definition all people with AIDS are classified as group CDC IV. Conversely not all people with clinical syndromes from group CDC IV come under the surveillance case definition of AIDS. Appendix B to this chapter sets out the CDC classification for HIV infection, indicating the differences from the surveillance case definition. The CDC classification for children aged under 13 is shown separately.

The epidemiological projections in this report are based on epidemiological monitoring according to the CDC surveillance case definition. The health care projections are based on hospital cost-records, which are generally based on the clinical classification into CDC groups. In terms of the results of the scenario analysis, the use of differing definitions of AIDS for epidemiological projections and for the consequences for health care is not of major significance.

1.3.3 Spread of HIV

Since the screening of blood supplies has been introduced HIV can only be transmitted by riskful encounters with an HIV-infected person. Studies of the spread of HIV therefore need to take account of the incidence of risk behaviour, possible HIV transmission routes and seroprevalance. In the scenario project this has been done by means of a detailed breakdown into *identifiable groups with a risk of HIV infection*.

In this context the literature often refers to "risk groups". We are aware that there is a certain sensitivity about using this term, because the concept of risk group can unintentionally and unfairly arouse the impression that homosexuality or hard-drug use necessarily involve a risk of contracting HIV. Where possible we will refer to sub-epidemics, patient groups, men who have sex with men, etc. In certain cases, however, the concept of "risk group", in the neutral epidemiological sense of the word, cannot be avoided.

On the basis of data from epidemiological studies, the HIV/AIDS epidemic may best be approached as a complex of related sub-epidemics. In the Netherlands the AIDS epidemic started in 1982 among men who have sex with men, while in 1985 it was encountered among injecting drug users (IDU). In 1990 these were still the most affected groups: as at 1.1.1991, 1,358 of the 1,516 (i.e. 89%) of the people with AIDS reported to the Chief Medical Inspectorate of Public Health fell into the patient groups of homo/bisexual men (N = 1,223), IDU (N = 116) or homo/bisexual IDU (N = 19). Epidemiological research has also revealed differences in seroprevalance among men who have sex with men, IDU and men and women with heterosexual partners only (Van Griensven, 1989; Van den Hoek, 1990; Hooykaas et al., 1989). On the basis of the available data it would therefore appear appropriate to draw a distinction between groups that are already heavily hit by the epidemic and groups that have the potential to be hit on a large scale.

With a view to the spread of HIV it would also appear appropriate to draw a distinction between the incidence of risk behaviour and possible HIV transmission routes. The ultimate spread of HIV infections is determined by the *number of partners* with whom, or the *size of the sexual network* within which, an HIV infected person has *riskful encounters*. In addition the spread of AIDS needs to be approached in terms of the *possible transmission routes* of the virus and "*bridges*" that connect sexual networks or figurations with one another (Darrow et al., 1986; Straver and Van Stolk, 1988; McClumeck et al., 1989; Van der Vliet, 1990; Van Zessen and Straver, 1991). The shared use of injection equipment is of relevance for the spread of HIV among IDUs, while theoretically the spread of HIV among the entire Dutch population is possible by means of high-risk sexual behaviour. Examples of "bridges" or "links" between subpopulations are injecting drug users actively engaged in commercial sex work or the sexual partners of HIV-infected persons.

1.4 Methodology of scenario research

Scenario studies have been conducted in the Netherlands under the auspices of the STG since 1983. To date scenario studies have been carried out on ageing, cardiovascular diseases, accidents, mental health care and mental health, and chronic diseases (STG, 1985; 1986; 1988; 1990; 1991).

First and foremost, these scenario-based projections are intended *to promote discussion* about elements of health care. In addition, the projections in the form of scenarios are designed to contribute towards "the anticipatory capacity of government policy in the longer term" (STG, 1987). The results of scenario studies have been incorporated in strategic policy documents such as *Towards the Year 2000* and the *Basic Document on Health Care*. It should be emphasized that scenario research is *exploratory and based on personal opinion rather than predictive in nature*. The definition of a scenario employed by the STG is:

> "A scenario describes how a particular image of the future may be arrived at from the present situation ... via a series of possible developments, with the aim of obtaining greater insight into the underlying mechanisms and the possibility of influencing those processes" (Hoogeveen and Brouwer, 1989).

The central elements of a scenario study emerge in this definition:
1. A definition of the initial situation, or "baseline analysis", by a description and interpretation of the present state of affairs and current trends.
2. The exploration of a number of final projected situations, including alternatives to the one considered most probable, together with the determination of its effects (i.e. exploratory scenarios).
3. The formulation of goals and specification of paths or strategies for achieving those goals, including the advantages and disadvantages associated with path and strategy (i.e. strategic scenarios).

The most commonly employed methods in scenario research are literature studies, the consultation of experts, a survey of final projected situations by means of mathematical simulations and statistical analysis. In tackling the problem being addressed by this study, we have followed the methodology customarily employed in scenario research.

1.4.1 *Exploratory and strategic scenarios*

In scenario research two types of scenarios may be distinguished, which feature in this project: exploratory scenarios and strategic scenarios. An exploratory scenario forms the starting point for the analysis stemming from the present day. The baseline analysis is used to explore the end-situations that will result if present trends continue unchanged. Alternative exploratory scenarios examine the impact of "intervening" developments. In the case of AIDS intervening developments might include a relapse into unsafe behaviour among gay men or a substantial spread of HIV among the heterosexual population.

Strategic scenarios are in a certain sense the complement of exploratory ones. The starting point for the analysis is not the present day but a goal towards which one wishes to work, after which the pros and cons of the various strategies for achieving that goal are examined. The formulation of goals and the description of the effects, costs and benefits of strategies are conducted against the background of the reference scenario.

The scenario project into the consequences of AIDS follows the above methodology. It starts with a definition of the concepts, the identification of the factors that affect the HIV/AIDS incidence and prevalence and a survey of areas in which AIDS and the AIDS epidemic could have a potential impact. These aspects have already been briefly examined in the introduction and the definition of the problem in the previous section. The problem analysis resulted in the development of a *conceptual model*, which acted as a guideline for the activities in the project. The conceptual model for this project is discussed in section 1.6. Before then we examine the way in which the consequences of AIDS are handled in the project and the specific nature of a scenario project concerned with a communicable disease in which behaviour is the central determinant.

1.5 *Sociocultural and economic impact of AIDS*

The AIDS scenario project has broad terms of reference, with the projections of epidemiological trends providing the reference point. In determining the impact of AIDS it is not always possible to assume a direct link between the scale and the consequences of the epidemic. This applies particularly to the sociocultural impact of AIDS, e.g. with respect to AIDS and discrimination against people with HIV/AIDS, since the latter is not directly related to the spread of HIV but is attributable to such factors as fear of infection and tolerance towards gay men, drug users and prostitutes.

In tackling the project we were aware that it is sometimes all but impossible to draw a dividing line between the epidemiology and the sociocultural context, and that behaviour and the context in which it is set can influence one another. The prevention of risk-producing sexual behaviour and injection drug use cannot, for example, be viewed in isolation from the sociocultural influences on sexuality, partner change, the use of contraceptives (including condoms) or prevailing values and norms towards injection drug use. The advent of AIDS and the activities being undertaken for its control will have an effect not only on risk behaviour but also on the social context. In tackling the project we have cut through this Gordian knot by selecting a number of relevant topics, themes and angles. In making this selection we have been guided by (1) the international literature on the social impact of AIDS and the relevance for the Dutch situation of the topics dealt with in the literature, (2) the legal/ethical debate prompted by AIDS in the Netherlands and (3) the social background that must be described or outlined in order to answer the questions being addressed by the project. It clearly proved worth examining the following overlapping topics: socio-sexological aspects; sexually transmitted diseases and HIV infection; drug use, drug users and drug assistance in the Netherlands; AIDS and gay emancipation; commercial sex work in the Netherlands; the reaction to AIDS, especially the legal/ethical framework; AIDS-control strategy - debate and choices; the impact of AIDS on the organization and structure of care and the organization and effects of preventive activities; and the consequences of AIDS for access to social facilities.

The economic consequences of AIDS have been expressed in terms of *monetary* and *non-monetary* costs. The project examines the costs of AIDS both *within and outside the health care system.* Within the health care system a distinction has been drawn between the effects for inpatient and outpatient health care, between somatic and psychosocial care, and between professional care and voluntary support and assistance. Outside the health care system we describe the programme costs, i.e the costs of prevention, testing, research, education and enhancement of expertise, while also paying due account to other costs, such as those arising from illness.

1.6 Scenarios for a communicable disease

The construction of scenarios may be advised in the event of (1) an open situation (2) that is governable and (3) in which discussion is possible about the appropriate approach and intervention strategies (De Vries, 1985). The relevant time-frame is the medium term. In the case of AIDS there is major uncertainty concerning the future epidemiological course, on the one hand because the behaviour responsible for the transmission of HIV is universal and subject to change while, on the other, the susceptibility to change also means that a further spread can be prevented. The path taken by the AIDS epidemic can be altered by a wide range of interventions. Options include divergent intervention strategies such as public information and promoting changes in behaviour, epidemiological monitoring, contact tracing and partner notification, isolation, tattooing, quarantine measures and the barring of foreign visitors or introduction of compulsory HIV testing for persons getting married. In addition the course of the epidemic will be influenced by measures to safeguard the quality of blood supplies and by research in the medical and biological field.

As far as the screening of blood donations is concerned there is a general consensus that this is an effective strategy for preventing HIV infections. On the other points discussion and choices are possible concerning the appropriate strategy. What constitutes a good approach in the medium term will depend among other things on the *epidemiological trend*. Different instruments and resources will be deployed if an epidemic is on the point of breaking out rather than if it is expected to taper off.

Furthermore, the evaluation of interventions and goals is indissolubly bound up with the *social and legal/ethical admissibility and desirability* of particular strategies. It is possible to come up with all sorts of ostensibly effective control strategies that would be at variance with the civil rights enshrined in the constitution or that would cut across societally desirable reactions towards AIDS. One of the considerations in selecting a strategy will be the extent to which the desire to avoid undesirable discrimination against HIV-infected persons and to preserve privacy and the integrity of the body are explicitly regarded as guiding principles.

With respect to goals it is not just a matter of desirability but also of feasibility. The history of combating sexually transmitted diseases indicates that notions of eradicating AIDS or bringing about a universal and permanent change in behaviour belong to the realms of utopia rather than reality.

Grosso modo the scenario project "The Sociocultural and Economic Impact of AIDS for Society" corresponds with other scenario projects. In certain respects, however, it differs totally, in that the project is concerned with a disease that can be transmitted by risk behaviour, which has major consequences for the development and interpretation of scenarios. In the case of exploratory scenarios this means that not only do the probable courses of the HIV/AIDS epidemic, as based on present trends, need to be explored but that account needs also to be taken of hard to predict but theoretically feasible epidemiological developments. Examples include an increase in HIV infections due for example to a reversion to risk behaviour, or the introduction of HIV among groups that have so far escaped largely unscathed.

With behaviour as the central variable a certain degree of uncertainty is inevitable. Future-oriented research is possible only within certain margins and without confining the projections in advance to a certain time-frame. The exploratory scenarios concerned with the *non-exclusion* of epidemiological trends relate to potential developments taking place at a particular but unspecified time. Such projections are conducted not for their realism but to illustrate the major changes to which potential, i.e. not inconceivable developments could give rise. In such surveys, which are largely conceptual in nature, there would be little point in specifying a time-frame.

The differences between the AIDS scenario project and other such projects are almost greater when it comes to the role of strategic scenarios. Communicable diseases and the control of infectious diseases are indissolubly linked: in principle there is no difference between the desirable and the necessary final projected situation in the future. The aim of strategic scenarios in this project is therefore in principle a fixed datum: in order to keep the impact of AIDS within bounds, HIV infection must be prevented as far as possible. Of relevance is whether this goal can be realized, how effective the AIDS control must be and what choices in AIDS control are possible and societally admissible.

1.7 Underlying conceptual model

In order to provide a framework for tackling the project and for the construction of scenarios a conceptual model has been drawn up. This conceptual model is a schematic and, in the interests of manageability and analytical discrimination, simplified representation of the most important elements and their interrelationships in the scenario analysis.

The central elements in the model are *HIV infection* and the *progression* to *AIDS*. These epidemiological elements are also placed as a whole in a larger compartment. Risk *behaviour* is the central determinant of infection and the spread of HIV. *Prevention* is aimed at the avoidance of HIV infection. In the Netherlands this amounts to public information and education and the promotion of behavioural changes. The development of the epidemiological and a part of the sociocultural aspects relate to the incidence/prevalence of HIV and

AIDS and the efforts to bring about a change in behaviour through preventive measures.

Figure 1.1 **Conceptual model for scenario analysis of the sociocultural and economic impact of AIDS.**

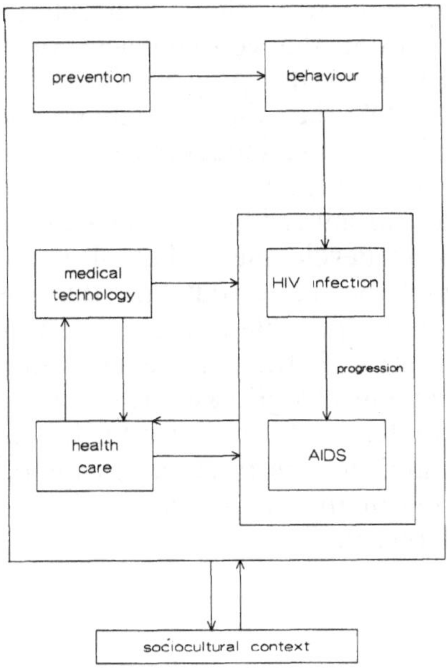

Medical Technology is used in order to alleviate the suffering due to HIV infection by efforts to improve the treatment of symptoms. Medical technology also covers research into a vaccine or a definitive anti-viral therapy. Apart from the HIV incidence itself, medical technology therefore also affects the care. By *Care* is meant all the activities undertaken in the care, support and counselling of people with AIDS. Care is a matter of mutual interaction: the demand and requirement for care for people with HIV and AIDS influences the delivery of care while the latter in turn affects the demand for care. Care also exerts an effect on medical technology: as clinical experience is gained greater possibilities will be opened up in diagnosis and treatment.

As noted in the previous section there is a continuing interaction between society and the epidemic taking place within it. This mutual interaction has been shown graphically by the two-way relationship between the *sociocultural context* and the other compartments in the model.

1.8 Summary

The scenario project "The Sociocultural and Economic Impact of AIDS for Society" has broad terms of reference. Projections of future trends in the HIV and AIDS epidemic, broken down where possible into sub-epidemics and transmission and distribution routes, are conducted in conjunction with their sociocultural and economic consequences. Apart from the consequences of the epidemic for health care and prevention the project also takes account of the societal context of AIDS, i.e. the continuing interaction between epidemiological trends and the influences on and reactions towards those trends from within society. A specific feature of this scenario project into a disease transmitted by risk behaviour is that it needs to examine not just likely developments but also a number of future situations that cannot be ruled out. In the case of the latter projections it is not always possible to set a time-frame in advance. In addition, the exploratory and strategic scenarios in a scenario project concerned with a communicable disease match up closely.

A conceptual model has been drawn up for the development of the baseline analysis and the construction of exploratory and strategic scenarios. The working method and associated choices are discussed in more detail in Chapter 2.

References

Bindels, P.J.E., J.T.L. Jong, M.J.J.C. Poos, A. Leentvaar-Kuijpers, J.C. Jager, R.A. Coutinho
Het epidemiologisch beloop van AIDS in Amsterdam, 1982-1988
Nederlands Tijdschrift voor Geneeskunde, 134 (1990), 8, 390-394

Council of State and Territ. Epidemiol., AIDS Program, Center for Infectious Diseases, Centers for Disease Control (CDC)
Classification System for Human Immunodefiency Virus (HIV) Infection in Children Under 13 Years of Age
MMWR, 36 (1987a), 225-235

Council of State and Territ. Epidemiol., AIDS Program, Center for Infectious Diseases, Centers for Disease Control (CDC)
Revision of the CDC Surveillance Case Definition for Acquired Immunodefiency Syndrome
MMWR, 36 (1987b), (suppl., no. 1S), 1-15

Darrow, W.W., E.M. Gorman, B.P. Glick
The Social Origins of AIDS: Social Change, Sexual Behavior, and Disease Trends
In: D.A. Feldman, T.H. Johnson, *The Social Dimensions of AIDS*, Praeger, New York, 1986, 95-107

Ende, M.E. van der, A.C.M. Kroes, J. Buitenwerf, C.L. van der Poel
AIDS door HIV-2 in Nederland
Nederlands Tijdschrift voor Geneeskunde, 134 (1990), 10, 495-497

Friedland, G.H., R.S. Klein
Transmission of the Human Immunodefiency Virus
New England Journal of Medicine, 317 (1987), 18, 1125-1135

Geneeskundige Hoofdinspectie van de Volksgezondheid (GHI)
GHI bulletin; De diagnose AIDS
Staatstoezicht op de volksgezondheid, Rijswijk, 1987

Geneeskundige Hoofdinspectie van de Volksgezondheid (GHI)
AIDS-diagnosis registration reports
continuous registration

Griensven, G.J.P. van
Epidemiology and Prevention of HIV-infection among homosexual men.
UvA, Amsterdam, 1989, academisch proefschrift

De Gruttola, V., G.R. Seage III, K.H. Mayer, C.R. Horsburgh jr.
Infectiousness of HIV between male homosexual partners
Journal of Clinical Epidemiology, 42 (1989), 9, 849-856

Hoek, A. van der
Epidemiology of HIV Infection among drug users in Amsterdam
Rodopi, Amsterdam, 1990, dissertation

Hochheimer, E.H., A.M. Heijnen, L. Wigersma (red.)
HIV-wijzer voor de huisarts; losbladig informatiesysteem voor de huisarts
Stichting Aanvullende Dienstverlening, Amsterdam, 1989

Holmberg, S.D., C.R. Horsburgh jr., J.W. Ward, H.W. Jaffe
Biological Factors in the Sexual Transmission of Human Immunodeficiency Virus
Journal of Infectious Diseases, 160 (1989), 1, 116-125

Hoogeveen, R.T., J.J.L.M. Brouwer
Scenario's in de volksgezondheid: Inleiding in de methodiek van de STG
Jan van Arkel, Utrecht, 1989

Hooykaas, C., J. van der Pligt, G.J.J. van Doornum, M.M.D. van der Linden, R.A. Coutinho
Heterosexuals at risk for HIV: differences between private and commercial partners in sexual behavior and condom use
AIDS, 3 (1989), 525-532

Houweling, H., R.A. Coutinho
Epidemiological and public health aspects of AIDS and HIV infection: current concepts.
RIVM, Bilthoven, 1989, report nr. 528900001

Lifson, A., N. Hessol, G.W. Rutherford, P. O'Malley, L. Barnhart S. Buchbinder, L., Cannon, T. Bodecker S., Holmberg, J. Harrison, L. Doll
Natural history of HIV infection in a cohort of homosexual and bisexual men: Clinical and immunological outcome, 1977-1990
Presentation at *VI international conference on AIDS*, San Francisco, 1990

Mann, J.M.
Global AIDS into the 1990s; An address presented 4 June 1989 at the V international Conference on AIDS Montreal Canada
WHO, Geneva, 1989

McClumeck, N., H. Taelman, P. Hermans, P. Piot, M. Schoumacher, S. De Wit
A cluster of HIV-infection among heterosexual people without apparant risk factors
New England Journal of Medicine, 322 (1989), 1460-1462

Reinking, D.P.,F.M van den Boom,, J.C. Jager, M.J.Postma
De sociaal-culturele en financieel-economische gevolgen van AIDS voor de samenleving: voorstudie
STG/NcGv/RIVM, Rijswijk/Utrecht/Bilthoven, 1989

Scenariocommissie Vergrijzing, vakgroep Planning en Beleid RUU
Ouder worden in de toekomst; scenario's over gezondheid en vergrijzing 1984 - 2000
Jan van Arkel, Utrecht, 1985

Scenariocommissie Hart- en Vaatziekten, Wils Systeem Analyse B.V.
Het hart van de toekomst, de toekomst van het hart; scenario's over hart- en vaatziekten 1985-2010
Bohn, Scheltema & Holkema, Utrecht/Antwerpen, 1986

Stuurgroep Toekomstscenario's Gezondheidszorg (STG)
Structuur en opdracht
STG, Rijswijk, 1987

Scenariocommissie Ongevallen en Traumatologie, Instituut Maatschappelijke Gezondheidszorg EUR
Ongevallen in het jaar 2000; scenario's over Ongevallen en Traumatologie 1985-2000, deel 1, hoofdrapport
Bohn, Scheltema & Holkema, Utrecht/Antwerp, 1988

Scenariocommissie Geestelijke Volksgezondheid en Geestelijke Gezondheidszorg, Onderzoeksteam Nederlands centrum Geestelijke volksgezondheid, R.V. Bijl, M.A. Janssen, E. Ketting, J.D. Kroon
Zorgen voor geestelijke gezondheid in de toekomst; toekomstscenario's geestelijke volksgezondheid en geestelijke gezondheidszorg 1990 -2010
Bohn, Scheltema & Holkema, Utrecht/Antwerp, 1990

Scenariocommissie Arbeid en Gezondheid
Arbeid, gezondheid en welzijn in de toekomst; toekomstscenario's arbeid en gezondheid 1990-2010
Bohn, Stafleu van Loghum, Houten/Antwerp, 1991

Straver, C.J., A. van Stolk
De kans op verbreiding van AIDS onder de Nederlandse bevolking
Maandblad Geestelijke volksgezondheid, 43 (1988), 4, 379-394

Tweede Kamer der Staten Generaal (TK, 1985)
Het verworven immuun deficiëntiesyndroom
Tweede Kamer der Staten Generaal, vergaderjaar 1985-1986, 19218, nrs. 1-2

Vliet, R.W.F.
Seksuele netwerken onder Nederlandse scholieren
In: T. Vogels, R. van der Vliet, *Jeugd en Seks; gedrag en gezondheidsrisico's bij scholieren*
SDU Uitgeverij, The Hague, 1990, 117-131

Vries, H. de
Planning, toekomstonderzoek en scenario's
Beleid & Maatschappij, 1985, 4, 94-101

Zessen, G.J. van, C. Straver
De mogelijke verspreiding van HIV onder de Nederlandse bevolking
In: G.J. van Zessen, Th. Sandfort (red.), *Seksualiteit in Nederland; Seksueel gedrag, risico en preventie van AIDS*, Swets & Zeitlinger, Amsterdam/Lisse, 1991, 205-224

Appendix A

'Surveillance case' definition of AIDS

This appendix contains criteria for the diagnosis of AIDS, as given in CDC (1987) en GHI (1987). The criteria relate to the 'revised' diagnosis. This revision - in essence a broadening - of the diagnosis took effect in the USA on the 1st of September 1987 and has also been adopted by WHO. As compared to the old criteria one of the changes made relates to the fact that in some specific cases it is now possible to diagnose AIDS in combination with a negative laboratory HIV-test result. Beside it the criteria applied to children below 13 years of age have changed.

I AIDS is diagnosed in case of Pneumocystis carinii in combination with a negative HIV-test result if no other causes for the immune deficiency, excluding diseases for being indicators of AIDS[3], are present.

II In combination with a doubtful laboratory HIV-test result (or absence of a test result) and no other causes for the immune deficiency, excluding diseases for being indicators of AIDS[1], are present the following diseases are indicators of AIDS:

- specific types of candidiasis,
- cryptococcosis, extrapulmonary,
- cryptosporidiosis with diarrhoea persisting > 1 month,
- cytomegalovirus disease of specific organs in a patient > 1 month of age,
- specified consequences of herpes simplex virus infection,
- kaposi's sarcoma affecting a patient > 60 years of age,
- lymphoma of the brain (primary) affecting a patient < 60 years of age,
- LIP/PLH complex affecting a child < 13 years of age,
- disseminated infection by e.g. Mycobacterium kansasii,
- Pneumocystis carinii pneumonia,
- progressive multifocal leukoencefalopathy, and
- toxoplasmosis of the brain affecting a patient > 1 month of age.

III With laboratory evidence of HIV infection one or a combination of the following diseases lead to the diagnosis of AIDS:

- a combination of recurrent and multiple infections in a child < 13 jaar (e.g. meningitis),
- disseminated coccidioidomycosis,
- specific consequences of cytomegalovirus infection,

---

[3] a. an immunosuppresive/cytotoxic therapy which started < 3 months before the indicator disease is diagnosed,
b. specific diseaeses, diagnosed < 3 months after the indicator disease is diagnosed (e.g. Hodgkin's disease and lymphocytic leucaemia), and
c. a genetical determined (e.g. congenital) immunodeficiency syndrome, not characteristic for HIV infection.

- HIV encefalopathy (also called AIDS dementia or subacute encephalitis due to HIV),
- disseminated histoplasmosis,
- isosporiasis with diarrhoea persisting > 1 month,
- kaposi's sarcoma,
- primary lymphoma of the brain,
- other non-Hodgkin's lymphoma and certain histological types (Burkitt, immunoblastic sarcoma),
- any disseminated mycobacterial disease not caused by M. tuberculosis,
- extrapulmonary tuberculosis door M. tuberculosis,
- certain disseminated mycobacterial infections,
- recurrent Salmonella septocaemia (not by S. typhi),
- HIV wasting syndroom ('slim disease'), and
- all indicator diseases under II.

Appendix B.1

CDC classification for HIV infection

CDC I
Acute infection with HIV. Symptoms resemble those of influenza. Seroconversion develops after three weeks to six months (this latent period is also known as the window phase). Antibodies against HIV then develop. This phase is also known as Seroconversion Syndrome.

CDC II
Asymptomatic infection. The individual is seropositive but has no outward manifestations of disease.

CDC III
Lymphadenopathy syndrome (LAS)/Persistent Generalized Lymphadenopathy (PGL). A chronic lymph node swelling of at least two non-inguinal lymph node stations occurs. These last for more than three months and the swelling must also be caused by HIV infection and must not provide grounds for classifying the patient in group IV.

CDC IV

a. Constitutional syndromes. This classification is employed in the event of fatigue/malaise + fever lasting longer than one month, or of diarrhoea lasting longer than one month or of an involuntary weight loss of 10% of body weight, caused in all three cases only by HIV infection. CDC IVa is also referred to as HIV Wasting Syndrome.
b. Neurological syndromes. This classification is employed in the event of neurological diseases, e.g. dementia or myelopathy or peripheral neuropathy, without any concurrent condition apart from HIV to explain the symptoms in any of the three cases. CDC IVb is also referred to as AIDS dementia complex.
c-1. Secondary infectious disease(s) from the list of the AIDS surveillance definition, including Pneumocystis carinii pneumonia.
c-2. Secondary infectious disease(s) from the following list: oral hairy leukoplakia, multidermatomal herpes zoster, recurrent Salmonella bacteriaemia, nocardiosis, Epstein-Barr virus, tuberculosis and oral candidiasis.
d. Secondary cancers give rise to classification in IVd. The forms of cancer are those from the CDC surveillance case definition for AIDS.
e. In the absence of symptoms attributable to HIV infection and not referred to above patients are classified as IVe.

In contrast to the comments on groups I, II, III and IV it should be noted that within group IV, double classification and transitions in all directions are possible.

Appendix B.2

CDC classification for HIV infection among children aged under 13

Class P-0 Indeterminate infection.
This includes prenatally infected children and children in whom the state of infection is indeterminate.

Class P-1 Asymptomatic infection.

a. Normal immune function.
b. Abnormal immune function.
c. Immune function not tested.

Class P-2 Symptomatic infection.

a. Non-specific findings.
b. Progressive neurological syndrome.
c. Chronic interstitial pneumonia.
d. Secondary infection(s).
   - d-1 Secondary infectious disease(s) from the list of the CDC surveillance case definition for AIDS.
   - d-2 Recurrent serious bacteriological infections.
   - d-3 Other specified secondary infectious diseases.
e. Secondary cancers.
   - e-1 Specified secondary cancers from the list of the CDC surveillance case definition for AIDS.
   - e-2 Other cancers that could be secondary to HIV infection.
f. Other diseases possibly attributable to HIV infection.

2 Scenario construction

2.1 *Introduction*

Does the new, communicable disease of AIDS constitute a threat to public health? What implications does AIDS have for public health, what sort of funding is required, and how can the ostracism of and discrimination towards affected individuals be prevented? And by way of logical extension, how can the danger of AIDS be averted by means of prevention and public information, infectious-disease control and research? These questions briefly summarize the subjects for this scenario analysis. Looking to the future there is uncertainty with respect to the epidemiology, the incidence of risk behaviour and the effects of prevention, care and medical technology and the social impact of AIDS. This chapter discusses the working method adopted for the scenario construction in more detail.

2.2 *Scenario construction*

2.2.1 *Subjects for scenario analysis*

The subjects for scenario analysis derive from the conceptual model in Chapter 1: *HIV/AIDS incidence, behaviour control, care and medical technology and the sociocultural context.*

The starting point for the projections and predictions is provided by the reference scenario, in which the epidemiological, economic and sociocultural consequences of AIDS are examined in conjunction. This scenario, which arises directly from the epidemiological, economic and sociocultural baseline analyses, explores the impact of developments in the incidence of AIDS. Projections are also carried out in sub-areas. The subjects for scenario analysis are introduced and briefly discussed below.

A central theme in studies of the future incidence and prevalence of HIV/AIDS is *risk behaviour and the effect of prevention.* We examine the epidemiological course of HIV and AIDS, differentiated according to high-risk sexual contact, injection behaviour and HIV transmission routes within and between groups with an identified risk of infection: men with multiple male partners, injecting drug users, commercial sex workers and their clients and men and women with multiple heterosexual partners.

Sooner or later each HIV-infected person will seek medical

care. The results of epidemiological projections can therefore be translated into consequences for health care. The studies concerning *care and medical technology* are broken down into the demand for care in the various sectors of care. A further breakdown in terms of institutes and disciplines is employed: inpatient and outpatient care, somatic and psychosocial care, and care and support by professionals and voluntary workers. In determining the impact of AIDS on care we take account of changes in and influences on care from medical technology. Relevant in this respect are projections of the consequences of improved diagnosis and treatment by means of biomedical research and accumulated expertise in the treatment of symptoms. The treatment of manifestations of disease thereby becomes briefer, more efficient and more effective, thus prolonging the life expectancy of people with AIDS and increasing the interval between hospital admissions. A concrete development in medical technology that could have a major impact on care and the demand for care in the near future is early intervention, i.e. the commencement of treatment at the earliest possible stage in the progression to AIDS. Among other things the aim here is to defer the onset of AIDS for as long as possible, to prolong life expectancy, improve the subjective well-being of the patient and prevent opportunistic infections (GR, 1990; NCAB, 1990). Account needs also to be taken of the consequences of care substitution, which can lead among people with AIDS to an increasing requirement for (intensive) home care (SCP, 1990).

The projections of the impact of AIDS also take account of the *social context* of AIDS and AIDS control. A distinction may usefully be drawn here between the social context within which the AIDS/HIV epidemic is developing and the consequences associated with the reaction to AIDS. With respect to the social consequences there remains the as yet unresolved question of insurance. It should also be noted that dilemmas arise if early intervention becomes a reasonable alternative: if life is prolonged by early intervention how does this square with the obligation to disclose HIV-positive status when applying for certain forms of insurance? As far as the social context of the AIDS epidemic is concerned it is relevant to examine the considerations on which the present AIDS control strategy and the organization of care are based. By way of extension alternative strategies may be explored in terms of their social and legal/ethical desirability and admissability.

2.2.2 *Types of scenarios*

In Chapter 1 a distinction was drawn between *exploratory* and *strategic scenarios*. The reference scenario is an example of an exploratory scenario based on the assumption that no fundamental changes take place in relation to the baseline analysis. In addition likely and potential epidemiological trends and the consequences of developments in care and medical technology are examined by means of exploratory scenarios. In line with these and in some cases indissolubly bound up with them, strategic scenarios are drawn up with a view to exploring the ways in which desirable and feasible final projected situations could be achieved and the resources this would require. A scenario analysis for AIDS might include strategies aimed at preventing new HIV infections or guaranteeing a high standard of care. The main points of departure and assumptions for the exploratory and strategic scenarios are discussed in the next two sections.

2.2.2.1 *Exploratory scenarios*

The *reference scenario* examines the impact of AIDS on the assumption that the trends in the baseline analyses continue unchanged. In order to provide an impression of the scope for intervention by means of information and education and the promotion of changes in behaviour, and taking account of the target-setting nature of AIDS control, part of the reference scenario has been separated off. In this subscenario we have explored the impact of AIDS that will unavoidably occur due to developments in the first decade of the HIV epidemic. Specifically, this means the impact of the HIV epidemic during the period 1979-1989. This subscenario provides an *underestimate* of the consequences of HIV/AIDS; it is *not a best-case variant* of the reference scenario. The reference scenario calculates the economic consequences of the identified epidemiological trends and the latter are discussed in relation to the social context of AIDS. The reference scenario therefore examines the epidemiological, economic and sociocultural aspects of AIDS in the year 2000.

The reference scenario is based on the assumption that no fundamental changes will take place in relation to the current situation. Specifically, this means among other things that we are assuming a concentration of the HIV epidemic within the groups of "men who have sex with men" and "injective drug users", with little risk of an independent epidemic among the heterosexual population. Similarly it has been assumed that no changes take place with respect to care, medical technology and the social context. The survival period of people with AIDS has, for example, been held constant and a relapse into risk behaviour has been ruled out.

In surveys of alternative final projected situations we examine which changes in relation to the reference scenario are due to intervening developments in the following areas: (1) behaviour and the effectiveness of prevention, (2) care and medical technology, and (3) the social context of AIDS. In behavioural scenarios we explore the consequences for the HIV epidemic of an increase in risk behaviour among men who have sex with men, possible alternative developments in the HIV epidemic among IDUs and the spread of HIV infection within the heterosexual population in general and the world of commercial sex work. With respect to care and medical technology another element of the reference scenario has been varied, by (among other things) taking account of the consequences of a prolonged survival period among people with AIDS or changes in the delivery of care. Changes in the social context of the epidemic are key elements in scenarios in which alternative strategies for AIDS control and the organization of care are described.

2.2.2.2 *Strategic scenarios*

Bailey (in preparation) has distinguished three basic types of strategic scenarios for AIDS scenario analysis: (1) an integral AIDS-specific policy, (2) a health care provision policy, in which AIDS control takes place within the framework of STD or infectious disease control, and (3) a laissez-faire policy, under which resources are made available at moments of acute crisis. The Netherlands has opted in favour of the first of the these approaches, i.e. an integral AIDS-specific control policy, as set out in the Policy Document on AIDS Policy (TK, 1987).

Concrete policy principles were formulated in the Policy Document with respect to prevention, care and research, while extra resources were made available in each area. As part of a review of the structure and organization of government policy a National AIDS Control Committee (NCAB) was set up, while the Policy Document also set government policy against the background of individual civil rights and the social responsibilities of government. Particular issues in this respect are HIV-antibody testing and the constitutional provisions protecting privacy and guaranteeing the integrity of the body.

As far as HIV/AIDS prevention is concerned the emphasis is on public information and education and promoting behaviour changes. With respect to care the underlying aims are to reduce hospitalization to the minimum, to promote the systematic transfer of knowledge and experience and, wherever possible, to fit the care of people with AIDS into normal health care provision.

The reference, behaviour and care/medical technology scenarios are implicitly based on an integral AIDS-specific control policy. The scenarios accordingly provide an impression of the extent to which AIDS-control goals can be realized in an epidemiological, preventive and social sense. Discussion is possible about the ways in which these goals should be achieved and the resources to be deployed. In the strategic scenarios we survey the options for *AIDS control* and the organization of *care for people with HIV-infected and AIDS*. In both these policy areas we have compiled two alternative strategies, which are discussed in terms of their consequences for epidemiological monitoring, prevention and care. In the case of the strategic scenarios for AIDS control we also examine the social and especially the legal foundation for the scenarios, while in the discussion of the care strategies we examine considerations that might justify changes in organization and extra attention to the care and support of people with AIDS and HIV. It should be emphasized that this element of the scenario analysis is subjective in nature; surveying the advantages and disadvantages of AIDS control and care strategies forms a part of this project, but a judgement as to the best AIDS control and care strategies does not.

2.2.2.3 Survey of types of scenarios and subject-areas for scenario analysis

The starting point for the scenario analysis is provided by the reference scenario (Chapter 6). This scenario examines the epidemiological, economic and sociocultural aspects of the AIDS epidemic and the epidemic of HIV. The reference scenario is exploratory in nature, although it also contains a clearly strategic component in that this scenario also establishes a framework for assessing the effectiveness, costs and benefits of current AIDS control. In Chapters 7 and 8 we examine intervening developments in the fields of behaviour, care and medical technology. These scenarios are primarily exploratory in nature. On the basis of the social context of AIDS and the AIDS epidemic, two alternative strategic scenarios are discussed in Chapter 9. Elements of the reference scenario are varied in Chapters 7-9. The above is shown schematically in Table 2.1, together with the chapters in which the various scenarios have been developed.

Table 2.1 Exploratory and strategic scenarios: subject-areas and assumptions

Exploratory scenarios	Subject-area/assumption	Chapter
- Reference scenario	Consequences of AIDS/ HIV epidemic in socio-cultural and economic respects given unchanged trends	6
Alternative exploratory scenarios:		
- Behaviour scenarios	Intervening development: risk behaviour and effects of prevention	7
- Care and Medical Technology Scenarios	Intervening development: improved treatment possibilities	8
Strategic scenarios		
- Social context	AIDS control options Care structure options	9

2.2.3 Parameters and indicators for scenario analysis

Table 2.2 sets out the parameters and indicators that have been selected for the scenario analysis in the epidemiological, sociocultural and economic fields.

The parameters are independent variables used for determining the scale and impact of the HIV/AIDS epidemic. The scenarios are generated by varying the values of the parameters. The consequences of AIDS are expressed in terms of indicators; these form the dependent variables in the analysis. An indicator may express the impact of AIDS in either quantitative or qualitative terms. Quantification is possible with respect to the epidemiology and the economic aspects, while the analysis of the sociocultural aspects of AIDS is largely qualitative. The indicators consist of the subject-areas covered by this analysis.

Table 2.2 **Parameters and indicators for scenario analysis**

	Parameters	Indicators
Epidemiology		
Behaviour	Group size	HIV incidence/
	Risk behaviour	prevalence
	Number of partners	- epidemic in its entirety
	Effects of prevention	- sub-epidemics
		AIDS incidence/
Progression	Incubation time	prevalence :
	Survival period	- epidemic in its entirety
		- sub-epidemics
		Case fatality
		PYLL
Economics	Relative costs	Patient-related:
	- Inpatient v. outpatient	Bed need:
	- Specialist v. non-specialist	- hospitals
	- Voluntary v. professional	- nursing homes
		Hospital costs:
		- medical treatment
		- hospital care
		- AZT (and prophylaxes)
		Nursing home costs
		District nursing costs and hours
		Home help costs and hours
		Intensive home care costs and days
		GP costs and consultations
		Costs of ambulant mental health care
		Hours of buddy help
		Non-patient-related:
		Number and costs of tests
		Costs of other prevention
		Research costs
		Costs of other programmes
Sociocultural	Socio-sexological aspects	Attitudes towards sexuality/sexual behaviour
	AIDS-control options	Knowledge of and attitudes towards AIDS
	Organization/ structure of care	Primary prevention v. alternative strategies
	Legal/ethical aspects	Importance of individual civil rights
	Societal response	Discrimination/ tolerance
		Access to social facilities

The working method may be illustrated with the aid of an example. In the chapter devoted to scenarios on care and medical technology we explore the effects of early intervention. In relation to the reference scenario it has been assumed that, as a intervening development, the progression to AIDS is delayed. In relation to Table 2.2 this means that the parameter "incubation period" is varied. The impact of early intervention translate themselves in terms of an increase in the prevalence of AIDS, demand for specific care, increased testing and intensified debate concerning access to social facilities. Translated into indicators this means: the AIDS prevalance, indicators concerning the demand for care and the number of tests, and considerations with respect to access to social facilities. The other parameters and indicators listed in Table 2.2 remain as in the reference scenario.

2.3 *Model-building*

Mathematical simulations are designed to show policy-makers at an early stage how the impact of the epidemiology of the HIV/AIDS epidemic may develop. The lack of information, for example on seroprevalence, risk behaviour and the effects of prevention, means that it is difficult to predict or approximate the future course of the AIDS epidemic. Mathematical simulations are therefore also designed to close the gap between the specification of data requirements and the available data (IOM/NAS, 1988).

In selecting the mathematical models for the scenario analysis we have, in the light of the above, opted in favour of models geared to predictions in the short term and models based on the spread of HIV. The second type of models may have been for medium to long-term projections. Other factors in the selection of models have included the available surveillance systems and the available data from epidemiological and socio-scientific AIDS research (PccAo, 1990). The more closely a model approximates reality the more complex the model tends to become and the more data are required for meaningful applications. A usable model strikes a balance between a minimal reduction of reality and practical application. More complex models might be used if more research data were to be become available. These might include models relating to network analysis and models for the spread of HIV that also incorporate the modelling of the immunological process.

2.3.1 *Mathematical modellingand scenario analysis*

In the construction of scenarios, epidemiological courses are generated with the aid of mathematical modelling at two levels (Jager et al., 1989):

(1) statistical modelling of available data, on the basis of the MIDAS empirical models (Heisterkamp et al. 1989) and the back-calculation method (Jager et al., 1990a; Hay, 1989);

(2) dynamic population models (Van Druten and Jager, 1991).

Table 2.3, taken from Jager et al., (1989), shows the selected models listed in terms of application. The notes to the table describe the applications of the selected models in scenario analysis. For the mathematical structure of the models we would refer to the appendix at the end of this chapter.

There is a fundamental difference between the various types of models (Cox et al., 1988). Process models take explicit account of the transmission mechanism which determines the course of the epidemic (Bailey 1988, in preparation; Bailey and Estreicher, 1987; Anderson, 1988, 1989; Dietz, 1988; Isham, 1988; Hyman and Stanley, 1988). The empirical models are based on statistical methods, which may be applied to data on the incidence of AIDS (Morgan and Curran, 1986; Downs et al., 1988; Healy and Tillet, 1988; Cox et al., 1988; Brookmeyer and Damiano, 1989).

Table 2.3 **Mathematical models according to their applications in scenario analysis** (taken from: Jager et al., 1989).

Nature of model	Main application	Model
Empirical models	- Description - Reconstruction - Short-term forecasting - Extrapolation	Heisterkamp et al., 1989 Jager et al., 1990a Hay, 1989
Process modelling (multi- or single group approach)	- Description - Reconstruction - Simulation - Sensitivity analysis - Specification of data needs - Hypothesis generation	Van Druten and Jager, 1991 Van Druten et al., 1988

2.3.1.1 MIDAS

MIDAS (Modelling Incidence and Delay Adjustment Simultaneously) is a statistical model which, after adjustment for delays in reporting, is used for forecasting the AIDS incidence/prevalence in the short term (Heisterkamp et al., 1988ab, 1989, in preparation). In conjunction with the back-calculation method and on the basis of the postulated incubation-period distribution, MIDAS may also be used to arrive at an estimate of the number of HIV-infected persons. In combination with curve-fitting techniques a reconstruction of the course of the HIV epidemic may then be made. This curve, which has been used in this project to show the HIV epidemic up to 1989, provides the starting point for long-range studies of the HIV/AIDS incidence.

MIDAS may be used not just to analyse the epidemic in its entirety but may also be applied to risk groups. In this report it has been used to chart the epidemiological trend among men who have sex with men. In addition it is possible to draw a distinction in terms of the degree of progression to AIDS in applications based on the CDC stages. Such applications are particularly relevant for long-range studies of the demand for care[1]. Simulations have also been conducted with MIDAS on a modest scale.

2.3.1.2 Process modelling

Process modelling relates to the spread of HIV within and between core groups and is used especially in relation to the behaviour scenarios in Chapter 7. In process modelling simulation techniques are used on the basis of assumptions concerning the epidemiological trend within a group. Process modelling can be effectively applied to individual groups, such as the AIDS epidemic among men who have sex with men and IDUs. *Multi-group* modelling provides insight into the possible spread of HIV between core groups and is an instrument for describing the effect of intervention strategies aimed at behavioural change. Multi-group modelling, among other things, enables epidemiological trends for the spread of HIV via heterosexual contact to be determined (Van Druten and Jager, 1991).

---

1 Hypotheses concerning infectiousness form another relevant area. The risk of transmission of HIV through risk behaviour is thought to be greater around the point of infection with HIV, immediately before diagnosis with AIDS and among people diagnosed with AIDS, i.e. in CDC stages I, III and IV. During the (often lengthy) asymptomatic state, i.e. CDC stage II, infectiousness is by contrast thought to be lower. Since this is one of the many hypotheses concerning infectiousness we have not included it in the scenario analysis. Infectiousness is examined in more detail in Chapter 3.

Figure 2.1 **Multi-group model: the HIV epidemic as resulting from overlapping subepidemics in sex subgroups, possible contacts between and within groups and the transmission routes unprotected anal (a) and vaginal (v) intercourse and needle sharing (n).** (Source: Van Druten and Jager (1991)).

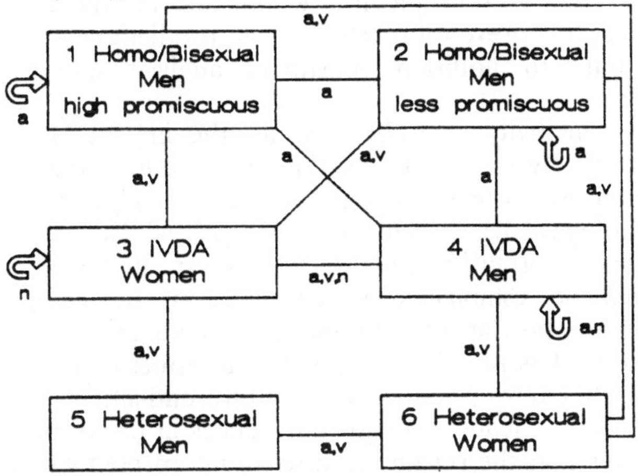

The basis of the model we have used is shown in Figure 2.1. In this model the AIDS epidemic is approached as the result of a number of overlapping epidemics in subgroups. The figure shows possible contacts between and within groups for the following transmission routes: unprotected anal intercourse (a), unprotected vaginal intercourse (v) and the shared use of needles by IDUs. For each subgroup values are required in this model for the following parameters: (1) group size, (2) number of partners with whom there is risk contact, (3) seroprevalence and (4) the risk of transmission of HIV. Interventions, such as an effect of prevention, are expressed by changes in the parameters. These parameters are included as parameters for scenario analysis in Table 2.1.

The multi-group model is a closed model. This means that no account is taken of the inflow of new susceptibles and the progression to AIDS and/or mortality. In order to prevent any distortion of the results to which this might be attributed, the model is used for studying the *beginning* of an epidemic within and between certain core groups, for example heterosexual men and women. These may be short and medium-term projections. In later stages of the epidemic the model may be used for short-term studies, for example among men who have sex with men and IDUs.

2.3.2 *Goals of mathematical modelling*

Mathematical models are used for various purposes. Reference has already been made to the description and reconstruction of the epidemiological trends to date, seroprevalence estimates, description of the spread of the epidemic within and between groups, including the effect of prevention, short-term predictions and medium-term projections. In addition sensitivity analysis and simulations are possible.

A sensitivity analysis examines the impact of a change in the parameters. By for example varying the group size and condom use it is established which changes have the biggest impact on the epidemiological trend. Sensitivity analysis is also used in the absence of precise information on the parameters. In these circumstances it can then be established which value of an unknown parameter provides the best approximation of the epidemiological trend to date. In addition it is possible to explore the effect of varying the value of imprecisely known parameters on future end-situations. If variation of the parameters leads to major differences in the results of projections, this means that the results need to be interpreted with caution.

As the concept of simulations implies, these are *approximations* rather than exact representations of reality. Simulations on the basis of process and multi-group modelling are aimed at exploring and tightening hypotheses concerning the future course of HIV.

2.3.3 *Linkage of model-building and socio-economic data*

In the construction of scenarios on the impact of AIDS the results from mathematical epidemiological models need to be linked up with the results of socio-scientific and economic research (Jager et al., 1988, 1989, 1990b, 1991ab; Dijkgraaf et al., 1990; Leidl, 1989, 1990; Leidl et al., in preparation, Brookmeyer and Liao, 1990). Figure 2.2 schematically sets out the procedure for such linkage. Depending on the model used an HIV/AIDS incidence figure is obtained that can be expressed in terms of HIV/AIDS prevalence and lethality. This involves a combination of data on the progression to AIDS and the survival period after diagnosis with AIDS (i.e. progression of the disease). In a succeeding stage data from socio-scientific and economic research are linked up with these results (i.e. the health care system). By way of illustration the following areas are included in Figure 2.2: health care services (need for hospital beds) and demography (Potential Years of Life Lost; PYLL). In a calculation on an *incidence-basis* the consequences for the PYLL are assigned to the year to which the incidence of deaths relates. Determinations of the

need for beds and the costs are made in this report on a *prevalence-basis*: the burden of AIDS on hospital beds and budgets, etc., is assigned to the year in which these consequences actually occur (see for example Hellinger (1990) for an approximation of the costs in the USA on incidence-basis).
The consequences of AIDS are measures in terms of indicators, as has been shown in Table 2.1.

Figure 2.2 **Impact assessment of the HIV/AIDS epidemic by linking epidemiological data and information on demography and health care services utilisation.**

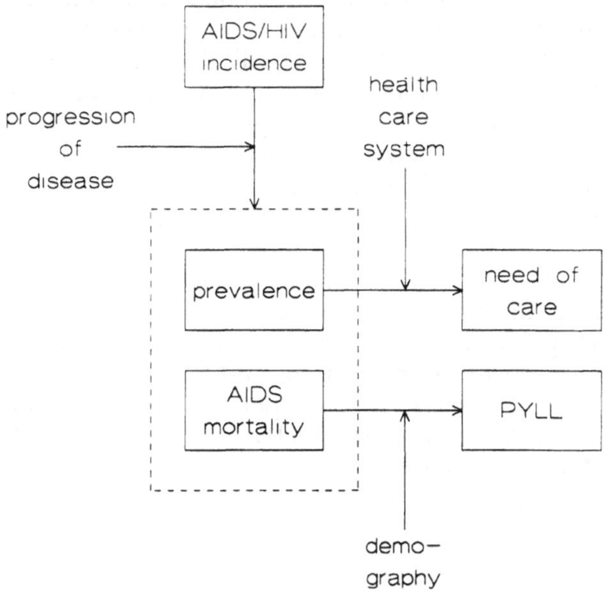

2.4 Commentary

The framework for scenario analysis described in this Chapter enables the consequences of AIDS and the advantages and disadvantages of various intervention strategies to be described in a large number of areas. Our working method has been presented on the basis of an introduction of the selection of subject-areas for scenario analysis. The description of the impact of AIDS to date is examined in detail in the baseline analyses (Chapters 3, 4 and 5).

The scenarios that have been introduced are a selection that can be *expanded as desired. The baseline analyses provide the building blocks, for example when it comes to the respective AIDS risks for ethnic minorities, young people and health-care providers.

The baseline analyses also provide a frame of reference for refining the parameters. Examples include incorporating the possible influence of such factors as age, life events and mobility on the incidence and prevalence of HIV. This chapter therefore also provides an initial framework that can be refined as desired for analysing the consequences of AIDS.

2.5 Summary

This chapter examines the working method for the construction of scenarios. Apart from a reference scenario based on the continuation of present trends, a number of alternative scenarios have been drawn up in which we explore cross-cutting developments in the following sub-areas of the reference scenario: risk behaviour and the effectiveness of prevention, care and medical technology and the social context of AIDS. The latter scenarios have been designated as strategic and the remaining ones as (largely) exploratory. For the purpose of the scenario analysis a number of parameters and indicators have been selected in the epidemiological, economic and sociocultural fields. The impact of AIDS has been determined on the basis of indicators we have drawn up. For the purpose of scenario analysis we have made use of mathematical models at two levels: statistical modelling and process modelling. The possible applications of the models range from a description and reconstruction of the epidemic to date to short-term predictions and long-term projections.

The method presented is regarded as a methodological framework for the scenario analysis of AIDS that is capable of being expanded and refined as required.

References

Anderson, R.M.

The Role of Mathematical Models in the Study of HIV Transmission and the Epidemiology of AIDS

Journal of Acquired Immune Deficiency Syndromes, 1 (1988), 241-256

Anderson, R.M.

Editorial review; Mathematical and statistical studies of the epidemiology of HIV

AIDS, 3 (1989), 333-346

Bailey, N.T.J.

Review of available and required data for applied modelling of HIV/AIDS, with special reference to assisting public health decision-making

Génève, 1988, consultant's report to the global programme on AIDS World Health Organization

Bailey, N.T.J.

Operational modelling of HIV/AIDS to assist public health policy making and control.

In: J.C. Jager, E.J. Ruitenberg (eds.), *AIDS Impact Assessment; Modelling and Scenario Analysis*, RIVM/Bilthoven, in preparation

Bailey, N.T.J. J. Estreicher

Implications of stochastic variations in HIV/AIDS modelling

In: J.C. Jager, E.J. Ruitenberg (eds.), *Statistical Analysis and Mathematical Modelling of AIDS*, Oxford University Press, Oxford, 1988

Brookmeyer, R., A. Damiano

Statistical methods for short term projections of AIDS incidence

Statistics in Medicine, 8 (1989), 23-44

Brookmeyer, R., Jiangang Liao

Statistical Modelling of the AIDS Epidemic for Forecasting Health Care Needs

Biometrics, 46 (1990), 1151-1163

Cox, D., R.M. Anderson, A.M. Johnson, M.J.R. Healy, V. Isham, A.D. Wilkie, N.E. Day, O.N. Gill, A. McCormick

Short-term prediction of HIV Infection and AIDS in England and Wales; report of a working group

Her Majesty's Stationery Office, London, 1988

Dietz, K.

The dynamics of spread of HIV-infection in the heterosexual popualtion

In: J.C. Jager, E.J. Ruitenberg (eds.), *Statistical Analysis and Mathematical Modelling of AIDS*, Oxford University Press, Oxford, 1988

Downs, A.M., R.A. Ancelle, J.C. Jager, S.H. Heisterkamp, J.A.M. van Druten, E.J. Ruitenberg, J.B. Brunet
The statistical estimation, from routine surveillance data, of past, present and future trends in AIDS incidence in Europe
In: J.C. Jager, E.J. Ruitenberg (eds.), *Statistical Analysis and Mathematical Modelling of AIDS*, Oxford University Press, Oxford, 1988, 1-16

Druten, J.A.M. van, Th. De Boo, J.C. Jager, S.H. Heisterkamp, R.A. Coutinho, E.J. Ruitenberg
AIDS prediction and intervention
Lancet, 1986a, 12, 852-853

Druten, J.A.M. van, Th. De Boo, J.C. Jager, S.H. Heisterkamp, R.A. Coutinho, E.J. Ruitenberg
Een model voor de voorspelling van het epidemiologisch verloop van AIDS onder homosexuelen met verhoogd risico
Tijdschrift voor Sociale Gezondheidszorg, 64 (1986b), 8, 279

Druten, J.A.M. van, Th. de Boo, J.M. Bos, J.C. Jager, S.H. Heisterkamp, H. Houweling
Verspreiding van HIV infectie in een cohort homosexuelen voordat gevallen van AIDS worden waargenomen
Tijdschrift voor Sociale Gezondheidszorg, 65 (1987), 7, 192-193

Druten, J.A.M. van
Comment on Dr. Isham's paper
In: V. Isham *Mathematical modelling of the transmission dynamics of HIV infection and AIDS: a review*, Journal of the Royal Statistical Society, series A, 151 (1988), 5-49

Druten, J.A.M. van, Th. de Boo, A.G.M. Reintjes, J.C. Jager, S.H. Heisterkamp, R.A. Coutinho, J.M. Bos, E.J. Ruitenberg
Reconstruction and prediction of spread of HIV infection in populations of homosexual men
In: J.C. Jager, E.J. Ruitenberg (eds.) *Statistical Analysis and Mathematical Modelling of AIDS*, Oxford University Press, Oxford, 1988a, 52-76

Druten, J.A.M. van, J.C. Jager, S.H. Heisterkamp
HIV infection dynamics in linked risk groups
In: M.H. Gail en N.L. Johnson (coordinators), *Proceedings of The American Statistical Association, sesquicentennial invited paper sessions*, 1989a, CH XVI, 622-641

Druten, J.A.M. van, J.C. Jager, M.J.J.C. Poos, S.H. Heisterkamp, R.A. Coutinho, E.J. Ruitenberg

HIV-infecties: een multigroep transmissie model
Tijdschrift voor Sociale Gezondheidszorg, 67 (1989b), 4, 40-41

Druten, J.A.M. van, A.G.M. Reintjes, J.C. Jager, S.H. Heisterkamp, M.J.J.C. Poos, R.A. Coutinho, M.G.W. Dijkgraaf, E.J. Ruitenberg
HIV infection dynamics and intervention experiments in linked risk groups
Statistics in Medicine, 9 (1990), 721-736

Druten, J.A.M. van, J.C. Jager
AIDS: Statistical analysis and mathematical modelling of the acquired immunodeficiency syndrome (AIDS); with a view to scenario-analysis
Rapport van de Katholieke Universiteit Nijmegen (KUN) en het Rijksinstituut voor Volksgezondheid en Milieuhygiëne (RIVM), RIVM-rapportnummer 958501004, June 1991

Druten, J.A.M. van, M.J.J.C. Poos, J. Hendriks, J.C. Jager
HIV epidemics in linked risk groups; a move to exploratory scenario-analysis
In: J.C. Jager, E.J. Ruitenberg (eds.), *AIDS Impact Assessment; Modelling and Scenario Analysis*, RIVM/Bilthoven, in preparation

Dijkgraaf, M.G.W., J.C.C. Borleffs, J.C. Jager, M.J.J.C. Poos, J.T.L. Jong, A.J.P. Schrijvers
National Projections of Hospital Costs of Patients with AIDS in The Netherlands
Presentatie op *VI International Conference on AIDS*, San Francisco, 1990

Hay, J.W.
Econometric issues in modelling the costs of AIDS
Health Policy, 11 (1989), 125-145

Healy, M.J.R., H.E. Tillet
Short-term extrapolation of the AIDS epidemic
Journal of the Royal Statistic Association, 155 (1988), 50-65

Health Council (GR)
Vroege medische interventies bij personen die met het AIDS-virus zijn geïnfecteerd
GR, The Hague, 1990, no. 16

Heisterkamp, S.H., J.C. Jager, A.M. Downs, J.A.M. van Druten, E.J Ruitenberg
Statistical estimation of AIDS incidence from surveillance data and the link with modelling of trends
In: J.C. Jager & E.J. Ruitenberg (eds.), *Statistical Analysis and Mathematical Modelling of AIDS*, Oxford University Press, Oxford 1988a

Heisterkamp, S.H., J.C. Jager, J.A.M. van Druten, A.M. Downs
The use of Genstat in estimating the expected numbers of cases of AIDS adjusted for reporting delays
Genstat Newsletter, 21 (1988b), 4-18

Heisterkamp, S.H., J.C. Jager, A.M. Downs, E.J. Ruitenberg, J.A.M. van Druten
Correcting reported AIDS incidence: a statistical approach
Statistics in Medicine, 8 (1989), 963-976

Heisterkamp, S.H., B.J. de Haan, J.C. Jager, J.A.M. van Druten, J.C.M. Hendriks
Short and middle term projections of the AIDS/HIV epidemic by a dynamic model with an application to the risk-group of homo/bisexual men in Amsterdam
Statistics in Medicine, 1991, submitted

Heisterkamp, S.H., A.M. Downs, M.J.J.C. Poos
MIDAS: A PC-program for adjusting reported AIDS data and short term projections
In: J.C. Jager, E.J. Ruitenberg (eds.), *AIDS Impact Assessment; Modelling and Scenario Analysis*, RIVM/Bilthoven, in preparation

Hellinger, F.J.
Forecasting the Number of AIDS Cases: An Analysis of Two Techniques
Inquiry, 27 (1990), 212-224

Hyman, J.M., E.A. Stanley
Using mathematical models to understand the AIDS epidemic
Mathematical Biosciences, (1988), 90, 415-473

Institute of Medicine / National Academy of Sciences (IOM/NAS)
Confronting AIDS; update 1988; executive summary
National Academy Press, Washington DC, 1988

Isham, V.
Mathematical Modelling of the Transmission Dynamics of HIV Infection and AIDS: a review
Journal of the Royal Statistic Association, 151 (1988), I, 5-49

Jager, J.C., M.J. Postma, J.C.C. Borleffs, E.J. Ruitenberg
Combining epidemiological models and economic information
Presentatie op *Conference on The Economic Impact of HIV Infection*, McGill University, Montreal 1988

Jager, J.C., M.J. Postma, F.M. van den Boom, D.P. Reinking, J.C.C. Borleffs, S.H. Heisterkamp, J.A.M. van Druten

Epidemiological models and socio-economic information: Methodological aspects of AIDS/HIVscenario analysis
In: D. Schwefel, R. Leidl, J. Rovira, M.F. Drummond (eds.), *Economic aspects of AIDS and HIV infection*, Springer Verlag, Berlin, 1989, 262-281

Jager, J.C., M.J.J.C. Poos, H. Houweling, C.A. Postema, R.A. Coutinho
Prognose aangaande HIV-infectie en AIDS-epidemie in Nederland op basis van wiskundige analyse
Nederlands Tijdschrift voor Geneeskunde, 134 (1990a), 51, 2486-2491

Jager, J.C., M.J.J.C. Poos, H. Houweling, C.A. Postema, R.A. Coutinho
Short term scenarios on the socioeconomic impact of AIDS on society
Presentatie op *VI International Conference on AIDS*, San Francisco, 1990b (FD121)

Jager, J.C., M.J. Postma, R. Leidl, B. Majnoni d'Itignano, A.E. Baert
AIDS impact scenarios: questions for the years to come
AIDS, 4 (1990), 11, 1166-1167

Jager, J.C., M.J.J.C. Poos, M.J. Postma, B.J. de Haan, S.H. Heisterkamp, D.P. Reinking, F.M.L.G. van den Boom
Use of epidemiological models for socioeconomic AIDS impact scenarios illustrated by data on the Netherlands
Presentatie op *VII International Conference on AIDS*, Florence, 1991b (TUD58)

Leidl, R.
Scenarios linking epidemiology and economics: possible impacts of drug treatment of HIV-infected in the FRG
Presentatie op *V International Conference on AIDS*, Montreal, 1989, (WHO16)

Leidl, R.
Model-Based Scenarios to Describe Economic Impacts of AIDS: The Role of Case-Mix
In: D. Schwefel, R. Leidl, J. Rovira, M.F. Drummond (eds.), *Economic Aspects of AIDS and HIV Infection*, Springer-Verlag, Berlin 1990

Leidl, R., M.J. Postma, M.J.J.C. Poos, J.C. Jager, B. Majnoni d'Intignano, A.E. Baert
Construction of socioeconomic impact scenarios based on routine AIDS surveillance data
In: J.C. Jager, E.J. Ruitenberg (eds.), *AIDS Impact Assessment; Modelling and Scenario Analysis*, RIVM/Bilthoven, in preparation

Lifson, A., N. Hessol, G.W. Rutherford, P. O'Malley, L. Barnhart, S. Buchbinder, L. Cannon, T. Bodecker, S. Holmberg, J. Harrison, L. Doll

Natural history of HIV infection in a cohort of homosexual and bisexual men: Clinical and immunological outcome
Presentation at *VI International Conference on AIDS*, San Francisco, 1990

McCormick, A.
Estimating the size of the HIV epidemic by using mortality data
Phil Trans R Soc Lond; B, 325 (1989), 163-173

Morgan, W.M., J.W. Curran
AIDS: current and future trends
Public Health Reports, (1986), 101, 459-464

Nationale Commissie AIDS bestrijding (NCAB)
Vroegtijdige interventie bij personen met een HIV-infectie
NCAB, Amsterdam, 1990

Programma Coördinatie Commissie AIDS onderzoek (PccAo)
Inventarisatie AIDS onderzoek in Nederland
PccAo, The Hague, 1990

Sociaal en Cultureel Planbureau (SCP)
Sociale en Culturele Verkenningen 1990
SCP, Rijswijk, 1990

Solomon, P.J., S.R. Wilson
Accomodating Change Due to Treatment in the Method of Back Projection for Estimating HIV Infection Incidence
Biometrics, 46 (1990), 1165-1170

Tweede Kamer der Staten Generaal (TH, 1987)
Nota inzake het AIDS-beleid
Tweede Kamer der Staten Generaal, vergaderjaar 1987-1988, 19218, nr. 8-9

Appendix

Statistical and mathematical methods

The projections for the HIV/AIDS incidence are based on two types of statistical modelling:

I trend analysis

II back-calculation method

In addition simulations are carried out with the aid of a mathematical model:

III the multi-group model.

The various methods are discussed below.

I Projections of the AIDS incidence by means of trend analysis

In trend analysis a functional relationship is postulated for the incidence of AIDS over time. Projections of the AIDS incidence are conducted by extrapolation of that relationship. The trend analyses are based on a statistical procedure (MIDAS), developed by the National Institute for Health and Environmental Protection (RIVM) and the WHO Collaborating Centre on AIDS in Paris (Heisterkamp et al., 1988a; 1988b; 1990; in prep.; Downs et al., 1988).

MIDAS has been developed for correcting for lags in reporting and for short-term predictions. Various functional relationships for the AIDS incidence may be assumed for the extrapolation. Use has been made of the reported AIDS incidence figures for the past six years. Extrapolation of the AIDS incidence (corrected for reporting delays) according to the function:

(1) A(t) = A * exp(B*t);

Where: A(t) = AIDS incidence per half year,
A = parameter,
B = parameter,
t = time.

The doubling-period is the period that must elapse for the half-yearly incidence of AIDS to double. This may be derived simply from parameter B in (1) (Heisterkamp et al., 1988). The doubling-period (b), expressed in years, then becomes equal to:

(2) b = ln(2)*6 / B.

(1) may now be rewritten as:

(3) A(t) = A * exp((ln(2)*6*t) / b)

The doubling-time has been increasing since the start of the epidemic (Jager et al., 1990). For this reason it was decided to explore a situation of decreasing growth in the AIDS incidence in the reference scenario. To do so parameter b has been made dependent on time (b(t)):

$$(4)\quad A(t) = A * \exp((\ln(2)*6*t) / b(t))$$

A linear increase of b(t)has been assumed; projection of the AIDS incidence follows from the estimation of the course of the AIDS epidemic according to the relationship:

$$(5)\quad A(t) = A * \exp((\ln(2)*6*t) / (c+d*t))$$

Where: c = parameter,
d = parameter.

II Estimation of the HIV incidence; the back-calculation method

The method by which it is estimated how many persons have probably become infected is known as the back-calculation method. This method is based on the incubation-time distribution and "counts back" to the most probable HIV incidence, given the AIDS incidence. As in the case of trend analysis the reported AIDS incidence provides the basis for calculation. Estimates of the HIV incidence are then used for projections of the AIDS incidence.

Studies of the incubation-time distribution indicate that the attack rate of AIDS in the first two years after infection with HIV is low (Lifson et al., 1990). This means that the AIDS incidence up to and including 1990 provides little reliable information on the HIV incidence in 1990 en 1989. Estimates of the HIV incidence are therefore confined to the period up to and including 1988.

The AIDS incidence is a function of the HIV incidence and the incubation-period distribution. The AIDS incidence in year t, A(t), amounts to:

$$(6)\quad A(t) = \sum_{\Theta=0}^{t} P(\Theta) * I(t-\Theta)$$

Here $P(\Theta)$ equals the probability of AIDS Θ years after the year in which the HIV infection took place; I(t) equals the HIV incidence in year t. I(t) shows the HIV incidence for persons who ultimately also contract AIDS. We are assuming that 100% of people infected with HIV end up developing AIDS. Among other things this means that we do not take any account of any mortality due to pre-AIDS disease (McCormick, 1989).

With respect to the incubation-period distribution we have assumed a three-stage model (Figure 2.3). The model is characterized by constant transition chances from the one compartment to the next. Using this model has a number of advantages. The various compartments may be interpreted as CDC stages (MMWR, 1987ab). In addition the consequences of early intervention may be straightforwardly modelled by interpreting stage 2 as the asymptomatic stage.

The parameters of this three-stage compartment-model have been estimated with the aid of the data on the incubation-period distribution from the San Francisco City Clinic Cohort Study (Lifson et al., 1990). Reasonable values for the residence times in the three stages were: one year, nine years and one year (Table 2.4).

Figure 2.3 **Progression to AIDS, modelled according to two alternatives: the 1-9-1 model and the 1-10-1 model.**

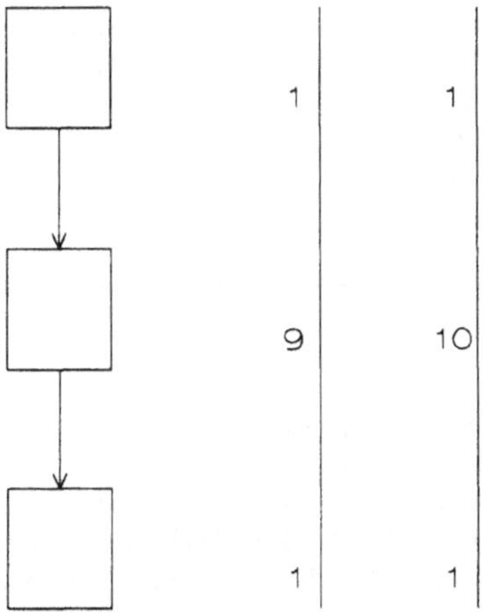

Figure 2.3 indicates these residence times, together with an alternative of 1 year, 10 years and 1 year. The alternative is an example of lengthening the asymptomatic (CDC II) stage by one year. This model application is conducted in scenario analysis into the consequences of early intervention (chapter 8).

The solution of (6) can result in negative figures for the HIV incidence in certain years. For this reason a definite positive function is assumed for the HIV incidence (I(t)). Two functional relationships are examined: quadratic exponential and logistical. In the projection conducted for the subscenario of the reference scenario we have assumed a functional relationship when using the back-calculation method (Jager et al., 1990). This is not the case for the remaining projections (Hay, 1989).

The analyses with the aid of the back-calculation method for the reference scenario are based on a constant incubation-time distribution. Any consequences of early treatment with AZT and PCP prophylaxes for the length of the incubation period are investigated in the care scenario into the consequences of early intervention (Chapter 8). The lengthening of the incubation period has been related in the literature to the calculation of negative figures for the incidence of HIV-infections (Hellinger, 1990; Solomon and Wilson, 1990; Heisterkamp et al., 1991, submitted).

Table 2.4 **Cumulative distribution of the incubation period in the San Francisco City Clinic Cohort Study (Lifson et al., 1990) and according to the 1 - 9 - 1 model (see text).**

	Lifson et al. (1990)	1 - 9 - 1 model
AIDS after 2 years	1%	1%
AIDS after 4 years	8%	9%
AIDS after 6 years	20%	23%
AIDS after 8 years	37%	38%
AIDS after 9 years	43%	46%
AIDS after 10 years	51%	53%
AIDS after 11 years	54%	59%
AIDS after 15 years	-[1]	78%
AIDS after 20 years	-[1]	90%

[1] no data available

The back-calculation method may be applied in order to determine the associated HIV incidence in the trend analysis of the AIDS incidence. In the reference scenario the HIV incidence before and after 1988 is determined with the aid of 'fast back-calculation' (Hay, 1989). The HIV incidence after 1988 is determined by calculating back from the AIDS incidence up to and including 2000 according to the trend analysis.

The subscenario of the reference scenario is based on the cumulative incidence of HIV up to and including 1988 as estimated by means of the back-calculation method. On this basis the AIDS incidence has been projected to the end of the year 2000. This forward-calculation also has been done with the aid of formula (6), with the incubation-time distribution according to the 1-9-1 model.

III *Multi-group model*

The HIV/AIDS epidemic is a resultant of various overlapping sub-epidemics. In order to analyse the interaction between sub-epidemics the multi-group model has been developed (Van Druten, 1988; Van Druten et al, 1986a; 1986b; 1987; 1988a; 1988b; 1989; 1990; Van Druten and Jager, 1991). The model distinguishes six groups:

1 males with numerous multiple male partners;
2 other males with multiple male partners;
3 injecting drug using women;
4 injecting drug using males;
5 males with multiple female partners;
6 women with multiple female partners.

The model generates the structure for modelling the spread within and between groups. It is also possible for a different "label" to be attached to the groups. The spread from and to the commercial sex world has for example been analysed with the aid of the multi-group model. Groups 3 and 6 in the model are then designated as IDU and non-IDU commercial sex workers.

Figure 2.1 (see 2.4.1.2) portrays the three main transmission routes:
- anal sexual intercourse (a),
- vaginal sexual intercourse (v),
- shared use of injection equipment (n).

The model contains a large number of parameters, which follows logically from the six groups and the three transmission routes. The parameters are linked up with the HIV incidence by means of the transmission matrix, T_{ij}. T_{ij} indicates a 6 x 6 matrix; t_{ij} indicates one element in this matrix (row i, column j).

The matrix summarizes the parameters of the three transmission routes within and between the six different groups.

The HIV incidences at point t ($dI_i(t) / dt$) are:

$$(7)\quad dI_i(t) / dt = t_{ij} X_i(t)\, I_i(t) / N_i + \sum_{j \neq i} t_{ij} X_i(t)\, I_j(t) / N_j$$

Where: $i = 1, ..., 6$
$X_i(t)$ = number of susceptible persons in group i
$I_i(t)$ = number of infected persons in group i
N_i = group size of group i
t_{ij} = transmission parameter ("transmission potential" of j to i)

The multi-group model is in essence an incidence model.

The parameters t_{ij} ($i = 1, ..., 6$ and $j = 1, ..., 6$) together form the transmission matrix T_{ij}. Each t_{ij} is a combination of underlying parameters, namely three for each of the three transmission routes (a,v,n):

f_{ij}^a = fraction of persons in group i with partners in group j with whom there is anal intercourse
f_{ij}^n = ditto, but with whom needles are shared
f_{ij}^v = ditto, but with whom there is vaginal intercourse

k_{ij}^a = number of new partners per unit of time (e.g.: year) of a person in group i with partners in group j, with whom there is anal intercourse
k_{ij}^n = ditto, but with shared needle use
k_{ij}^v = ditto, but with whom there is vaginal intercourse

b_{ij}^a = risk of infection via anal intercourse per partnership if person in group i is infected and person in group j is susceptible
b_{ij}^n = ditto, but through shared needle use
b_{ij}^v = ditto, but through vaginal intercourse

The relationship between parameters and element t_{ij} of the transmission matrix T_{ij} is:

$$(8)\quad t_{ij} = \sum_{m=a,n,v} b_{ij}^{m} * k_{ij}^{m} * f_{ij}^{m}$$

Because the number of partners of persons from group i in group j must be equal to the number of partners of persons from j in group i, it follows:

$$(9)\quad f_{ij}^{m} * N_i * k_{ij}^{m} = f_{ij}^{m} * N_j * k_{ij}^{m}$$

for m = a, n, v

These are the subsidiary conditions of the model. The model as formulated above provides the basis for an open model, that is a model which includes inflow of susceptibles and outflow (due to AIDS and death).

Part II Baseline analyses

3 Baseline analysis HIV/AIDS in the Netherlands: 1982-1991

3.1 Introduction

In terms of public health, the 1980s will undoubtedly go down as the AIDS decade. The new disease has attracted widespread interest. Hardly any self-respecting scientific journal or popular magazine has failed to include an article on the AIDS epidemic. The annual number of epidemiological, socio-scientific, legal/ethical and economic articles and commentaries on AIDS in the Netherlands has even exceeded the annual incidence of the disorder. In the literature studies conducted for the baseline analysis in this project, over 2000 books, articles, reports studies and lectures (some in Dutch but most in English) were encountered on AIDS and its impact.

This chapter discusses the main findings from literature studies in the socio-epidemiological field and their consequences for scenario analysis. The sociocultural and economic aspects of HIV/AIDS in the Netherlands are discussed in Chapters 4 and 5 respectively.

3.2 HIV/AIDS in the Netherlands

The working document "Socio-epidemiological aspects of HIV/AIDS in the Netherlands: 1982-1990" (Reinking et al., 1990) provides an interim survey of data drawn from epidemiological and socio-scientific research into the HIV/AIDS epidemic in the Netherlands. The reference date in the working document is March 1990. This section summarizes the working document and brings it up to date, where possible to 1.1.1991. Apart from a survey of developments in the HIV/AIDS incidence and prevalence for the epidemic as a whole and general data on infectiousness and developments in the incubation period, this section provides a survey for each sub-epidemic.

3.2.1 Incidence and prevalence of AIDS

Diagnosed cases of AIDS have been notified to the Chief Medical Officer of Health (GHI) since the start of the epidemic. Table 3.1 provides a survey of notifications up to and including 31.12.1990, broken down by patient group.

Table 3.1 **People with AIDS by patient group and year of diagnosis, 1982-1990** (GHI, 1991).

	1982	1983	1984	1985	1986	1987	1988	1989	1990	Totaal
Homo/bisexual males	2	17	29	58	117	186	250	300	264	1223
IDU	-	-	-	1	6	16	32	32	29	116
Homo/bisexual males and IDU	-	-	-	1	2	6	7	2	1	19
Haemophilia patients/blood products	-	-	-	1	-	3	5	6	6	21
Blood transfusions	2	2	1	2	3	5	4	6	3	28
Heterosexual contact	-	-	1	1	4	17	14	26	25	88
Mother-child transmission	-	-	-	-	-	1	3	1	2	7
Other	1	-	-	-	4	5	6	9	4	29
Total	5	19	31	64	136	239	321	382 (394)[1]	334 (443)[1]	1531 (1652)[1]

* Anticipated number of people with AIDS after adjustment for delays in reporting.

In practice not all people with AIDS are immediately notified to the GHI but there is a lag-effect, which may be calculated on the basis of the reporting pattern in previous years (Heisterkamp et al., in preparation). Up to and including 31.12.1990 a cumulative number (including the lagged response) of 1,652 AIDS diagnoses are expected. Figure 3.1 shows the results of the estimated lag-effect. The figure indicates that approximately a third of the AIDS incidence in 1989A is reported in 1989B or later. The figure indicates further that on the basis of the reporting pattern for 1990B an AIDS incidence of 215 may be anticipated, of which over half has been reported. The number of people with AIDS adjusted for late notification is also shown in brackets in Table 3.1.

Figure 3.1 **Reported and expected incidence of AIDS per half-year (A = first half-year, B = second half-year) by period of diagnosis.**

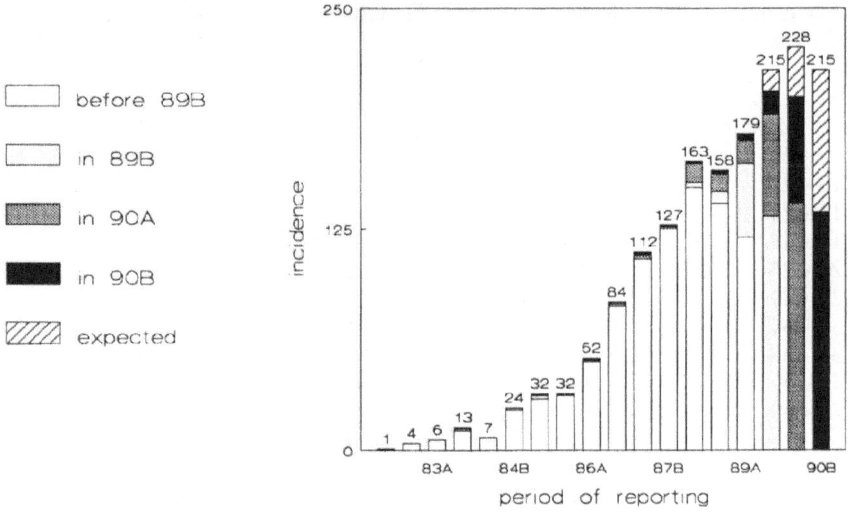

As may be seen from Table 3.1 nearly 80% of the notifications since 1987 have related to gay or bisexual men. The other notifications relate largely to the IDU and heterosexual-contact categories. It may also be seen that there are a number of sequential epidemics: among heterosexuals and IDUs, for example, the AIDS epidemic started a year later than it did among men who have sex with men.

The majority of the notifications stem from Amsterdam, namely 949 (62%), of which 784 (49%) relate to persons living in Amsterdam (GG&GD, 1991). Since 1987 roughly 50% of the notifications have related to persons living in Amsterdam. AIDS primarily affects men aged 25-50. Of the 1,531 notifications, 1,432 (94%) relate to men and 1,228 (80%) to men aged 25-50 (see Table 3.2). A total of 14 cases of AIDS among children aged under 13 has been reported. Broken down by risk factors this related to seven cases of mother-child transmission, seven cases where blood transfusions were the risk factor and one case in the "other/indeterminate" category.

The most frequently cited symptoms at the time of diagnosis with AIDS are an opportunistic infection (1,119 or 73%), Kaposi's sarcoma (198 or 13%) or a combination of the two (69 or 5%).

Table 3.2 **Distribution of AIDS cases by age and sex (cumulative as at 31.12.1990)** (GHI, 1991).

Age group (in years)	**Men**	**Females**	**Total**
0 - 11 months	2	3	5
1 - 4 years	1	4	5
5 - 9	4	-	4
10 - 12	-	1	1
13 - 14	-	-	-
15 - 19	1	1	2
20 - 24	39	11	50
25 - 29	185	25	210
30 - 34	281	22	303
35 - 39	321	10	331
40 - 49	431	10	441
50 - 59	129	7	136
60 +	38	5	43
Total	1432	99	1531

3.2.1.1 Doubling time

The doubling time is a measure of the speed at which an epidemic is spreading: on the basis of the observed increase in the incidence of AIDS in a particular period it is determined how much time needs to elapse for the AIDS incidence to double. Figure 3.2 shows how the doubling time has changed, on the basis of (overlapping) periods of three years. The doubling time has been recalculated every six months.

It may be seen that the doubling time has been increasing since the early years of the AIDS epidemic, namely from nine months at the start of the epidemic to 52 months in the most recent three-year period. The doubling time among homosexual or bisexual men is at present 49 months and among IDUs as long as 158 months. The AIDS epidemic is currently spreading more rapidly among men who have sex with men than among IDUs. Classified by region it may be seen that the doubling time in Amsterdam is 58 months, compared with 45 months outside Amsterdam.

Figure 3.2 **Doubling time in months calculated for overlapping, successive periods of three years (A = first half year; B = second half year).**

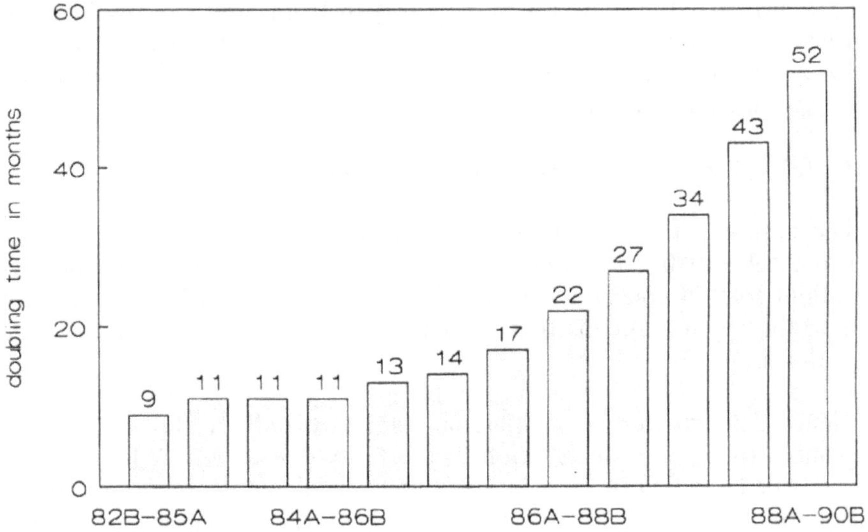

3.2.1.2 Lethality

The lethality due to AIDS is not precisely known. The CBS (Central Bureau of Statistics) cause-of-death statistics up to 1.1.1990 records 560 cases of AIDS as the primary cause of death (CBS, 1991a). This figure relates to Dutch residents, i.e. individuals whose names appear on the population register. Up to 1.1.1990, 1,150 of the 1,197 people with AIDS known to the GHI were living in the Netherlands. Assuming that all persons living in the Netherlands are included in the population register the lethality at that point would be nearly 50%, namely 560 deaths out of 1,150 patients. On the other hand it is also known that there were 250 patients at that time of non-Dutch nationality. It is not known what proportion of these were included in the population register in the Netherlands. The Amsterdam GG&GD reported a lethality of 53% among 784 AIDS patients living in Amsterdam as of 1.1.1991 (without adjustment for notification delays).

3.2.1.3 *Survival time*

The survival time of AIDS patients has been rising for a number of years. Bindels et al. (1991) report an increase in the average survival time among AIDS patients in Amsterdam from nine months in 1982-1985 to 16 months in 1987 and 22 months for those diagnosed in 1989. The rise in the survival time is attributable to improved and earlier diagnosis and better treatments.

3.2.1.4 *Potential Years of Life Lost (PYLL)*

The number of Potential Years of Life Lost (PYLL), as derived from Haenszel (1950), is often taken as an indicator for the indirect patient-related consequences of disease. The use of PYLL instead of mortality figures means that account is also taken of age at the time of death.

Figure 3.3 provides a comparison (standardized for the size of age groups) of the age distribution of mortality due to AIDS, lung cancer and suicide (ICD 162; ICD E950-959; Leidl et al., in preparation). For the purposes of international comparability, lung-cancer and suicide mortality figures from 1985 have been used (CBS). The age distribution upon death from AIDS in the Netherlands is based on the GHI data as at 1.1.1991 (Table 3.2), as also used in other epidemiological model simulations, and an assumed age-independent survival time of 18 months. Figure 3.3 indicates that AIDS affects younger people than do lung cancer and suicide.

Figure 3.4 shows the number of PYLL per death due to AIDS, lung cancer, suicide, road accidents (ICD E810-819) and infectious diseases (ICD 001-139) in the Netherlands, West Germany and France. Apart from the mortality figures for AIDS, the figures relate to 1985 and derive from the Central Bureau of Statistics (Netherlands), the Statistisches Bundesamt (W. Germany) and the Institute National de la Santé et de la Recherche Médicale (France). The mortality due to AIDS arises from the incidence in the period 1982-1990 and an assumed average survival time of 18 months. The average number of PYLL per AIDS-related death in the Netherlands is estimated at 33.7 years. This virtually corresponds with the PYLL figure for West Germany and France. The average PYLL per death due to AIDS is comparable with the PYLL per fatal road accident.

Figure 3.3 **Standardized (for size of the age interval) distribution of mortality due to AIDS, compared with mortality from lung cancer and suicide (1985).** Sources: GHI and CBS.

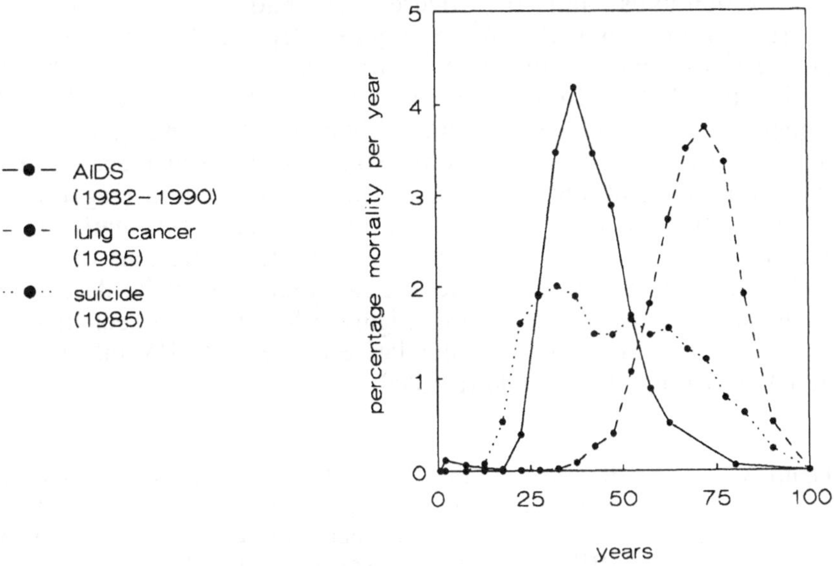

Figure 3.4 **Number of PYLL per death due to AIDS (1982-1990) in three countries; compared with four other causes of death (1985).** Sources: see text.

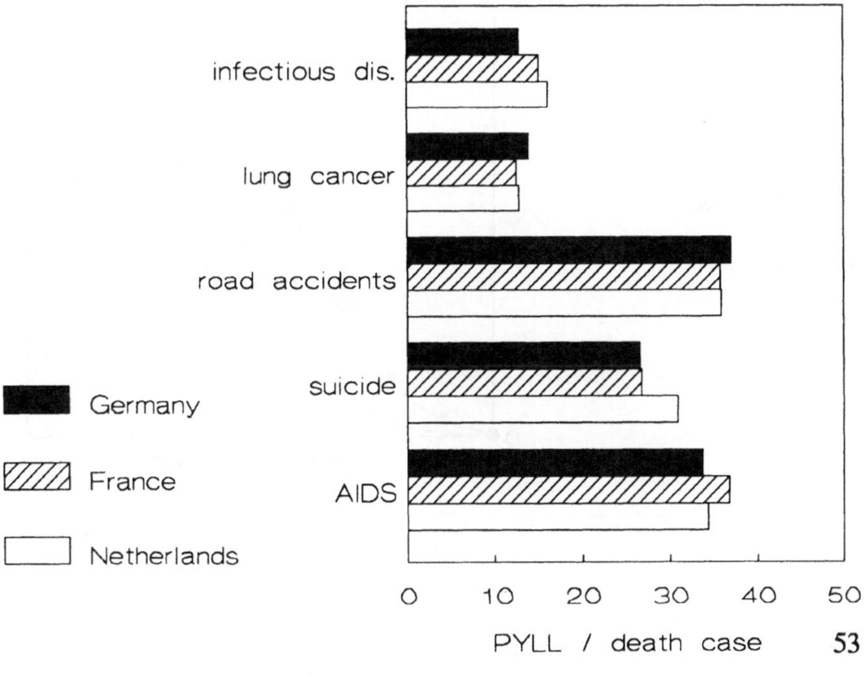

3.2.2 *Incidence and prevalence of HIV infections*

There are no data on the total number of HIV-infected persons in the Netherlands and the figure has had to be derived by approximation from the AIDS figures. By combining the AIDS notifications adjusted for late reporting and data on the incubation-period distribution from research in the USA (Lifson et al., 1990; Longini et al., 1989) an estimate is obtained of the number of HIV-infected persons. Figure 3.5 shows estimates of the incidence of HIV infections with the aid of this back-calculation method (Jager et al., 1990). Estimates are shown based on two different mathematical functions for the trend in the incidence of HIV infections up to and including 1988. Infections in the last two years cannot be determined by means of this method. From Figure 3.5 it may be seen that the most recent estimates of the cumulative number of HIV infections as at 1.1.1989 range from 6,000 to 8,000.

Figure 3.5 **Results of the back-calculation method: yearly and cumulative HIV-incidence. Baseline: on the basis of Lifson et al. (1990) and the quadratic exponential function for HIV incidence. Alternative A: the logistic instead of quadratic exponential function for HIV incidence. Alternative B: on the basis of Longini et al. (1989) instead of Lifson et al. (1990).**

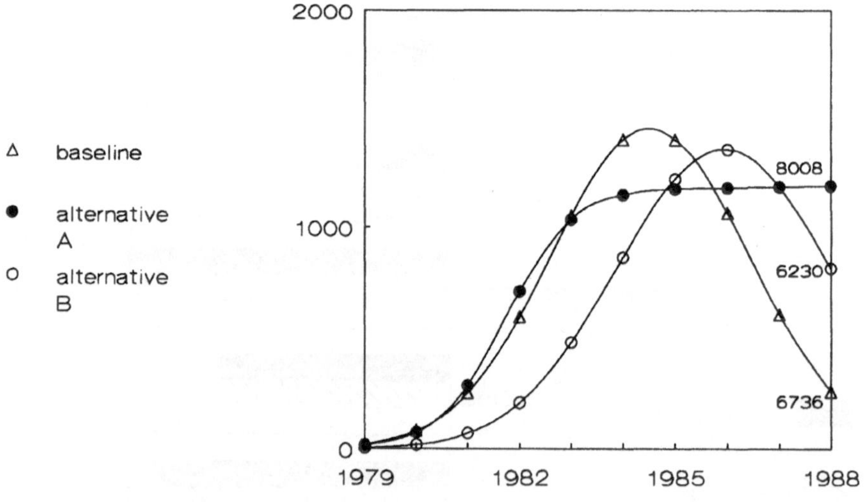

3.2.3 *Factors influencing the incidence and prevalence of HIV/-AIDS*

The principal risk factors for HIV infection are high-risk sexual contact, especially receptive anal intercourse, and the shared use of injection equipment among hard-drug users (Van Griensven and Coutinho, 1988; Turner et al., 1989). As far as sexual behaviour is concerned, the incidence of high-risk sexual contact, the number of sexual partners and the effects of preventive measures (including condom use) are therefore significant variables in this project. Of importance for the transmission of HIV is the risk of infection associated with high-risk contact between an HIV-infected person and a non-infected person. For the scale and distribution of the epidemic the relevant factors are the size of these groups of seropositives, those susceptible and the transmission routes by which the virus spreads within sexual figurations (Straver and Van Stolk, 1988). The same applies to injection behaviour: instead of risk-taking sexual behaviour read risk-taking injection behaviour.

3.2.3.1 *Infectiousness*

On the basis of the international literature it is not possible to arrive at a clear-cut determination of infectiousness. Differences per transmission route emerge from the international literature: Ward et al. (1989) found an transmission probability of > 50% from receiving a blood transfusion; Wiley et al. (1989) determined the transmission probability *per unprotected vaginal intercourse* between a seropositive man and a non-infected woman at 0.14%, although in some cases the probability rose to nearly 100%; on the basis of a cohort study among men who sex with men in Amsterdam, Van Griensven (1990) determined the risk of transmission *per partner* with whom there was anal intercourse at 4%.

In general the risk of transmitting HIV by means of sexual intercourse is lower than the 22-25% risk of passing on a sexually transmitted disease such as gonorrhoea (Holmberg et al., 1989). There are however factors that radically affect the low risk of HIV infection. Holmberg et al., 1989) cite three relevant biological factors:

- The infectiousness of the HIV-infected person, depending among other things on the stage of progression to AIDS.
- Differences in characteristics of the virus that affect the virulence.
- Differences in susceptibility to an HIV infection, including a history of STDs (see also: The European Study Group, 1989). It must be concluded that the infectiousness of HIV is variable

and cannot be precisely determined (Friedland and Klein, 1987; Houweling and Coutinho, 1989).

3.2.3.2 *Incubation time distribution*

With respect to the incubation time, defined as the interval between HIV infection and diagnosis with AIDS, we have, in line with the international literature, followed the San Francisco City Clinic Cohort Study. This study relates to 489 primarily gay men whose date of seroconversion is known with reasonable accuracy (Table 3.3). Whether the incubation time distribution applies for all people with AIDS aged over 13 is as yet not clear.[1] There are indications to suggest an equal or shorter incubation-period distribution among drug users (Rezza et al., 1990; Gorter et al., 1990). There is also some evidence to suggest a link between the age of HIV infection and the length of the incubation period: the older one is at the point of infection the shorter the incubation period (Goedert et al., 1989; Weiss et al., 1990).

Table 3.3 Cumulative distribution of the incubation period in the San Francisco City Clinic Cohort Study (Lifson et al., 1990).

AIDS after 2 years	1%
AIDS after 4 years	8%
AIDS after 6 years	20%
AIDS after 8 years	37%
AIDS after 9 years	43%
AIDS after 10 years	51%
AIDS after 11 years	54%

95% confidence interval after 11 years: 49-59%

3.2.3.3 *Group size and geographical distribution*

Other factors determining the size of an epidemic are group size and geographical distribution. The group size provides an indication of the maximum scale that the epidemic can assume within a group.

[1] Among persons aged under 13, who fall under the differing definition for paediatric AIDS, the progression to AIDS is much faster. Oxtoby et al. (1991) estimate the risk of developing AIDS among infants at over 20% during the first year of life and over 10% in each succeeding year. Evans et al. (1991) found comparable results among children who became HIV-positive as a result of a blood transfusion.

Separate concentration on Amsterdam would appear justified for a combination of reasons: the concentration of drug users in the capital (De Zwart, 1990), the differences in seroprevalence among hard-drug users within and outside Amsterdam (De Haan et al., 1991) and the function performed by Amsterdam as a meeting and social centre for gay men (Bakker en Schuyf, 1985). In addition there is the correlation between degree of urbanization and the incidence of prostitution and STDs (Miltenburg et al., 1988; Boutellier, 1987).

Caution is in order when it comes to determining group size. It needs to be borne in mind that a gay identity or drug use does not automatically involve a risk of contracting AIDS: the former may have no sexual partners or be HIV-negative and mutually monogamous, while the latter may not inject or share injection equipment. Moreover, restricting oneself to gay men as a core group may lead to an underestimation of the total groupsize. There are men who have sex with men that do not identify themselves as gay. The geographical distribution also needs to be qualified to some extent because the Netherlands is a small country with good domestic and international communications.

The figures in Table 3.4 on groups with a possible HIV risk are chiefly estimates. Part of the table is also derived from percentage estimates (see the notes to the table).

As far as possible, an indication has been provided for each group covered by the scenario study as to the proportion with multiple contacts, i.e. more than one sexual partner a year. No information on this point was found for gay men. In the case of the heterosexual population the figures are based on British research, which corresponds closely with a recently published Dutch study (Van Zessen and Sandfort, 1991). In the case of hard-drug users the numbers injecting have been shown. On the basis of the ages of people with AIDS and STDs, an age limit of 20-45 has been set in Table 3.4 for groups with unprotected sexual contact as a risk factor. No age limit has been set for the clients of commercial sex workers. Studies indicate that the age of commercial sex workers' clients varies considerably, the average being around 40 (Kinnell, 1989; Van Mens, 1989).

Table 3.4 **Group size of eight groups with an identified risk of HIV infection.**

Group	Size	Source
Gay men		
Total (20-45 years)	± 125.000 [1]	Van Zessen, 1990, estimate based on Houwelingen et al., 1987
Amsterdam	± 25.000	
Risk behaviour	unknown	
Hard-drug users		
Total	15.000 - 20.000	De Zwart, 1989, estimate
Amsterdam	5.500 - 7.500	Buning, 1990, estimate
Rotterdam	± 3.500	Toet and Van der Ven, 1989, estimate
Injectors		
Amsterdam	± 2.500	Buning, 1990, estimate
foreign users	± 1.500 [2]	ditto
Dutch users	± 800 [2]	ditto
ethnic minorities	± 75 [2]	ditto
Heterosexual males		
Total (20-45 years)	± 3.000.000	CBS, 1991b
≥ 2 partners througout life	± 1.800.000 [3]	based on: Johnson et al., 1989
≥ 2 partners in last year	± 300.000 [3]	ditto
Heterosexual women		
Total (20-45 years)	± 3.000.000	CBS, 1991b
≥ 2 partners throughout life	± 1.200.000 [4]	based on: Johnson et al., 1990
≥ 2 partners in last year	± 150.000 [4]	ditto
Commercial sex workers (CSWs)	15.000 - 20.000	NCAB, 1990a, estimate
sidewalk	1.500 - 2.000 [5]	ditto
window	4.500 - 6.000 [5]	ditto
club	4.500 - 6.000 [5]	ditto
Drug using CSWs		
Amsterdam	500 - 1.000	Buning, 1990, estimate of daily number
Clients of CSWs		
At any point	600.000 [6]	Boutellier, 1987, estimate
Regular clients	± 100.000 [6]	ditto

1 Derived from the estimate: 4% of the population is gay.
2 Derived from the estimate: 70% injection use among foreign users, 30% among Dutch users and 5% among users from ethnic minorities.
3 Derived from the estimate: 60% have 2 of more sexual partners during their entire life and 10% have had 2 or more partners in the last year.
4 Derived from the estimate: 40% have 2 or more sexual partners during their entire life and 5% has had 2 or more partners during the last year.
5 Derived from the estimate: 10% of the commercial sex workers work in sidewalk - prostitution, 30% in window prostitution en 30% in club prostitution.
6 Derived from the estimate: 20% of the males have ever had sexual contact with a prostitute and 3% have regular contact.

3.3 *HIV/AIDS by sub-epidemic*

3.3.1 *Men who have sex with men*

A reconstruction based on two cohorts of men with multiple male partners indicated that the HIV epidemic had probably started among this group in 1979. The Amsterdam cohort study revealed evidence of a rapidly rising incidence of HIV in the early 1980s, reaching 7% in 1985. After 1986 behavioural changes saw a rapid decline in the HIV incidence to 1% in 1989. Cumulatively the cohort study revealed a seroprevalence rising from 32% in 1984-1985 to 42% in 1989 (Van Griensven, 1989). In 1990 an increase in the HIV incidence was once again detected in the cohort (Van den Hoek et al., 1990a). No seroprevalence surveys were conducted outside this cohort of men who have sex with men. Because the cohort is not representative of gay men in general it is possible to make no more than cautious statements about the cause of the HIV epidemic among this group.

As in the US and Australia, a spectacular change in behaviour was observed in this cohort study during the period 1986-1989. In particular, the change of behaviour took the form of fewer partners and less anal intercourse with non-regular partners. Greater use of condoms was also observed, especially among seropositives having sexual contact with multiple partners (Van Griensven, 1989; Connell and Kippax, 1989; Martin et al., 1989). On the basis of the figures for the STD incidence in Amsterdam it is probably fair to speak of a large-scale change in behaviour among gay men (Van de Laar et al., 1990; Fennema et al., 1989; Wigersma et al., 1989). A survey conducted among the readers of the *Gay*-magazine (Gay-krant) also indicated that 90% (N = 522) intended in future to avoid all or most risks (Tielman and Polter, 1989). This could be regarded as the first step on the path towards a change in the social environment in which safe sexual behaviour is the social norm, resulting in a permanent change in behaviour (Stall et al., 1988). That point has not however yet been reached.

3.3.1.1 *Behavioural change*

The most significant reaction to date in relation to the risk of HIV and AIDS would appear to be the decline in anal intercourse (Turner et al., 1989). Among seroconverters in the Amsterdam cohort a peak in anal intercourse with multiple partnes was observed around the time of infection. After seroconversion, anal intercourse falls to the level of some years before, while the number of partners and condom use remains more of less unchanged (Kuiken et al., 1990). De Wit et al. (1991) conclude that apart from an increase in unsafe sexual contacts, irregular or inexpert use of condoms is a possible cause of the rise in the number of HIV infections in 1990.

An important question for long-range studies concerns the comprehensiveness and consistency of the behavioural change. On the basis of the data to date it would appear realistic to assume that AIDS has had consequences for sexual behaviour, that a proportion of people still have risk behaviour, and that there is a diversity of behaviour, whereby some people enter into higher-risk behaviour for limited periods. In a study of US cohorts (N=1,122) O'Reilly et at. (1990) found a relapse of 4%, i.e. higher reported unprotected intercourse in a follow-up survey conducted six months after first measurement. St. Lawrence et al. (1990) observed no consistent change in behaviour over a period of 16 months among 40% of the participants in a behavioural change programme (N=68).

Projections based on simulations can, however, only be interpreted qualitatively on this score. Assumptions need for example to be formulated about the percentage of gay men with multiple partners and the incidence of unsafe sexual encounters. As far as the number of partners is concerned it appears reasonable to assume that gay men with multiple partners generally have more partners than heterosexual males (Miller et al., 1989). With respect to the motives for risk-taking sexual contact a complex of individual and environment-related factors are associated with risk behaviour: age, education, sexual contact with steady or casual partners, knowledge of one another's serostatus, being in love, excitement, estimation of personal capacity for safe sex, attitudes within the social environment to the use of condoms, the availability of condoms, consumption of alcohol and the existence of people with AIDS in the immediate environment (O'Reilly, 1990; St. Lawrence et al., 1990; Pollack et al., 1990; Stall et al., 1990; Dallas, 1990; Martin et al., 1989; Ekstrand et al., 1989; Grant, 1989).

3.3.1.2 AIDS prevention directed towards men who have sex with men

The large-scale change in behaviour among men who have sex with men has been due at least in part to a large number of targeted information and prevention activities. In the Netherlands the campaigns have generally been initiated by organizations working for or representing gay men: the COC, the Ancillary Services Department (SAD) and the Schorer Foundation. The campaigns have been conducted in conjunction with the Health Information and Education

Agency (Buro GVO) in Amsterdam and the Steering Group for AIDS information for gay set up by the National Commission for AIDS Control (NCAB) in 1987.

The first information campaign was set up in 1983. The COC distributes printed information material developed and produced by the Buro GVO Amsterdam, such as posters, leaflets, booklets and postcards, at gay meeting places. COC also organizes information evenings. *AIDS-info* is an information sheet that has been produced since 1984 and is distributed free of charge in gay and other places of entertainment and via the *GAY*-magazine. The SAD issued guidelines for safer sex in the same year. Information and education was later organized by means of group activities, such as the Safe Sex Video Show, and workshops on condom use and safer sex. Since 1989 the information and education activities have become more outreaching, small-scale and aimed at the individual. The emphasis in the information is placed to a greater extent on the promotion of personal responsibility for safer sexual behaviour. Without departing from the prevention advice of avoiding anal intercourse, attention is also devoted to the effective use of condoms for those who continue to use that technique. A special campaign for this purpose was set up in 1991 (NCAB, 1989a, 1991).

3.3.1.3 Points of concern

Apart from transmission via homosexual contacts account must also be taken of HIV transmission by men with bisexual behaviour. Few and for the purposes of scenario analysis inadequate data are available from Dutch studies on males with both male and female sexual partners. It would appear clear that a substantial proportion of men who have sex with men have at some stage in their lives had female partners, e.g. before discovering their gay identity, and that there may be 10,000-15,000 married men who have sex with men in the Netherlands (Deenen and Van Naerssen, 1988; Haverkos et al., 1989; Gijs et al., 1989).

3.3.2 Hard-drug users

In the case of hard-drug users various HIV-transmission routes need to be taken into account. The shared use of injection equipment - in the form of lending syringes or the technique of "front loading" (Grund and Kaplan, 1990)[2] - appear the most important transmission

---

[2] Front loading is a technique in which drugs are distributed to other syringes from a single syringe in which the plunger has been drawn back and the needle removed.

route (Van den Hoek, 1990). In addition allowance needs to be made for transmission to partners through sexual contact and transmission by commercial sex workers.

3.3.2.1 Shared use of injection equipment

As in other countries there is evidence in the Netherlands of the rapid spread of HIV after its introduction in the population of hard-drug users (Des Jarlais et al., 1990; Skidmore et al., 1990). The Netherlands differs, however, appreciably from other countries in terms of the low percentage - 30% - of injectors among hard-drug users and the virtual lack of injectors among Moluccan, Surinamese, Moroccan and Antillian drug users (Van Gelder and Sijtsma, 1988ab; Buning, 1990; Blom and Janssen, 1987; EC Concerted Action on Assessment of AIDS/HIV Prevention Strategies, 1991). By way of comparison, the estimated proportion of injectors among "heroin tourists" is 70% (Korf, 1987; Buning, 1990). There is also a lack of "shooting galleries" for shared drug use (Des Jarlais et al., 1986). In the Netherlands people mainly take drugs "at home" or "alone" - although this does not of course rule out the borrowing/lending of syringes and needles (Van den Hoek, 1990). Van Haastrecht (personal communication, 1991) found indications of a rapid increase in the incidence of HIV in Amsterdam in 1983-1984. Since 1986 seroprevalence has stabilized at around 30%, although infections are still occurring (Van Haastrecht et al., 1991a). In so far as data are available from point-prevalence studies (in some cases conducted sometime ago), the seroprevalence outside Amsterdam is less than 10%. This difference in seroprevalence is not explicable in terms of differences in risk behaviour between IDU within and outside Amsterdam (Van Limbeek et al., 1987; Barends, 1988; De Haan et al., 1991).

In the reconstruction of the course of the HIV epidemic and the progression to AIDS among IDUs the impact of HIV-related mortality and morbidity and that of HIV infections among foreign IDUs need to be taken into account (Selwyn et al., 1989). These factors can affect the anticipated number of people with AIDS.

In response to the HIV/AIDS epidemic among IDUs, large-scale syringe exchange projects have been set up in the Netherlands. In August 1990 there were 126 places where syringes could be exchanged, of which 14 in Amsterdam (NIAD, 1990). The projects differ in terms of scale, working methods and coverage. In the four largest cities 1.2 million syringes were handed out in 1989, of which 820,000 in Amsterdam and 250,000 in Rotterdam (Buning, 1990; NCAB, 1990b). It is difficult to put a figure on the proportion of drug users reached by the syringe distribution system since the frequency of injection is highly variable, depending among other things on earnings, detention, whether people use mainly cocaine or heroin and periods in which there is temporarily no use (Grapendaal, 1989, Hoekstra et al., 1985; Swierstra, 1990). There are indications to suggest that it is rare for the type of use to change during a drug career: drug users are either mainly injectors or mainly smokers (Gossop et al., 1989). On the basis of the average frequency of injection in the non-representative cohort of hard-drug users in Amsterdam, the coverage of the low-threshold syringe exchange in Amsterdam and Rotterdam would be less than 50% (Hartgers et al., 1989; NCAB, 1990b). By way of comparison, the coverage of the less low-threshold methadone clinics amounts to around 70% (NVC, 1990).

3.3.2.2 Sexual contact

HIV can also be transmitted among and from IDUs by sexual contact. Here a distinction may be drawn between commercial sex contacts and private contacts. An estimated 80% of female IDU enter into prostitution at some point in their addiction career, while there are thought to be some 500 drug-dependent commercial sex workers working daily in Amsterdam (Buning, 1990). Foreign hard-drug addicts, in particular, are said to be largely dependent for their income on the sex industry, in the broadest sense of the word (Korf, 1987)[3].

Commercial sex workers themselves state that their contacts take place almost without exception using a condom; few if any instances of anal intercourse are reported. On the other hand it may be noted that commercial sex workers with a pressing need for drugs can be persuaded to have unprotected intercourse, that there is unprotected intercourse with regular clients and that the incidence of STD among drug-dependent commercial sex workers indicates that the contact is not always protected. Condoms are used less frequently with private partners (Van den Putte, 1986; Van Gelder and Van Roekel, 1989; Van den Hoek, 1990; Miller et al., 1989).

Hard-drug users and drug-dependent commercial sex workers are sometimes described as socially isolated individuals having little more than brief business contacts with other users. There are, for example, said to be few contacts between heroin tourists and Dutch

---

[3] Apart from prostitution as such the study in question also mentions work in peepshows, topless bars and live-shows: 40% of the female and 10% of the male heroin tourists (N=382) named the sex industry as their primary source of income (Korf, 1987).

users, and Surinamese and Moroccan users involved in small-scale dealing are said to look down on degenerate Dutch injecting addicts (Van Gemert, 1988; Van den Berg and Blom, 1987; Janssen and Swierstra, 1982). The Amsterdam cohort study of hard-drug users, however, reports that 50% have a steady sexual partner, that there are numerous changes of partner and that the majority have an STD history. Of these partners roughly half were also IDUs (Van den Hoek, 1990). As in Britain, knowledge of serostatus led to fewer partners and greater condom use (Donoghoe et al., 1989). Anal intercourse was barely reported.

Although only a small number of people with AIDS have so far become infected through sexual contact with an IDU, the risk profile means that there is every reason to conduct studies into the potential for HIV to be spread by sexual contact with IDUs. The spread of HIV to persons not sharing injection material is a particular risk factor in commercial sex work.

3.3.2.3 HIV/AIDS prevention aimed at IDUs

In order to prevent the spread of HIV among IDUs a number of prevention campaigns have been started up, initiated by drug clinics, the government and private initiative. These include the NCAB, the GG&GD Amsterdam, the Netherlands Institute for Alcohol and Drugs (NIAD), the Netherlands Federation of Junkie Unions (FNJB) and the Medico-Social Heroin Users Service (MDHG). The prevention policies are designed to reduce risk behaviour by means of information and education on safer drug use and safer sexual contact, by the setting up and expansion of facilities such as syringe-exchange schemes and the provision of condoms. The national project "AIDS and Drug Policy" run by the NIAD includes information campaigns and syringe exchange projects. At the regional and local level small-scale efforts can be found in which HIV/AIDS prevention workers try to reach various groups such as drug using commercial sex workers, prisoners or etnic minorities who are IDU and private sexual partners of IDUs.

The large-scale provision of written information on infection risks, safer injecting and safer sexual contact, in the form of leaflets, brochures and stickers, got under way in 1984. Since 1990 information has also been provided on cleaning syringes with bleach. Among other things the information activities have come in for criticism with respect to the distribution of the information material and the extent to which it fits in with IDUs' perceptions. On the other hand, there is little interest among hard-drug users in AIDS information material (De Loor, 1991).

Condoms are distributed by means of a large number of syringe exchange and methadone programmes. Generally hard-drug users tend to make little use of such facilities as condoms have to be asked for especially and the need for their use is not yet generally accepted (NCAB, 1989a, 1990b). Large quantities of condoms are sold in the "living-room" projects conducted for sidewalk prostitutes (Kleinegris, 1990). HIV/AIDS prevention appears to be inducing a change in behaviour among IDUs, although 20% continue to lend or borrow syringes. Counselling would appear an essential element in promoting safer injecting behaviour (Van den Hoek, 1990; Hartgers 1990), personal communication). It may be noted that nearly all syringes are returned and that the availability of syringes does not appear to lead to an increase in drug injection (Buning, 1990). The syringe-exchange programme has come in for criticism with respect to its availability and accessibility and focus on risk-laden moments (De Loor, 1991). The popularity of syringe exchange has continued to increase and would appear an effective supplement to AIDS information. There has also been an increasing trend to supply various kinds of syringes specially adapted for heroin or cocaine (Van Doorninck, 1991, personal communication).

3.3.2.4 Points of concern

In projections of the future epidemiological trend among IDUs it is important to draw a distinction between the various HIV transmission routes. In this respect the effect of HIV/AIDS prevention as well as the seroprevalence and distribution of risk behaviour are of particular importance. Equally as much risk behaviour was detected among IDUs in The Hague as in Amsterdam, although the seroprevalence was very low (De Haan et al., 1991). In view of the spread of HIV among IDUs in other countries, where peaks in the spread of HIV appear to be associated with the point at which HIV was first introduced in various towns, more may yet lie in store for Netherlands (Skidmore et al., 1989). An alternative explanation is that, along the same lines as London, the hitherto low seroprevalence outside Amsterdam is related to a concentration of risk contacts within a certain section of the population (Coleman and Curtis, 1988). The likely influx of new users is also important. Dutch estimates of the number of hard-drug users have remained constant for a number of years and the average age of hard-drug users in touch with outreach facilities has been rising (Buning, 1990). It is unclear whether this means that the scale of the hard-drug problem is waning or whether the drug service and hence also the HIV/AIDS prevention network is having difficulty in establishing contact with new, young users, such as young people from the second generation of ethnic minorities - while it may well be that it is precisely these young, new users who are apt to exhibit risk behaviour (Friedman et al., 1989). Another point of concern is the international mobility of drug users and the spread of HIV (Bisset et al., 1989; Van den Hoek, 1990).

3.3.3 Heterosexuals

The general opinion is that to date, there appears to be no question of an independent epidemic among the heterosexual population in the Netherlands. The probability of such an epidemic in the future is also regarded as unlikely (Bonneux en Houweling, 1989; Luijckx et al., 1988). Indications for a low spread of HIV among the heterosexual population include a seroprevalence of less than (and in some cases much less than) 1% encountered in surveys conducted among heterosexuals with numerous changing sex partners and among pregnant women and in blood-bank screening, and the traceability to known risk groups of a high proportion of the people with AIDS with heterosexual contact as the risk factor (Van der Linden et al., 1990; Dudok de Wit, 1989; Van Lith et al., 1989; Coutinho et al., 1989, 1990). These are however point-prevalence studies conducted among non-representative groups. Apart from these indications a growing group of people with AIDS has been identified in recent years with heterosexual contact as the sole risk factor, part of the population is exposing itself to STDs and hence to HIV, and there has been a rise in the incidence of syphilis among heterosexuals. Neither seroprevalence screening among groups with an STD risk nor anonymous screening is conducted in the Netherlands, although support is given for anonymous screening on a voluntary basis among visitors to STD outpatient clinics (GR, 1990; TK, 1991). The initial results of anonymous screening in the US and the UK provide grounds for further research into the role of heterosexual transmission in certain geographical areas (Ades et al., 1991; Tappin et al. 1991; Coutinho, 1990).

3.3.3.1 Sexual behaviour

Among the trends in sexual behaviour in Western countries identified in studies are the fact that the age of first sexual intercourse among young people is falling (in the Netherlands it averaged 17.4 years in 1989) and that differences in partner change between men and women have been steadily diminishing over the past 20 years. Constants in sexual behaviour are: an average 12% of the population has more than one sexual partner a year, and a small percentage has more than five; sexual contact is tied up with close relationships; heterosexuals with multiple partners are often serially monogamous, i.e. they have a series of successive, often brief, intimate relationships; condoms are not very popular as a contraceptive; an estimated 20% of males have had sexual relations with a commercial sex worker at some point in their lives, and approximately 5% in the past year; fewer than 10% of sexually active young people have ever had anal intercourse (Kooij et al., 1983; Van de Rijt et al., 1987; De Vroome et al., 1988; Vogels and Van der Vliet, 1990; Johnson et al., 1989; Miller et al., 1989; Van Zessen, 1991, Boutellier, 1987). As discussed in more detail in Chapter 4, AIDS appears to have led to a change in emphasis in sexual behaviour and the way it is approached. A number of heterosexual subpopulations with, at first glance, an above-average HIV/AIDS risk are examined below: STD clients, commercial sex workers and their clients and non-commercial sexual partners.

3.3.3.2 Sexually transmitted diseases (STDs)

Due in part to the greater openness towards sexuality/homosexuality and the availability of oral contraceptives, the incidence of STD has risen sharply among young adults since the end of the 1960s. The STD incidence among commercial sex workers and their clients has remained more constant (Mooij, 1990)[4]. The incidence of syphilis and gonorrhoea reached a peak at the end of the 1970s. In 1985 the STD incidence for gonorrhoea was 25.3 per 10,000 inhabitants and for syphilis approximately 1, with major differences between the large cities and rural areas (Miltenburg et al., 1988). A sharp decline of over 20% a year, due in part to the impact of the HIV/AIDS-STD campaigns, has occurred nationwide since 1985 (Van de Laar et al., 1990; Leenaars et al., 1989; GHI, 1990). In Amsterdam a decline was already observed in the early 1980s (GG & GD, 1990).

An increase in syphilis was however noted in Amsterdam in 1987 and nationally in 1989, much of which must be attributed to heterosexual males (Van den Hoek et al., 1990b; GHI, 1990). An increase in the number of visitors to STD clinics was also noted in 1989, following a decline from 1983 among gay and from 1987 among heterosexual males (Van Haastrecht et al., 1991b). Classified by STD risk groups it emerges that the increase in STDs since the 1960s is primarily attributable to gay men and young heterosexuals and the fall

---

[4] Foreigners or ethnic minorities have traditionally been identified as risk groups for STDs (GR, 1986). Mooij (1990) cites Bijkerk, who notes imperfections in the STD surveillance in the 1960s: both tourists and migrants were classed as foreigners. An increase in STD among foreigners does not therefore necessarily mean an increase in STDs among ethnic minorities.

in the 1980s primarily to a decline among gay men.

Also of importance for scenario analysis are the figures of recidivism among STD clients, which showed a sharp increase in the 1980s, i.e. in the face of a general trend towards more cautious behaviour a small group has persisted with risk behaviour (Mooij, 1990; Van de Laar et al., 1990).

3.3.3.3 HIV/AIDS prevention aimed at the general population

Initially HIV/AIDS prevention among the general population concentrated on a "passive/active" information policy. No information was provided on a large scale (passive), but if people had a need for information it was available (active). At the initiative of the WVC, the NCAB and the STD Foundation embarked on major publicity campaigns in 1987. The first multi-media information campaign was the "Flower with Bee" campaign, supported by TV spots, posters, leaflets and advertisements. The subsequent campaign conducted by the STD Foundation to change sexual behaviour was aimed at promoting the use and public acceptance of condoms. This was done by getting well-known Dutch people to say that "they" used them. This condom campaign formed part of a multi-year plan. Two follow-up campaigns were conducted: the "Safe Sex on Holiday" campaign in 1988, aimed primarily at adolescents, and the "Excuses" campaign of 1989, aimed at young people aged 18-25 and designed to eliminate misunderstandings and misconceptions about HIV/AIDS and other STDs. In 1988 the Ministry of Welfare, Health and Cultural Affairs (WVC) and the Ministry of Social Affairs organized the "AIDS and Work" campaign, which was designed to step up the information provided in various workplaces and to draw it together in an over-arching campaign. In the same year the WVC organized the campaign "AIDS and Young People" as a back-up for the information activities being conducted at schools among 13-17 year-olds. These campaigns were designed to make the information being provided to young people more generally known with a view to promoting the integration of AIDS control in society. During the subsequent publicity campaign conducted by the WVC, greater attention was paid by means of radio, TV and advertising to the prevention of discrimination and stigmatization of people with HIV/AIDS and the encouragement of involvement and public support (NCAB, 1988a, 1989, 1991).

The AIDS information campaigns have led to a high level of public knowledge about AIDS. An increasing number of people claim moreover to have adapted their behaviour in order to avoid HIV infection. The main form this has taken has been an increase in condom use (although not extending to 100% of high-risk contacts), monogamy and limiting the number of sexual partners. Little if any reference is made to changes in sexual techniques (De Vroome et al., 1990). Condoms are largely regarded by young people as a contraceptive; when females are on the pill there is less inclination to use condoms (Vogels and Van der Vliet, 1990). In response to the national AIDS information campaigns in 1987 sales of condoms rose by 20% to 25 million, of which 3% were used for anal intercourse, before dropping again slowly (with traditional peaks in the summer months) to the 1985 level (personal communication LRC Leerdam, 1991; personal communication).

3.3.4 Commercial sex work

Commercial sex workers and their clients are traditionally regarded as risk groups for STDs (GR, 1986a). In addition the spread of HIV among non-drug-dependent commercial sex workers appears to provide a good indicator of the spread of HIV among the heterosexual population (Padian, 1989). For the present there appears to be no suggestion in Western societies of any large-scale spread of HIV among non-drug-dependent commercial sex workers; the shared use of injection equipment among commercial sex workers appears to be the most significant risk factor for HIV (Piot and Laga, 1988, 1989; Hooykaas et al., 1989). On account of the large number of changing sexual contacts within the commercial sex world, however, the spread of HIV on a "zig-zag" basis is not inconceivable: an HIV-infected commercial sex worker can transmit the virus to a large number of clients, who in turn can infect further commercial sex workers (Van Gelder and Van Roekel, 1989).

3.3.4.1 Commercial sexual contacts

Projections for commercial sex work need to take account of numerous, sometimes virtually hidden manifestations of sex work. In the Netherlands there are estimated to be 15,000-20,000 prostitutes, including 1,300 men, working in sidewalk, window and club prostitution, through escort services and privately (NCAB, 1990a; Boutellier, 1987). Apart from female Dutch commercial sex workers there is a comparatively hard to reach, growing and highly mobile group of foreign commercial sex workers, some of them from the Dominican Republic and the Cape Verde Islands, in which countries HIV has spread to a certain extent among the heterosexual population (Brussa, 1987; Koenig, 1989; NCAB, 1990a). As far as the clientele of commercial sex workers is concerned it is estimated that nearly 20% of males visit a commercial sex worker at some point in their lives and that 3% of males do so regularly (Boutellier, 1987).

With respect to sexual contacts and condom use in commercial sex work there are only a few known surveys on sidewalk, window and club prostitution. It is possible that the number and types of contacts and condom use vary from one type of sex work to another: vaginal intercourse is less common in sidewalk prostitution than it is in clubs, since the former often takes the form of sex in the client's car. On the other hand unprotected sexual contact with drug-dependent commercial sex workers is more common in sidewalk prostitution. In sidewalk prostitution the number of sexual contacts is estimated at four to five largely protected contacts per day during a working week of four to five days. As many as 40 unprotected contacts per month are, however, also cited (Hooykaas et al., 1989, Van Mens, 1989; Van Gelder and Van Roekel, 1989).

Among attenders at Amsterdam STD outpatient clinics a sharp decline from an average of 35 to 15 contacts per month was observed between 1986 and 1988 (Van Haastrecht et al., 1991b). Unprotected sexual intercourse was said to be an individual matter between client and sex worker and to be more common with regular than casual clients. Factors included the avoidance of sex with drug-dependant commercial sex workers, clients' attitudes towards condoms, the mutual evaluations of clients and sex workers as to whether the other was "clean" or addicted, fear of STDs and HIV/AIDS and the level of payment (Van Gelder and Van Roekel, 1989). The surveys make little reference to anal intercourse (e.g. in prostitution with boys), although this was questioned by the experts consulted on two grounds: there is a reasonable sale of condoms for anal intercourse in commercial sex work, and furthermore there might be dissimulation (Van der Poel, 1989; Biersteker, 1990; personal communication; Tillemans, 1990; personal communication). Boy-prostitution and the commercial sex activities of male hard-drug users do not appear to have been a significant factor in the spread of HIV among gay men in Amsterdam, although it may be noted that US research suggests a high seroprevalence rate among male commercial sex workers (Van den Hoek et al., 1991; Coutinho et al., 1988; Elifson et al., 1989).

3.3.4.2 Non-commercial contacts

Little is known about the non-commercial contacts of clients and sex workers. Surveys conducted among commercial sex workers suggest a lack of any or an average of two private contacts every three months. Surveys among clients indicate that 25-50% have sexual relations solely with commercial sex workers (Van Mens, 1989; Hooykaas et al.,

1989; Van Gelder and Van Roekel, 1989).

3.3.4.3 HIV/AIDS prevention and commercial sex work

HIV/AIDS prevention in the sex industry is directed towards the commercial sex workers themselves, clients and the operators. As a follow-up to the large publicity campaigns an experimental "condom promotion campaign" was conducted in the sex industry in 1988. The impact was, however, almost entirely confined to organized commercial sex work: foreign sex workers were barely reached. Clients responded positively to the campaign (Biersteker, 1989).

Since commercial sex workers are not an easily reached group, the working group on STDs and prostitution (1987) has called for the integrated provision of HIV/AIDS information/prevention and curative treatment of STDs. With this in mind the follow-up campaign "Safe sex - no worries" was started up in 1990. During the same period the GG & GD Amsterdam provided cassettes for foreign commercial sex workers with AIDS information in various languages, since written material was not getting through. The STD Foundation and the NCAB have also started up information projects for foreign commercial sex workers (NCAB, 1990a).

In a number of places special "living room projects" have been set up for sidewalk prostitutes, in which AIDS information and education are also provided. Apart from sales of condoms training is also provided on the correct use of condoms and on ways of inducing clients to use them (NCAB 1988b; Kleinegris, 1990).

Apart from the general publicity campaigns, commercial sex workers are also approached at a more individual level. The working group "Client and Prostitution" (the prostitutes' representative organization) and the STD Foundation, for example, from time to time conduct campaigns to distribute free condoms and leaflets and stickers. Efforts are also made to convey the "safe sex message" to operators with a view to reaching commercial sex workers and their clients.

Little is known about the effect of HIV/AIDS prevention. The impression is that Dutch commercial sex workers are well informed and that condoms are widely used. The incidence of risk contacts is attributable to other factors as discussed in section 3.2.4.1. No data are available on the effect among foreign women.

3.3.4.4 Points of concern

Knowledge of the role of sex tourism in the spread of HIV and about clients from ethnic minorities is confined to impressions. Organized sex tourism in the Netherlands seems not to occur on any scale. The research data do not indicate whether clients from ethnic minorities have difficulties with condom use on religious or cultural grounds, or whether sex workers have racial prejudices or fear to loose Dutch clients (Biersteker, 1989, 1990, personal communication).

3.4 Other groups at risk for HIV/AIDS

3.4.1 People with haemophilia

Some 13% (162) of the 1,250 people with haemophilia in the Netherlands have become seropositive from treatment with HIV-infected blood (Rosendaal et al., 1987). Since the introduction of the HIV-antibody test in 1985 infection with HIV by means of this transmission route can be virtually excluded: all blood donations are screened and all blood products undergo heat treatment. No further spread of HIV among this group is expected.

By international standards a comparatively low percentage of people with haemophilia in the Netherlands are HIV-infected. In the US an estimated 70% of such patients are seropositive. Causes of the comparatively low seroprevalence include the careful preparation of blood products; the non-commercial operation of blood banks; the low dependence on imported blood; and the possible effect of an early call to donors with a possible AIDS risk not to donate blood (Smit and Rosendaal, 1989; Van Aken, 1990, personal communication).

Nevertheless, these have been testing times for people with haemophilia: the advent of AIDS has seriously eroded the improved methods of treatment and the highly improved medical and social situation[5].

With respect to people with haemophilia there is also the question of the transmission of HIV to sexual partners and of perinatal AIDS. Without ancillary risk factors such as drug use and an STD history the chance of sexual transmission, even given a large number of unprotected vaginal contacts, appears small (Van der Ende et al., 1988; Andes et al., 1989). As far as maternal-foetal transmission is concerned a significant question concerns the extent to which an HIV or AIDS diagnosis will lead to a decision not to have or to postpone having children (Smit, 1987).

---

[5] Apart from physical suffering there is also the tension, depression, anxiety, fear and sense of guilt among people with haemophilia (HIV-infected and otherwise) and especially their parents and loved ones (Rosendaal et al., 1987; Rosendaal et al., 1988; Agle et al., 1987).

The Netherlands Association of Haemophiliac Patients (NVHP) and the treatment centres provide information for people with haemophilia. The NVHP has issued a booklet entitled "Haemophilia and AIDS, 55 questions and answers for patients, parents and carriers".

3.4.2 Health care workers

A group at potential risk for acquiring HIV is workers in health care and paramedical professions through accidental needle stick injuries or cuts. Both internationally and in the Netherlands this has led to a special emphasis on, and recommendation of, preventive measures as also taken to safeguard against other communicable diseases, such as Hepatitis B (GR, 1986b). The literature indicates that to date, the risk in practice is very low (Marcus et al., 1988; Klein et al., 1988; Leentvaar-Kuijpers et al., 1989)[6].

With respect to the risks for health care workers, seroprevalence is of particular importance in future explorations since a large-scale spread of HIV would also mean a higher risk of HIV infection in health care work. In this respect the geographical distribution of HIV is also a relevant factor; if HIV infection tends to be concentrated in certain parts of the country, e.g. the centres of large cities, as in the US (Turner et al., 1990), health care workers responsible for looking after patients in these regions will be at above-average risk.

3.4.2.1 HIV/AIDS prevention aimed at health care workers

Advisory reports by the Standing Committee on AIDS of the Health Council and by such bodies as the basic health care services, the Academic Medical Centre and the National Commission for AIDS Control (NCAB) have devoted special attention to the need to inform medical/paramedical staff. The Ancillary Services Association (SAD) has developed a special HIV/AIDS manual to assist general practitioners. As part of the "AIDS and Work" campaign an information film was made for nursing staff. Teleac, Dutch Educational Televicion, has developed a course aimed at people professionally involved in the provision of care and information.

In 1989 the attitudes of doctors towards AIDS was measured in

---

[6] At the same time, AIDS has led to varying reactions among health care workers, such as anxiety, negative attitudes towards core groups and a debate about the practical necessity and legal/ethical admissability of routine testing in the event of operations (Lodewijkx, 1989; Hamman-Konings et al., 1988; Storosum et al., 1990; Kelly et al., 1987; Meijler, 1988; Roscam Abbing, 1988).

three hospitals with a high, medium and low prevalence of AIDS. The majority of the doctors proved concerned about the possibility of being contaminated with HIV by a patient; their extensive factual knowledge about the risk of infection did not eliminate concern and fear (Storosum et al., 1990).

3.4.3 Persons from lower socio-economic classes

Increasing attention is being paid internationally (e.g. in the US) to the spread of HIV and AIDS among men and women from minority or underprivileged groups and of HIV/AIDS among young people, generally in connection with drug use and prostitution. The consequences for maternal-foetal AIDS are also noted in this context. In many cases these are young men and women from underprivileged groups in large urban centres (Miller et al., 1990). Holmes (1989) points to the explosive increase in STDs among the lower socio-economic classes in the US in the 1980s, especially among blacks and hispanics, while the STD incidence among the white middle classes fell substantially during the same period.

So far AIDS in the Netherlands has been largely confined to males and studies among pregnant women indicate that perinatal AIDS (e.g. among female IDUs) is not as yet a substantial problem. There are no data in the Netherlands on the spread of HIV among ethnic minorities. As far as STDs are concerned, a steady increase in the number of Turkish heterosexual males was observed in Amsterdam in the 1980s, in contrast to other Dutch and ethnic groups (Van Haastrecht et al., 1991b). On the basis of recent research the HIV/AIDS risk for young Dutch people may be regarded as small. Further research into the HIV/AIDS and STD risk among young people from the second ethnic minority generation is in the process of preparation (Vogels and Van der Vliet, 1990).

3.4.3.1 HIV/AIDS prevention aimed at persons from lower socio-economic classes

Poorly educated people and children of non-Dutch origin are less well informed about AIDS and HIV/AIDS prevention (Vogels and Van der Vliet, 1990). There are grounds for believing that linguistic problems, cultural differences and the level of education mean that the publicity campaigns do not reach ethnic minorities properly. Since 1988, special information and prevention activities have been organized for the largest groups, namely Surinamese, Moroccan, Turkish and Antillean immigrants. The aim in doing so is to bring the problem of sexuality and HIV/AIDS out into the open, to increase the level of understanding, to focus attention on the importance of HIV/AIDS prevention and to eliminate unnecessary fears of infection (NCAB, 1988c, 1990cd).

These activities have been incorporated into the existing migrant TV and radio programmes. In addition the AIDS hotline has been providing information in Turkish and Moroccan since 1989 and courses are provided in order to train public information officers in their own language. A high proportion of the initiatives taken in the field of AIDS information and education for migrants has been conducted by the NCAB, which appointed a special coordinator for the purpose in 1989.

No research has been conducted among Dutch immigrants into their knowledge of, attitudes towards and behaviour in respect of sexuality and AIDS. The extent of this behaviour and the effects of AIDS information are therefore unknown.

3.4.4 Mother-child transmission

As of 1.1.1991, 15 children aged under 13 had been diagnosed as having AIDS. Among seven children this was the result of mother-child transmission. Broken down by risk factor of the mother there were two instances of injecting drug use and two of heterosexual contact. Seroprevalence research among pregnant women continues to suggest a low seroprevalence (Van Lith et al., 1989; Coutinho et al., 1989, 1990).

3.4.4.1 Information concerning maternal-foetal AIDS

Information activities on maternal-foetal AIDS centre around the personal responsibility of the woman. Women who are HIV-positive are advised to avoid getting pregnant, while they are also provided with the necessary information for taking a decision about pregnancy and/or abortion (NCAB, 1989b).

At present maternal-foetal AIDS is not a problem in the Netherlands. Changes in the epidemiological trend among women or changes in attitudes towards pregnancy among people with HIV could, however, change this situation.

3.5 Summary

This socio-epidemiological part of the baseline analysis provides a survey of the HIV/AIDS epidemic between 1982 and 1991. Apart from a presentation of key data on the epidemic in its entirety a number of subepidemics have also been examined. A reconstruction has examined the most important factors that have so far determined the scale and spread of the HIV/AIDS epidemic. The analysis has concentrated especially on the necessary data for analysing likely and possible epidemiological trends. Key data such as group size, risk contacts and the number of partners have been identified for each group and special areas of concern for the projections have been identified. A number of groups for whom the spread of HIV/AIDS is of special concern have also been examined, namely people with haemophilia, health care workers and possible future core groups.

To date the HIV/AIDS epidemic in the Netherlands has been largely concentrated among men who have sex with men and among IDUs. Receptive anal intercourse and the shared use of injection equipment are the leading risk factors. An independent epidemic among the heterosexual population is not regarded as particularly probable, although due consideration needs to be given to groups who expose themselves to the risk of contracting a STD. A particularly important factor for the future spread is the extent to which changes in behaviour are consistent and lasting. The conclusion to emerge from the chapter is that a change in behaviour has taken place among groups with a high AIDS risk, although it is uncertain whether that change is consistent and lasting. In the case of the heterosexual population there appears to have been a less radical change in behaviour.

References

Ades, A.E., S. Parker, T. Berry, F.J. Holland, C.F. Davison, D. Cubitt, M.Hjelm, A.H. Wilcox, S.N. Hudson, M. Briggs, R.S. Tedder, C.S. Peckham
Prevalence of maternal HIV-1 infection in Thames Regions: results from anonymous unlinked neonatal testing
Lancet, 337 (1991), 1562-1565

Agle, D., H. Gluck, G.F. Pierce
The Risk of AIDS: Psychological Impact on the Hemophilic Population
General Hospital Psychiatry, 1987, 11-17

AIDS surveillance GG & GD Amsterdam
Aantal AIDS-patiënten gemeld vanuit Amsterdam tot en met December 1990
GG & GD Amsterdam, Amsterdam, 1991, kwartaaloverzicht nr. 7

Aken, W. van
personal communication, 1990

Andes, W.A., S.R. Rangan, D. Wulff
Exposure of heterosexuals of HIV and Viremia, Evidence for Continuing Risks in Spouses of Hemophiliacs
Sexually transmitted Diseases, 16 (1989), 2, 68-72

Bakker, E., J. Schuyf (red.)
Homoseksualiteit en de Media; verslag van een studiedag georganiseerd door Homo RTV Urania en Homostudies Utrecht
RUU, Interfacultaire werkgroep Homostudies, 1985

Barends, W.
Routinematig HIV-onderzoek in een Rotterdams methadonprogramma
Medisch Contact, 43 (1988), 2, 58-60

Berg, T. van den, M. Blom; Mr. A. de Graaf Stichting
Tippelen voor dope; levensverhalen van vrouwen in de heroïneprostitutie
SUA/Mr. de Graafstichting, Amsterdam, 1987

Biersteker, S.
Primaire preventie van aids/SOA in de prostitutie: projectplan en aanzet tot meerjarenplan
SOA-stichting, Utrecht, 1989

Biersteker, S.
personal communication, 1990

Bindels, P.J.E., M.J.J.C. Poos, J.T.L. Jong, J.W. Mulder, J.C. Jager, R.A. Coutinho,

Trends in mortality among AIDS patients in Amsterdam, 1982-1988
AIDS, 1991, accepted

Bisset, C., G. Jones, J. Davidson, B. Cummins, S. Burns, J.M. Inglis, R.P. Brettle
Mobility of injection drug users and Transmission of HIV
Lancet, 335 (1989), 44

Blom, M., O. Janssen
Molukse heroïnegebruikers in Nederland; een typologie van levensstijlen van Molukse heroïnegebruikers
RUG, Instituut voor Criminologie, 1987

Bonneux, L., H. Houweling
Is een epidemie van heteroseksueel overgedragen HIV-infectie mogelijk in Europa?
Nederlands Tijdschrift voor Geneeskunde, 133 (1989), 39, 1922-1926

Boutellier, J.C.J.
Enkele cijfers over prostitutie
Justitiële Verkenningen, 13 (1987), 1, 36-44

Brussa, L.
De buitenlandse prostituée
In: F. Belderbos, J. Visser (red.), *Beroep: Prostituée*, Utrecht, Stichting Welzijns Publicaties, 1987, 91-105

Buning, E.C.
De GG & GD en het drugprobleem in cijfers: deel IV
GG & GD Amsterdam, 1990

Centraal Bureau voor de Statistiek (CBS)
Vademecum Gezondheidsstatistiek
CBS, The Hague, 1991a

Centraal Bureau voor de Statistiek (CBS)
Statistisch zakboek 1990
CBS, The Hague, 1991b

Coleman, R.M., D. Curtis
Distribution of Risk Behaviours for HIV infection amongst Intravenous Drug Users
British Journal of Addiction, 83 (1988), 1331-1334

Connell, R.W., S. Kippax
Sexuality in the AIDS crisis: patterns of sexual practice and pleasure in a sample of Australian gay and bisexual men
The Journal of Sex Research, 27 (1990), 2, 167-198

Coutinho, R.A., R.L.M. van Andel, T.J. Rijsdijk
Role of male prostitutes in spread of sexually transmitted diseases and human immunodeficiency virus
Genitourinary Medicine, 64 (1988), 207

Coutinho, R.A., K. Boer, M.F. Schutte, W.J. van der Velde, D.K.F. Mulder, G.J.J. van Doornum
HIV-prevalentie bij zwangeren in drie poliklinieken in Amsterdam
Nederlands Tijdschrift voor Geneeskunde, 133 (1989), 19, 978-980

Coutinho, R.A., K. Boer, M.F. Schutte, W.J. van der Velde, D.K.F. Mulder-Folkerts, G.J.J. van Doornum
HIV-prevalentie bij zwangeren in en rond Amsterdam in 1989
Nederlands Tijdschrift voor Geneeskunde, 134 (1990), 26, 1264-1267

Coutinho, R.A.
Eerste resultaten van anonieme HIV-screening in de Verenigde Staten
Nederlands Tijdschrift voor Geneeskunde, 134 (1990), 45, 2173-2175

Dallas, M
Onveilige seks bij homomannen; een verkennend onderzoek naar omvang en achtergronden
RUU, Homostudies, 1990, publikatiereeks Homostudies Utrecht deel 17

Deenen, A., L. van Naerssen
Een onderzoek naar enkele aspecten van de homoseksuele identiteitsontwikkeling
Tijdschrift voor Seksuologie, 12 (1988), 105-116

Donoghoe, M.C., G.V. Stimson, K.A. Dolan
Sexual behavior of injecting drug users and associated risks of HIV infection for non-injecting sexual partners
AIDS Care, 1 (1989), 1, 51-59

Doorninck, M. van
personal communication, 1991

Dudok de Wit, C.
HIV-seropostieve bloeddonoren in 1988; epidemiologische mededelingen
Nederlands Tijdschrift voor Geneeskunde, 133 (1989), 10, 523

EC Concerted Action on Assessment of AIDS/HIV Prevention Strategies
Assessment of the AIDS/HIV Preventive Strategies; Annual Activity Report; period: april 1990 - march 1991
Institute of Social and Preventive Medicine, Lausanne, Switzerland, 1991

Ekstrand, M.L., R.D. Stall, T.J.Coates, L. McKusick

Risky sex relapse: the next challenge for AIDS prevention programs: The AIDS behavioral research project
Presentation at *V International Conference on AIDS*, Montreal, 1989 (TDO8)

Elifson, K.W., J. Boles, M. Sweat, W.W. Darrow, W. Elsea, R.M. Green
Seroprevalence of Human immunodeficiency virus among male prostitutes
New England Journal of Medicine, 322 (1989), 832-833

Ende, M.E. van der, P. Rothbarth, J. Stibbe
Heterosexual transmission of HIV by haemophiliacs
British Medical Journal, 297 (1988), 1102-1103

European Study Group
Risk factors for male to female transmission of HIV
British Medical Journal, 298 (1989), 886 - 890

Evans, J.L., E. Chapman, B. Caldwell, N. Luban
Clinical outcome of transfusion associated HIV in Children
Poster at *VII International Conference on AIDS*, Florence, 1991 (MC 3355)

Fennema, J.S.A., J.A.R. van den Hoek, A.J. Rijsdijk, M.M.D. van der Linden, R.A. Coutinho
Het vóórkomen van seksueel overdraagbare aandoeningen bij bezoekers van twee geslachtsziektenpoliklinieken in Amsterdam
Nederlands Tijdschrift voor Geneeskunde, 133 (1989), 4, 372-376

Friedland, G.H., R.S. Klein
Transmission of the Human Immunodeficiency Virus
New England Journal of Medicine, 317 (1987), 18, 1125-1135

Friedman, S.R., D.C. Des Jarlais, A. Neaigus, A. Abdul-Quader, J. Sotheran, M. Suffan, S. Tross, D. Goldsmith
AIDS and the new drug injector
Nature, 339 (1989), 333-334

Gelder, P. van, J.H. Sijtsma
Horse, coke en kansen; sociale risico's en kansen onder Surinaamse en Marokkaanse harddruggebruikers: I Surinaamse harddruggebruikers
UvA, Instituut voor Sociale Geografie, 1988a

Gelder, P. van, J.H. Sijtsma
Horse, coke en kansen; sociale risico's en kansen onder Surinaamse en Marokkaanse harddruggebruikers: II Marokkaanse harddruggebruikers
UvA, Instituut voor Sociale Geografie, 1988b

Gelder P. van, A. van Roekel (m.m.v. S. Altink, T. Laar)
Baltsen en Banen; interactiemomenten en veilige sextechnieken rond de

gedoogzone voor tippelprostitutie in Rotterdam
GGD-Rotterdam e.o., afd. epidemiologie, 1989, rapportnummer 59

Gemert, F. van
Mazen en netwerken; de invloed van beleid op de drugshandel in twee straten in de Amsterdamse binnenstad
UvA, Instituut voor Sociale Geografie, 1988

Geneeskundige Hoofdinspectie van de Volksgezondheid (GHI)
anonymous registration of AIDS diagnoses
continuous registration

Geneeskundige Hoofdinspectie van de Volksgezondheid (GHI)
registratie van SOA-meldingen
continuous registration

GG & GD Amsterdam
Geslachtziektenbestrijding GG en GD Amsterdam; jaarverslag 1989
GG & GD Amsterdam, Amsterdam, z.j.

Gijs, L., C. van Proosdij, C. Straver
Homoseksuele mannen in het huwelijk
Eburon, Delft, 1989, NISSO-studies 4

Goedert, J.J., C.M. Kessler, L.M. Aledort, et al.
A prospective study of HIV type 1 infection and the development of aids in subjects with hemophilia
New England Journal of Medicine, 321 (1989), 1141-1148

Gorter, R.W., K. Vranizan, A.R. Moss, B. Brodie, H. Wolfe
Progression of HIV disease in intravenous drug users
Poster op *VI International Conference on AIDS*, San Fransisco, 1990 (ThC644)

Gossop, M., P. Griffiths, J. Strang
Chasing the dragon: characteristics of heroin chasers
British Journal of Addiction, 83 (1989), 17, 899-900

Grant, P., R. Gold, M. Skinner, D. Plummer
Situational factors associated with, and rationalizations employed to justify unprotected intercourse in gay men
Presentation at *V International Conference on AIDS*, Montreal, 1989 (TDO7)

Griensven, G.J.P., R.A. Coutinho
Transmissiewijzen van het humaan immonudeficiëncyvirus
Nederlands Tijdschrift voor Geneeskunde, 132 (1988), 40, 1835-1842

Griensven, G.J.P. van
Epidemiology and Prevention of HIV-infection among homosexual men
UvA, Amsterdam, 1989, dissertation

Griensven, G.J.P. van, P.J. Veugelers, E.M.M. de Vroome, R.A. Coutinho, J.A.M. van Druten
Heterogeneity and fluctuations in homosexual behavior: implications for modelling the AIDS-epidemic
Presentation at *VI International conference on AIDS*, San Fransisco, 1990

Grapendaal, M.
De tering naar de nering; middelengebruik en economie van opiumverslaafden
Justitiële Verkenningen, 15 (1989), 5, 23-46

Grund, J.P.C., C.D. Kaplan
HIV-transmissie in het dagelijks ritueel van intraveneuze druggebruikers
Nederlands Tijdschrift voor Geneeskunde, 133 (1989), 17, 899-900

Haan, H.A. de, J.A.R. van den Hoek, H.J.A. van Haastrecht, C.W. van der Meer, R.A. Coutinho
Relatief lage HIV-prevalentie onder druggebruikers in Den Haag ondanks riskant spuitgedrag
Nederlands Tijdschrift voor Geneeskunde, 135 (1991), 6, 218-221

Haastrecht, H.J.A. van
personal communication, 1991

Haastrecht, H.J.A. van, J.A.R. van den Hoek, C. Bardoux, A. Leentvaar-Kuypers, R.A. Coutinho
The course of the HIV epidemic among Intravenous Drug Users in Amsterdam, The Netherlands
American Journal of Public Health, 81 (1991a), 1, 59-62

Haastrecht, H.J.A. van, J.A.R. van den Hoek, R.A. Coutinho
Aanwijzingen voor veiliger seksueel gedrag bij heteroseksuelen in Amsterdam onder invloed van AIDS.
Tijdschrift voor Sociale Gezondheidszorg, 69 (1991b), 1, 3-8.

Haenszel, W.
A Standardized Rate for Mortality Defined Units of Lost Years of Life
American Journal of Public Health, 40 (1950), 17-26

Hamman-Konings, G.M.J., G. ter Horst, M.J. van Hegten, J. Hoogstraten, G.M. Maritz, K.L. Meijer, Y.M. Meyland, Chr. van der Waag
AIDS en de Tandheelkundige praktijk: extern rapport
UvA, Sociale Tandheelkunde ACTA, Amsterdam, 1988

Hartgers, C., E.C. Buning, G.W. van Santen, A.D. Verster, R.A. Coutinho
The impact of the needle and syringe-exchange programme in Amsterdam on injecting risk behaviour
AIDS, 1989, 3, 571-576

Hartgers, C.
personal communication, 1990

Haverkos, H.W., W.J. Bukoski, Z. Amsel
The initiation of Male Homosexual Behavior
JAMA, 262 (1989), 4, 501

Health Council (GR)
Advies inzake Sexueel overdraagbare aandoeningen
GR, The Hague, 1986 /11 (1986a)

Health Council (GR)
AIDS problematiek in Nederland: richtlijnen voor groepsonderzoek en adviezen voor preventie
GR, The Hague, 1986 /22 (1986b)

Health Council (GR)
Verspreiding van het AIDS-virus in Nederland: methoden van onderzoek
GR, The Hague, 1990

Heisterkamp, S.H., A.M. Downs, M.J.J.C. Poos
MIDAS: A PC-program for adjusting reported AIDS data and short term projections
In: J.C. Jager, E.J. Ruitenberg (eds.), *AIDS impact assessment; modelling and scenario analysis*, RIVM/Bilthoven, in preparation

Hoek, J.A.R. van den
Epidemiology of HIV Infection among drug users in Amsterdam
Rodopi, Amsterdam, 1990 (dissertation)

Hoek, J.A.R. van den, G.J.P. van Griensven, R.A. Coutinho
Aanwijzingen voor toename van onveilig seksueel gedrag bij homoseksuele mannen in Amsterdam
Nederlands Tijdschrift voor Geneeskunde, 134 (1990a), 1229-1230

Hoek, J.A.R. van den, M.M.D. van der Linden, R.A. Coutinho
Increase of infectious syphilis among heterosexuals in Amsterdam: its relationship to drug use and prostitution.
Genitourinary Medicine, 66 (1990b), 31-32

Hoek, J.A.R. van den
personal communication, 1991

Hoekstra, J.C., R.R. van den Heuvel, T.J.B.M. Postma
Economische analyse van het heroïneprobleem
Tijdschrift voor Alcohol, drugs en andere psychotrope stoffen, 11 (1985), 3, 123-130

Holmberg, S.D., C.R. Horsburgh jr., J.W. Ward, H.W. Jaffe
Biological Factors in the Sexual Transmission of Human Immunodeficiency Virus
The Journal of Infectious Diseases, 160 (1989), 1, 116-125

Holmes, K.K.
HIV infection in the context of changing epidemiological patterns of sexually transmitted disease
Presentation at *V International conference on AIDS*, Montreal, 1989

Hooykaas, C., J. van der Pligt, G.J.J. van Doornum, M.M.D. van der Linden, R.A. Coutinho
Heterosexuals at risk for HIV: differences between private and commercial partners in sexual behavior and condom use
AIDS, 3 (1989), 525-532.

Houweling, H., J.C. Jager, R.A. Coutinho, H. Bijkerk, E.J. Ruitenberg
Epidemiologie van AIDS en HIV infecties in Nederland: huidige situatie en prognose voor de periode 1987-1990
Nederlands Tijdschrift voor Geneeskunde 131 (1987), 19, 818-824

Houweling, H., R.A. Coutinho
Epidemiological and public health aspects of AIDS and HIV infection: current concepts
Bilthoven, RIVM, 1989, rapport nr. 5289000001

Jager, J.C., M.J.J.C. Poos, H. Houweling, C.A. Postema, R.A. Coutinho
Prognose aangaande HIV-infectie en AIDS-epidemie in Nederland op basis van wiskundige analyse
Nederlands Tijdschrift voor Geneeskunde, 134 (1990), 51, 2486-2491

Janssen, O., K. Swierstra (m.m.v. E. van Barneveld)
Heroïnegebruikers in Nederland; een typologie van levensstijlen
RUG, Instituut voor Kriminologie, 1982

Jarlais, D.C. Des, S.R. Friedman, D. Strug
AIDS and Needle Sharing within the IV-Drug Using Subculture
In: DA Feldman, TH Johnson, *The Social Dimensions of AIDS*, Praeger, New York, 1986, 111-125

Jarlais, D.C. Des, S.R. Friedman, C. Casriel
Target Groups for Preventing AIDS among Intravenous Drug Users: 2. The Hard Data Studies

Journal of Consulting and Clinical Psychology, 1990, vol. 58, no. 1, 50-56

Johnson, A.M., J. Wadsworth, P. Elliot, L. Prior, P. Wallace, S. Blower, N.L. Webb, G.I. Heald, D.L. Miller, M.W. Adler, R.M. Anderson
A pilot study of sexual lifestyles in a random sample of the population of Great Britain
AIDS, 3 (1989), 135-141

Kelly, J.A., S.J. St. Lawrence, S. Smith, H.V. Hood, D.J. Cook
Medical students attitudes toward AIDS and homosexual patients
Journal of Medical Education, 62 (1987), 549-556

Kinnell, H.
Prostitutes, their clients and risks of HIV-infection in Birmingham
Department of Public Health Medicine, Birmingham, 1989

Klein, R.S., J.A. Phelan, K. Freeman, P.H.C. Schable, G.H. Friedland, N. Trieger, N.H. Steinbigel
Low occupational risk of human immunodeficiency infection among dental professionals
New England Journal of Medicine, 321 (1988), 86-90

Kleinegris, C.
Wil de echte preventiewerker nu opstaan?
Stichting HAP, Utrecht, 1990

Koenig, E.R.
International Prostitutes and Transmission of HIV
Lancet, 337 (1989), 782-783

Kooy, G.A. (sam.)
Sex in Nederland; het meest recente onderzoek naar mening en houding van de Nederlandse bevolking
Utrecht/Antwerp, Spectrum paperback, 1983

Korf, D.J.
Heroïnetoerisme II; resultaten van een veldonderzoek onder 382 buitenlandse dagelijkse opiaatgebruikers in Amsterdam
UvA, Instituut voor Sociale Geografie, 1987

Kuiken, C.L., G.J.P. van Griensven, E.M.M. de Vroome, R.A. Coutinho
Risicofactoren en sexuele gedragsverandering in voor HIV-antilichamen geseroconverteerde homosexuele mannen.
Tijdschrift voor Sociale Gezondheidszorg, 68 (1990), 329-334.

Laar, M.J.W. van de, J.A.R. van den Hoek, J. Pickering, G.J.P. van Griensven, R.A. Coutinho, H.P.A. van de Water
Dalende trend van gonorroe in Nederland: betekenis voor de

AIDS-epidemie?
Nederlands Tijdschrift voor Geneeskunde, 134 (1990), 13, 647-652

St. Lawrence, J.S., T.L. Brasfield, J.A. Kelly
Factors which predict relapse to unsafe sex by gay men
Poster at *VI International Conference on AIDS*, San Francisco, 1990 (FC725)

Leenaars, P.E.M., G.H. de Weert-van Oene, A.J.P. Schrijvers
Circuitkeuze van SOA-patiënten
Utrecht, SOA-stichting/RUU, 1989

Leentvaar-Kuijpers, A., J.N. Keeman, E. Dekker, M.M. Dekker, M.C. Ansink, R.A. Coutinho
HIV-beroepsrisico van snijdende specialisten en operatiekamermedewerkers in het Sint Lucas Ziekenhuis te Amsterdam
Nederlands Tijdschrift voor Geneeskunde, 133 (1989), 48, 2399-2391

Leidl, R. , M.J. Postma, M.J.J.C. Poos, B. Majnoni d'Intignano, J.C. Jager, A.E. Baert
Construction of socioeconomic impact scenarios based on routine AIDS surveillance data
In: J.C. Jager, E.J. Ruitenberg (eds.), *AIDS impact assessment; modelling and scenario analysis*, RIVM/Bilthoven, in preparation

Limbeek, J. van, L. Wouters, A.C. Hekker, A. Cramer
Een pilot studie naar het voorkomen van personen met anti-stoffen tegen HIV in hulpverleningsinstellingen voor drugverslaafden buiten de Randstad
FZA, Bilthoven, 1987

Linden, M.M.D. van der, F.W. van der Velde, C. Hooykaas, G.J.J. van Doornum, R.A. Coutinho
HIV-prevalentie onder heteroseksuelen met veel wisselende partners
Nederlands Tijdschrift voor Geneeskunde, 134 (1990), 28, 1361-1364

Lith, J.M.M. van, Tj. Tijmstra, G.H.A. Visser
De houding van zwangeren ten aanzien van het onderzoek op HIV-infectie
Nederlands Tijdschrift voor Geneeskunde 133 (1989), 25, 1273-1277

Lodewijkx, H.
Hercules en Hydra; een exploratief onderzoek naar belemmeringen in de AIDS-hulpverlening
Eburon, Delft, 1989, NISSO-studies 3

London Rubber Company (LRC), Leerdam
personal communication, 1991

Longini, I.M., W. Scott Clark, R.H. Byers, J.W. Ward, W.W. Darrow, G.F. Lemp, H.W. Hethcote

Statistical analysis of the stages of HIV infection using a Markov model
Statistics in Medicine, 8 (1989), 831-843

Loor, A. de
AIDS preventie voor druggebruikers begint niet bij de buren
Adviesburo drugs August de Loor, Amsterdam, 1991

Luijckx, B.J., G. Marsman, G. van der Rijt
AIDS en de risico's voor hetero's
Intermediair, 24 (1988), 6, 21, 23, 25, 31

Marcus, R., C.D.C. Cooperative Needlestick Surveillance Group
Surveillance of Health Care Workers exposed to blood form patients infected with the human immunodeficiency virus
New England Journal of Medicine, 321 (1988), 1118-1123

Martin, J.L., L. Dean, W. Hall
The impact of AIDS on the Gay Community: Changes in Sexual Behavior, Substance Use and Mental Health
American Journal of Community Psychology, 17 (1989), 3, 269-293.

Meijler, F.L.
Het testen op HIV-infectie in de cardiologie
Nederlands Tijdschrift voor Geneeskunde, 132 (1988), 31, 1445-1446

Mens, L.P.M. van
De invloed van de vrij veilig campagne op condoomgebruik door prostituanten
Maandblad Geestelijke volksgezondheid, 44 (1989), 7/8, 774-486

Miller, H.G., C.F. Turner, L.E. Moses (eds.)
AIDS The second decade
National Academy Press, Washington D.C., 1989

Miltenburg H.M.Th.M., M.E.M. Paalman, J.Th.N.M. Reus
Gonorroe in Nederland (en enkele beschouwingen over andere soa); verslag van een telefonische enquête onder behandelaars naar het voorkomen van gonorroe in 1985
Utrecht, SOA-stichting (i.s.m. project epidemiologie basisgezondheidsdiensten en GHI), 1988

Mooij, A.
De ziektes van de revolutie: Geslachtsziektes in Nederland vanaf de jaren zestig
In: G. Hekma, B. van Stolk, B. van Heerikhuizen, B. Kruithof (red.), *Het verlies van de onschuld; seksualiteit in Nederland*, Wolters-Noordhof / Amsterdams Sociologisch Tijdschrift, Amsterdam, 1990

Nationale Commissie AIDS Bestrijding (NCAB)
- *Werkplan voorlichting en preventie 1988*
  NCAB, Amsterdam, 1988a
- *Notitie AIDS en prostitutie*
  NCAB, Amsterdam, 1988b
- *Werkplan AIDS-voorlichting migranten*
  NCAB, Amsterdam, 1988c
- *Werkplan Voorlichting en Preventie 1989*
  NCAB, Amsterdam, 1989a
- *Notitie Kinderen, HIV-infectie en AIDS*
  NCAB, Amsterdam, 1989b
- *AIDS en prostitutie 1990*; bijgestelde notitie AIDS en prostitutie 1988 van de Nationale Commissie AIDS-Bestrijding en advies van de NCAB en de SOA Stichting aan de Vereniging van Nederlandse Gemeenten inzake gemeentelijk prostitutiebeleid
  NCAB, Amsterdam, 1990a
- *Het AIDS en drugsbeleid in Nederland*; de stand van zaken
  NCAB, Amsterdam, 1990b
- *AIDS-voorlichting aan migranten 1989 en 1990*
  NCAB, Amsterdam, 1990c
- *AIDS-voorlichting aan migranten 1991 en verder*
  NCAB, Amsterdam, 1990d
- *Werkplan Voorlichting en Preventie 1991*
  NCAB, Amsterdam, 1991

Nederlands Instituut voor Alcohol en Drugs (NIAD)
Spuitomruiladressen in Nederland
NIAD, Utrecht, 1990

Nederlandse Vereniging Consultatiebureaus voor Alcohol en Drugs (NVC)
LADIS 1988, jaarstatistieken uit het landelijke alcohol en drugs informatiesysteem
Utrecht, NVC, 1990

Oxtoby, M., R. Byers, R.J. Simonds, M. Rogers, R. Berkelman
Age at AIDS diagnosis for Perinatally-infected Children, United States
Presentation at *VII International Conference on AIDS*, Florence, 1991 (WC 36)

Padian, N.S.
Editorial review: Prostitute women and AIDS: epidemiology
AIDS, 2 (1988), 413-419

Piot, P., M. Laga
Prostitutes: a high risk group for HIV-infection
Sozial- und Präventivmedizin, 33 (1988), 336-339

Piot, P., M. Laga
Genital ulcers, other sexually transmitted diseases, and the sexual transmission of HIV
British Medical Journal 298 (1989), 623-624

Poel, S.C. van der
Jongensprostitutie in het AIDS-tijdperk
Maandblad Geestelijke volksgezondheid 44 (1989), 7/8, 787-799

Pollack, L., M.L. Ekstrand, R. Stall, T.J. Coates
Current reasons for having unsafe sex among gay men in San Fransisco: The AIDS behavioral research project
Poster at *VI International Conference on AIDS*, San Fransisco, 1990 (FC721)

Putte, B. van den
Harddruggebruikende straatprostituées en AIDS: een voorlichtingskundig onderzoek
UvA, 1986, doctoraalscriptie

O'Reilly, K.R., D.L. Higgins, C. Galavotti, J. Sheridan
Relapse from safer sex among homosexual men: evidence from four cohorts in the AIDS community demonstration project
Poster at *VI International Conference on AIDS*, San Fransisco, 1990 (FC717)

Reinking, D.P., F.M. van den Boom, M.J. Postma, J.C. Jager, E.J. Ruitenberg
Sociaal-epidemiologische aspecten van HIV/AIDS in Nederland: 1982-1990
STG/NcGv/RIVM, Rijswijk/Utrecht/Bilthoven, 1990

Rezza, G., A. Lazzarin, G. Angarano, A. Sinicco, A. Zerboni, R. Aiuti, R. Pristerà, B. Salassa, M. Barbanera, S. Gafà, L. Ortona, P. Costigliola, U. Tirelli, P. Pezotti
AIDS free time after seroconversion in injecting drug users and other risk groups
Poster at *VI International Conference on AIDS*, San Fransisco, 1990 (ThC647)

Rijt, G. van der, G. Marsman, J.B. Luijckx
Kennis over AIDS en weerstanden tegen condoomgebruik
In: J.H. Blans (red.), *AIDS, voorlichting en gedragsverandering*, Boom, Meppel/Amsterdam, 1987, 73-84

Roscam-Abbing, H.D.C.
Het testen op HIV-infectie in de cardiologie (reactie op F.L. Meijler)
Nederlands Tijdschrift voor Geneeskunde, 132 (1988), 37, 1707-1708

Rosendaal, F.R., C. Smit, I. Varekamp, A. Bröcker-Vriends, H. van Dijck, T.P.B.M. Suurmeijer, E. Briët
Hemofilie in Nederland 3; verslag van een in 1985 gehouden landelijk

onderzoek onder mensen met hemofilie
RUL/RUG, Leiden/Groningen, 1987, extra editie faktor, orgaan van de Nederlandse Vereniging van Hemofiliepatiënten

Rosendaal, F.R.
AIDS and haemophilia, a study among Dutch haemophiliacs on the psychosocial impact of the AIDS threat, prevalence of HIV-antibodies and the adoption of measures to prevent HIV transmission
Haemostasis, 18 (1988), 73-82

Selwyn, P.A., D. Hartel, W. Wasserman, E. Drucker
Impact of the AIDS epidemic on Morbidity and Mortality among intravenous Drug users in a New York City Methadone Maintenance Program
American Journal of Public Health, 79 (1989), 10, 1358-1363.

Skidmore, C.A., J.R. Robertson, A.A. Robertson, R.A. Elton
After the epidemic: follow up study of HIV seroprevalence and changing pattern of drug use
British Medical Journal, 300 (1990), 219-223

Smit, C.
Hemofilie en aids in Amerika, verslag van een studiereis
Amsterdam, NVHP, 1987

Smit, C., F. Rosendaal
Hemofilie en AIDS: een andere werkelijkheid
In: H. Vuijsje, R.A. Coutinho (red.), *Dilemma's rondom AIDS*, Lisse, Swets en Zeitlinger, 1989, 47-67

Stall, R., T.J. Coates, C. Hoff
Behavioral risk reduction for HIV infection among gay/bisexual men
American Psychologist, 43 (1988), 11, 878-885

Stall, R., M. Ekstrand, L. Pollack, T.J. Coates
Relapse from safer sex: The AIDS behavioral research project
Presentation at *VI international conference on AIDS*, San Francisco, 1990 (ThC108)

Storosum, J.J., H.N. Sno, H.F.A. Schalken, M. Nahuis, E.P. Meijer, J.A. Swinkels, L.J. Krol, S.A. Danner
Attituden van artsen ten aanzien van AIDS
Medisch Contact, 45 (1990), 25, 797-798

Straver, C.J., A. van Stolk
De kans op verbreiding van AIDS onder de Nederlandse bevolking
Maandblad Geestelijke volksgezondheid, 43 (1988), 4, 379-394.

Swierstra, K.
Drugcarrières: van crimineel tot conventioneel
Stichting drukkerij Regenboog, Groningen, 1990, academisch proefschrift

Tielman, R.A.P., S. Polter
Effect voorlichting over en preventie van AIDS bij homo-activisten en lezers van de Gay-krant
RUU, Homostudies, 1989, voorpublicatie vierde meting

Tillemans, G.
personal communication, 1990

Toet, J., A.P.M. van de Ven
Het RODIS uit de steigers; resultaten 1988
GGD-Rotterdam e.o., afdeling epidemiologie, Rotterdam, December 1989, rapport 65

Turner, C.F., H.G. Miller, L.E. Moses (eds.)
AIDS Sexual behavior and intravenous drug use
National Academy Press, Washington D.C., 1989

Tweede Kamer der Staten Generaal (TK, 1990)
Standpunt inzake het rapport van de Gezondheidsraad betreffende methoden van onderzoek naar de verspreiding van het AIDS-virus in Nederland
Tweede Kamer der Staten Generaal, vergaderjaar 1990 -1991, 19218, nr. 39

Vogels, T.R. van der Vliet
Jeugd en seks: gedrag en gezondheidsrisico's bij scholieren
SDU, The Hague, 1990

Vroome, E. de, Th. Sandfort, M. Paalman, R. Tielman
De ontwikkeling van kennis, houding en gedrag inzake veilig vrijen en AIDS; onderzoek onder de Nederlandse bevolking in het kader van de landelijke preventie campagnes: een vergelijking van 3 metingen
SOA-stichting, Utrecht, 1988

Vroome, E.M.M. de, M.E.M. Paalman, Th.G.M. Sandfort, M. Sleutjes, K.J.M. de Vries, R.A.P. Tielman
AIDS in the Netherlands: the effects of several years of campaigning
International Journal of STD & AIDS, 1990, 1, 268-275

Ward, J.W., T.J. Bush, H.A. Perkins, L.E. Lieb, J.R. Allen, D. Goldfinger, S.M. Samson, S.H. Pepkowitz, L.P. Fernando, P.V. Holland, S.H. Kleinman, A.J. Grindon, J.L. Garner, G.W. Rutherford, S.D. Holmberg
The natural history of transfusion associated infection with Human Immunodeficiency virus; factors influencing the rate of progression to Disease

New England Journal of Medicine, 321 (1989), 14, 947 - 952

Weiss, S.H., T.N. Denny, J. French, C.W. Klein, M.A. Jaffee, R. Altman
Increases risk of AIDS in older intravenous drug abusers and rates of HIV-seroconversion: 5-year follow up findings from the New Yersey (NJ) intravenous drug abuser (ivda) cohort study
Poster at *the VI international conference on AIDS*, San Fransisco, 1990 (ThC645)

Wigersma, L., H.A. Lemette, E.H. Hochheimer
Hulpvragen inzake geslachtsziekten en AIDS in de weekendpolikliniek voor homoseksuele mannen: ontwikkelingen 1983-1987
Nederlands Tijdschrift voor Geneeskunde, 133 (1989), 20, 1033-1035

Wit, J.B.F. de, E.M.M. de Vroome, T.G.M. Sandfort, G.J.P. van Griensven, R.A. Coutinho, R.A.P. Tielman
Stijging van de incidentie van HIV-infectie, het gevolg van een toename in onveilig seksueel gedrag?: Bevindingen in een cohort homoseksuele mannen in Amsterdam.
Tijdschrift voor Sociale Gezondheidszorg, 69 (1991), 1, 26-30.

Wiley, J.A., S.J. Herschkorn, N.S. Padian
Heterogeneity in the probability of HIV transmission per sexual contact: the case of male-to-female transmission in penile-vaginal intercourse
Statistics in Medicine, 8 (1989), 1, 93-102

Zessen, G.J. van
Sex en de levensloop
In: G.J. van Zessen, Th. Sandfort (red.): *Seksualiteit in Nederland: seksueel gedrag, risico en preventie van AIDS*, Swets & Zeitlinger, Amsterdam/Lisse, 1991, 35-58

Zwart, M.W. de
Alcohol, tabak en drugs in cijfers
Utrecht, NIAD, afdeling Onderzoek, 1989

4 Baseline analysis of sociocultural aspects of AIDS: 1982-1991

4.1 Introduction

As with epidemics in the past, the outbreak of the AIDS epidemic led to questions, reactions and debate within the health care system and society in general. Subjects that have come up, and continue to come up, in relation to AIDS include: the preservation of individual civil rights versus safeguarding public health, the responsibilities of the medical profession towards patients, the funding and organization of the care of AIDS patients and HIV-infected persons, debate about the correct control strategy, and the fear of a strong moral backlash towards AIDS and the consequences this could have for attitudes towards sexuality and public perceptions of people with AIDS, gay men and drug users.

A description and analysis of the impact of AIDS cannot therefore be confined to a survey of the incidence and prevalence, risk factors for infection and the implications for health care but must also examine the societal aspects of AIDS. Sections 4.1-4.4 of this chapter, which is based as far as possible on Dutch literature, examines societal developments in the field of sexuality, gay emancipation, hard-drug use and commercial sex work and changes in these resulting from AIDS. Sections 4.5-4.8 concentrate on the reaction to AIDS. We examine the characteristics of AIDS policy, the value attached to individual civil rights, the conflicting interests concerning HIV-testing, the organization and administration of HIV/AIDS prevention and initiatives in the care of people with HIV and AIDS.

4.2 Socio-sexological aspects

Socio-sexological studies provide insight into HIV transmission routes and the potential for infection. Such studies describe transitions and changes in the sexual scripts and interpersonal sexual networks spanning the period from childhood via adolescence and adulthood to old age. Broadly speaking a script for sexually active persons contains information on the "with whom, what, when, where and why" of sexual behaviour. The scripts are distinctly sociocultural in nature since sexual behaviour is determined not just by biological processes or age but also by attitudes towards sexual maturation, accepted and prohibited forms of sexual behaviour and relationships, which vary from society to society and change within societies (Gagnon, 1989). The sociocultural influences on sexual scripts range from the acceptance of homosexuality and attitudes towards the sexual roles of men and women to the social acceptance and practical availability of condoms.

Of particular importance for the risk of infection with HIV is the incidence of unprotected sexual contact, especially unprotected anal intercourse. The risk of HIV tends to be identified with traditional STD risk groups: males with multiple male partners, commercial sex workers (especially injecting drug users), their clients and young adults. Emphasis has also been placed in the Netherlands on the sexual experimental stage, i.e. the period in a person's sexual career characterized by a succession of sexual contacts within more or less exclusive relationships, on the group with any casual partners and the group with casual and regular sexual partners (Van Zessen and Sandfort, 1991).

By way of extension, determination of the networks in which unprotected sexual contact takes place provides insight into the spread of HIV infection among the population. The spread may take place by means of casual and regular partners or by means of a change in one's regular sexual partner. Apart from HIV infections within a network HIV may also spread between networks. Commercial sex workers and their clients, males with male and female sexual partners and the sexual partners of injecting drug users have been identified as possible "bridges" between the various networks (Straver and Van Stolk, 1988; Van Zessen en Straver, 1991; Piot and Laga, 1988).

Linking up the various life-cycle stages and relevant scripts of networks provides a highly variegated picture. In the rapidly changing Western societies we find *major individual differences* in personality development and personal histories, with *high mobility* and hence the *potential for highly ramified networks*, resulting in major differences within and between sexual scripts and sexual networks. For the possible spread of HIV this means that account needs to be taken of the marked differences in HIV risks within and between groups and with national and international transmission routes for the virus.

4.2.1 Sexual liberalization

A large-scale change in public attitudes towards marriage, the family and sexuality took place in a short space of time at the end of the 1960s. Key aspects of the new liberal sexual morality were the decoupling of sexuality and marriage and a greater openness towards and acceptance of individual differences in handling sexuality (Middendorp, 1974; 1975).

The rapid process of sexual liberalization has not been so much a sudden switch or sexual revolution as a culmination point in a much longer process of developments in attitudes towards the function of the family, the extension of the welfare state, greater mobility, a decline in social control and, in particular, the process of greater individual emancipation. Individuals increasingly take themselves as the yardstick and seek a high measure of freedom and responsibility in determining their own lives. Freedom and responsibility for determining and expressing sexuality are a key element in this process (Laeyendecker, 1988; Frenken, 1984a; Schnabel, 1990; Schmidt, 1990). A major practical factor in the break from traditional sexual morés was the introduction of reliable contraceptives in the 1960s. This led to a large increase in the use of condoms and especially oral contraceptives, which have continued to grow in popularity since their introduction in the 1960s (Frenken, 1984a; Verweij, 1989).

The discussion about sexual liberalization changed course in the 1970s. Sexual freedom was reappraised and a new concept was introduced: sexual responsibility. This switch in attitude was due in particular to the rising and increasingly influential women's movement. It became clear that in the field of sexuality, too, there existed inequality between men and women and that sexual violence (e.g. rape and incest) were and continue to be prevalent. Other developments from the 1970s include the marked rise in assistance sought by people for dealing with relational and sexuality problems and the increase in the number of STDs associated among other things with sexual liberalization and the introduction of oral contraceptives (Frenken, 1984b, 1987; Bijkerk, 1982; Schnabel, 1980; Mooij, 1990). The reappraisal to which this gave rise led to the exploration of a post-liberal sexual morality in which sexual freedom would be combined with an ethic of solidarity (Frenken, 1984a).

4.2.2 Sexuality: attitudes and behaviour

The dramatic changes in sexual morality have had implications for legislation, interpersonal relationships, attitudes towards sexual intercourse and the age of first sexual intercourse.

In the field of legislation the prohibition on the display and public sale of contraceptives was replaced in 1969 by a law on the free sale of contraceptives, while homosexual intercourse between an adult and a minor ceased to be a criminal offence (Kooij, 1975)[1]. With respect to later possibilities for HIV/AIDS prevention (i.e. the

[1] Another socially important but in this respect less relevant issue was that of abortion, which occupied centre-stage from the end of the 1960s. An international survey is provided in Ketting and Van Praag (1983).

promotion of condoms) and the sociocultural climate (i.e. political acceptance of homosexuality) there were important changes in the legislation on public morality[2].

In the field of sexual behaviour and multiple sexual partners, the sexual liberalization has been described as a "cultural symbolic revolution" (Schnabel, 1980, 1990) or a "revolution in talking about sex" (Frenken, 1984a). The literature notes a number of trends, some going back to the beginning of this century, whereby the age of first sexual intercourse is falling, people's sexual histories increasingly consist of a number of successive, exclusive intimate relationships and people are more prepared to enter into multiple sexual partners. The number of people with casual partners only, however, has remained small. Nor has there been a marked rise in the number of sexual partners throughout life. Like the pre-sexual liberalization era, sexual intercourse remains primarily bound up with an exclusive intimate relationship, although changing attitudes towards the nature and significance of partner relationships mean that such associations can be very short-lived. For the majority of the population the number of heterosexual partners during life has remained below ten. Anal intercourse does not appear widespread (Kooy, 1983; Vogels and Van der Vliet, 1990; Bolt, 1989; Johnson et al., 1989; Van Zessen and Sandfort, 1991).

A significant factor in determining the spread of HIV among the heterosexual population in general is the selective choice of partners. In general people select a partner from their own ethnic group of much the same age with a corresponding level of education. In this respect people's social lives are an important factor in bringing people together. Also relevant is the fact that individuals with several casual and casual or regular partners often have sexual partners who have several casual and/or regular partners as well (Van Zessen and Straver, 1991).

4.2.3 Impact of AIDS

Like the sexual revolution AIDS has not led to any switch in sexual behaviour or the incidence of multiple sexual partners among the population. As far as attitudes towards sexuality and sexual behaviour are concerned, AIDS and HIV/AIDS prevention have if anything led to greater openness rather than repression (Schnabel, 1989a; Schmidt,

---

[2] By way of supplement to the above we would also note major changes in the willingness to report sexual offences and in prosecution policy. Exhibitionism and, before 1970, fornication with minors, provide fewer grounds than before for prosecution while sexual violence (i.e. rape and incest) have become more liable to prosecution (Frenken, 1984b).

1990). Other than that AIDS is said to have had a possible effect on attitudes towards dealing with sexual freedom and responsibility, in that the AIDS information activities have added an extra dimension, namely protection against HIV infection and other sexually transmitted diseases (Schnabel, 1989a).

As far as the spread of HIV is concerned, Van Zessen and Straver (1991) conclude that in the short term the conditions for a substantial spread of HIV appear to be lacking: most people have a comparatively small number of partners, generally in successive and exclusive intimate relationships, the most common form of intercourse is vaginal and the sexual network structure is fairly unstable and fragmented. This means that on the one hand the HIV transmission routes are limited, while on the other HIV-infection is a real threat for a constantly changing part of the population. A slow spread of HIV remains possible, as do outbreaks on a small scale.

4.3 Gay emancipation, AIDS and discrimination

The late 1960s saw a breakthrough in the acceptance and recognition of homosexuality. Having previously been treated as a problem, disorder or abnormality, homosexuality became an accepted fact, with an appreciable increase in tolerance towards it (Groenendijk, 1987; SCP, 1988). The gay movement - now known as the Netherlands Association for the Integration of Homosexuality-COC (NVIH-COC) - which emerged as a national force in the 1960s also received increasing support for its drive for emancipation. In 1971, for example, the section specifically concerned with homosexual contact was dropped from the Public Morality Act of 1911 and the NVIH-COC received political recognition (Tielman, 1982). Since 1971 the political activities have been largely concerned with legislative measures to combat discrimination against homosexuality, e.g. by means of campaigns and initiatives to do with the Equal Treatment Act (Hoogma, 1990).

Among other things these initiatives and campaigns were based on the fact that the growth in tolerance towards homosexuality had not led to any decline in discrimination. The greater openness and visibility for example also led to greater violence against gay men, while there continue to be serious forms of discrimination against gay men (CRM, 1981; Dobbeling and Koenders, 1984; Dercksen and Van der Veen, 1990).

4.3.1 *The spread of HIV: threats to the individual and society*

In the Netherlands the epidemic of HIV infections and the AIDS epidemic have largely centered on men who have sex with men. For this group the AIDS epidemic represented a threat in various respects: it was possible to become infected oneself; in the short term a radical change in behaviour was required in order to counter the further spread of HIV; and within society there was the danger of discrimination against gay men because AIDS could unjustifiably be equated with homosexuality or homosexual behaviour.

4.3.2 *Behavioural change*

Socio-sexological research has revealed that a proportion of the population of men who have sex with men was at high risk of HIV infection: the high incidence of anal intercourse, a large number of sexual partners and the substantial expansion in the 1970s of places of entertainment and places to meet where sexual contact was possible created the right conditions for a rapid spread of HIV infection. In addition the lengthy HIV incubation period meant that the HIV prevalence could reach significant proportions before the gravity of the situation had been recognized (Van Griensven, 1989; Van Zessen and Sandfort, 1991).

The, by international standards, tolerant climate towards homosexuality and the role played by Amsterdam as a national and international meeting-point for gay men render it likely that the spread of HIV in the Netherlands occurred largely via Amsterdam. When the threat posed by AIDS became clear this led, as seen in Chapter 3, to a large-scale change in behaviour among gay men in a brief period of time.

4.3.3 *Societal consequences*

By international standards the Netherlands has a well organized, active and politically influential gay movement which has mounted a wide variety of initiatives that later continued on a separate footing. The J.A. Schorer Foundation, for example, has existed since 1967, later evolving into a national agency for lesbians and gay men concerned with the provision of support and services and with prevention.

This has not been without importance when it comes to the public's reaction to AIDS. Since the beginning of the activities to combat AIDS and the first information and prevention campaigns, representatives of organizations of and for gay men have played an important part in drawing attention to AIDS and getting HIV/AIDS prevention under way, in the provision of help and in the debate about the way in which AIDS control should be tackled (De Rijk and Van den Boom, 1989)[3]. The tolerant public climate towards homosexuality meant among other things that representatives of the gay movement were recognized as discussion partners and were able to influence the form and content of AIDS control.

Contrary to initial fears, AIDS would not appear to have had any negative consequences in the Netherlands for gay emancipation. Tolerance towards homosexuality has remained high and AIDS has not provided grounds for any marked increase in discrimination against gay men (SCP, 1989; Dercksen and Van der Veen, 1990). Wigersma (1990) even suggests in this respect that "The enormous public attention to AIDS has probably promoted rather than undermined gay emancipation".

Van Den Boom et al. (1991a) note that the success of the efforts on the part of the gay movement have resulted in a somewhat paradoxical situation. By referring to the determinants of HIV transmission and an emphasis on sober AIDS information based on the facts, the gay community has succeeded in averting the danger that AIDS would be regarded as a gay disease. This does, however, entails the risk of denying the fact that AIDS will remain a problem for a long time for the gay community in general and sexually active gay men in particular. This danger could become more acute given a decline in political and public interest in AIDS prompted by large-scale behavioural changes among gay men, initial research successes in treatment methods and the absence of an independent epidemic among the heterosexual population.

4.4 Drug use and drug users in the Netherlands

The present hard-drug use problem arose in the early 1979s in the Netherlands when heroin became widely and cheaply available (Van de Wijngaart, 1990). In a short space of time the number of hard-drug users rose to an estimated 15,000-20,000 in 1984. This estimate has remained unchanged which, in combination with the rising ave-

---

[3] Of the various organizations that emerged in the field of information and assistance we may mention just two: the psychosocial AIDS Assistance Division (APHA) of the Schorer Foundation and the activities of the Ancillary Services Department (SAD), formerly the Homosexual Health Care Group Amsterdam. Concrete initiatives include the buddy projects of the Schorer Foundation and the HIV/AIDS manual for GP's developed by the SAD. For a survey of the activities of both organizations we would refer to De Rijk and Van den Boom (1989) and the annual reports of the Schorer Foundation and the SAD.

rage age of hard-drug users in contact with outreach schemes, leads one to assume that the problem of heroin use may have peaked in terms of scale (De Zwart, 1989; Van Es et al., 1990).

Significant developments in hard-drug use since the 1970s include the spread of such behaviour to Surinamese and Molluccan youth and, in the 1980s, to ethnic minorities such as Moroccan young people. An increasing level of polydrug use has also been observed. Apart from heroin there is widespread use of cocaine, which became available on a large scale in the 1980s[4]. The latter is important in relation to injection since intravenous cocaine use inquires more frequently injecting than heroin.

Based on the surveillance systems for drug care, hard-drug users appear to be concentrated in the big cities and the border regions. In addition there are three times as many drug-dependent males as females, and most users are aged 21-34, are unemployed, living alone or cohabiting and have a low level of education (NZR, 1990ab).

4.4.1 Consequences of the hard-drug problem for society

The consequences of the hard-drug problem for society are discernible in the field of law and order and the provision of support and guidance for users. We shall be concentrating on the consequences for health care and examine the underlying principles of government policy and the care and treatment of drug addicts and the reaction to AIDS.

4.4.1.1 Care and treatment of drug users in the Netherlands

By way of response to the increasing number of hard-drug users an extensive system of facilities for hospital, semi-hospital and out-of-hospital care and treatment has been developed in the Netherlands. Apart from a specific circuit consisting of Institutes for the Treatment of Drug-Dependance, Alcohol and Drugs Abuse Clinics and Drug-Dependence Clinics, care and treatment for hard-drug users are also provided within the general circuit of health care facilities and by means of private initiative. These include primary health care, general and teaching hospitals and their psychiatric departments and general psychiatric hospitals. The private initiatives are generally based on humanitarian (religious) motives and concentrate on specific groups

---

[4] Unlike heroin, cocaine is also frequently encountered among socially integrated users or users from non-deviant subcultures. Injecting cocaine is uncommon among this group of users (Bieleman et al., 1989; Cohen, 1990). In the US the use of crack is also related to behaviour entailing a high risk of HIV infection. In the Netherlands crack is thought to be used on a very small scale.

of users, such as foreign or Molluccan users or users with special problems (Jacobs and Bijl, 1991; NcGv, 1990).

Both the delivery of and demand for care rose appreciably in the 1980s (NZR, 1990ab). In the case of out-of-hospital care there has been a particularly notable increase in the number of participants in the methadone programme. Since 1984 methadone has been distributed to a reasonably constant number of at least 12,000 hard-drug users, of which an estimated 9,000 are in maintenance programmes and 3,000 in withdrawal programmes (NVC, 1990; Buning, 1990; Driessen, 1990).

This extensive network of methadone distribution programmes, in particular, means that an estimated 75% of hard-drug users are seen frequently. With respect to HIV/AIDS prevention this means that the majority of users can be reached comparatively easily. By contrast there are few contacts with young users in the second ethnic minority generation (Buning, 1990).

4.4.2 Drug use and drug users

Data are available in the Netherlands from social-scientific research into the economic aspects of drug use, such as the procurement and costs of hard drugs, the incidence of drug-related crime, the life-styles of drug users, networks and cultures/subcultures of users, mortality and the different stages and differences in duration of hard-drug careers. The incidence of injecting use, the AIDS/HIV incidence and the effects of prevention have already been discussed in Chapter 3. Here we examine a number of aspects of the careers and life-styles of drug users and government policy towards hard-drug dependence.

4.4.2.1 Addiction careers, morbidity and mortality

In terms of the duration of drug-dependence, short (average eight years) and long (up to 20 years) drug-dependence careers may be identified. Drug users in Rotterdam and Amsterdam generally fall into the latter category. In most cases users drop out of the drugs world after the age of 35. Drugs-related mortality, due among other things to overdoses, is around 10% after five years drug-taking, 15% after ten years and 20% after 20 years (Swierstra, 1990).

4.4.2.2 Life-styles and networks

Research has been conducted into lifestyles and networks among a large number of different groups of drug users: Dutch users, users outside the large cities, Molluccan users, drug-dependant commercial sex workers, Moroccan and Surinamese users and foreign users.

These studies provide indications of separate circuits of users and a hierarchically structured drugs culture, characterized by a complex system of drug-dependence relationships. Hard-drug users dealing on small scale occupy a particularly high place in the hierarchy, while the urban homeless, whose position is one of marked social isolation, occupy the lowest rung on the ladder. Contacts within the drugs world are generally brief, volatile and often related to the purchase and sale of drugs and, less commonly, to the use of drugs. Mutual dependence is encountered at the level of drug-dealing. Many small dealers, for example, use intermediaries, such as carriers and errand boys, who perform odd jobs in exchange for drugs (Haverkamp, 1984; Blom and Janssen, 1987; Gemert, 1988; Janssen et al., 1982; Van den Berg and Blom, 1987; Van Gelder and Sijtsma, 1988ab).

In connection with AIDS, foreign drug users or heroin tourists would appear to merit special attention. In Amsterdam there were thought to be over 2,200 foreign users - out of an estimated total of over 7,500 hard-drug users - of whom 70% were injecting users (IDUs) (Buning, 1990)[5]. The heroin tourists, who come to visit not the Netherlands but specifically Amsterdam, largely lead a vagrant existence and chiefly mix with others from their own country. Foreign users who settle in Amsterdam (temporarily or permanently) also come into contact with Dutch and Surinamese users (Korf, 1987).

These considerations provide the basis for the following hypothesis on the spread of HIV among IDUs: the existence of contact between to some extent separate circuits of users can lead to an abrupt increase in HIV infection among IDUs. The introduction of HIV within user networks or user generations rapidly leads to an explosive increase in HIV infections. Increases of this kind within geographical regions and user generations are known from the international literature (Skidmore et al., 1989; Turner et al., 1989) and provide a frame of reference for explaining differences in seroprevalence in various cities in the Netherlands that cannot be attributed to differences in risk behaviour (De Haan et al., 1991). The mobility of hard-drug users provides an explanation why HIV can spread between groups of users in various cities and countries (Van den Hoek, 1990;

[5] The GG & GD Amsterdam provides both quarterly and annual estimates of the prevalence of hard-drug users. On an annual basis some 3,560 users were thought to have visited Amsterdam in 1989 (some only briefly). The number of drug users in Amsterdam also varies considerably according to season, being highest in the summer months. The quarterly estimate of over 2,200 users is the mean of the four quarterly estimates (Buning, 1990).

Bisset et al., 1989).

4.4.2.3 Government policy

Under an amendment to the Opium Act in 1976, a distinction was drawn between soft drugs such as hemp products and hard drugs such as heroin and cocaine. The former were regarded as entailing an acceptable risk while hard drugs involved an unacceptable risk. The possession and use of soft drugs were subject to less severe penalties. In the case of hard-drug dependence a dual-track policy was adopted: the use of hard drugs was approached from a health viewpoint and drug dealing and trafficking in criminal terms.

Internationally, the Netherlands is regarded as a liberal country in terms of dealing with drug addiction. With respect to drugs legislation, adherence to international agreements and the penalties handed down in cases of drug trafficking or disturbances of public order, this image is unjustified (Van Atteveld, 1988; Hulsman, 1984).

4.4.3 Impact of AIDS

AIDS has not led to changes in the way the hard-drug problem is approached and tackled. AIDS and drugs policy has made use of the extensive circuit of outreach facilities, and use has been made of existing contacts with users and user organizations, such as the Federation of Junkie Unions (*Junkiebonden*) and the Heroin Users Medical/Social Department (MDHG). AIDS has not provided grounds in the Netherlands for a fundamental debate about the hard-drug problem or basic differences of opinion about the approach towards AIDS and drugs policy.

AIDS has led to a number of new initiatives and the expansion of existing provision. Examples include the large-scale introduction of syringe-exchange programmes, low-threshold facilities for reaching drug-dependent commercial sex workers and the introduction of a support project for the psychosocial support of HIV-infected addicts by volunteers (NIAD, 1990; NCAB, 1990a; Driessen et al., 1991).

The AIDS-related increase in mortality among drug users in the US has not been observed in the Netherlands (Selwyn et al., 1989; Cobelens et al., 1990). There has, however, been an increased HIV-infection-related morbidity among IDUs in Amsterdam, especially from pneumonia (Van den Hoek, 1991, personal communication).

4.5 *Developments in commercial sex work*

Since 1970 commercial sex work in the Netherlands has become larger in scale, more commercialized and more firmly entrenched. The "classical" forms of window, club and sidewalk prostitution were set up on a larger and increasingly commercial scale. New forms of commercial sex work arose, such as sex cinemas and sex shops offering prostitution and "homeworkers" advertising their services. New forms of commercial sex work also appeared on the scene: drug-dependent sex workers and foreign sex workers. A fourth development has been the increased mobility of sex workers; since the mid-1970s there has been a growing number of foreign sex workers in the Netherlands[6] (Stemvers, 1985, NCAB, 1988; Belderbos and Visser, 1987).

Prostitution in the Netherlands is illegal. According to criminal law this takes the form of the ban on brothels under Art. 250 of the Criminal Code, under which prostitution is a criminal offence. In practice, however, a blind eye has been turned for many years. There is at present a proposal to abolish Art. 250 of the Criminal Code,[7], meaning that the exploitation of prostitution would, within certain limits, no longer be a punishable offence. The municipalities would be given the scope to introduce legally valid measures, e.g. to cope with the nuisance factor and to improve the conditions of work and health situation commercial sex workers. The NCAB and the SOA Foundation recently submitted an advisory report on this proposed legislative amendment to the Union of Netherlands Municipalities, the burden of which is that unduly strict municipal regulation could damage the relationship of mutual trust between commercial sex workers and information or welfare workers and the ability to reach commercial sex workers under the HIV/AIDS prevention campaign (NCAB-SOA Foundation, 1990).

---

6 This group is also important in health terms: in many cases these are women living illegally in the Netherlands whom the health care system has difficulty in reaching. HIV infections among this group of sex workers can therefore remain undetected for a long time.

7 We may briefly summarize this long-standing debate. Those who favour the abolition of Art. 250 of the Criminal Code advance the following arguments: (i) that an administrative approach towards prostitution would work better than a criminal one. Prostitution is a permanent social phenomenon. Instead of combating prostitution the emphasis should be on the coercion and violence with which it is associated and the conditions of work and health situation of prostitutes should be improved; (ii) that prostitution should be recognized as a profession; (iii) that account should be taken of women's right to physical and psychological integrity and to decide for themselves.

4.5.1 *Impact of AIDS*

The possibility that AIDS could be spread by commercial sex work has been a consideration since an AIDS policy was first formulated and has provided the grounds for special efforts directed towards sex workers and their clients. No evidence has been found of any change in public attitudes towards prostitution and the way it should be approached. The effect of prevention campaigns is discussed in Chapter 3.

4.6 *The response to AIDS*

AIDS has led to all sorts of reactions and initiatives aimed at (1) countering the spread of HIV infection, (2) the care and support of HIV-infected persons, (3) research and research programming and (4) countering undesirable social consequences of AIDS.

The reaction to AIDS on the part of the Dutch government has involved the Ministries of WVC, Justice, Social Affairs and Employment and Defence. The policy is coordinated by the Ministry of WVC. In the field of policy support and advice and assistance a large number of bodies and committees have been set up, such as the National Commission for AIDS Control (NCAB), the permanent committee on AIDS of the Health Council, the AIDS Research Programme Coordination Committee (PccAo) of the Health Research Council (RGO) and the AIDS platforms set up to deal with regional policy. The key document with respect to the government's response is the Policy Document on AIDS Policy (TK, 1987) of State Secretary Dees, the substance of which is set out in section 2.1.2.2. A follow-up report by State Secretary Simons is expected in the spring of 1992. Other government policy documents and memoranda examined in this chapter relate to legal aspects of the use of HIV testing in research and medical examinations, the psychosocial care framework plan and the guidelines for HIV-testing in medical examinations for prospective employees (TK 1987ab, 1990abc).

The NCAB, set up in 1987 for a period of four years, is responsible for policy advice and executive activities ranging from the organization and operation of the AIDS Hotline to coordinating responsibilities in the field of AIDS information and the coordination of national policy with the activities of the AIDS platforms operating at regional level. The "NCAB internal evaluation 1987-1991" (NCAB, 1991b) contains a survey of the tasks, organization and working method, together with a list of advisory reports and publications by the NCAB. An external evaluation of the NCAB recently concluded that the organization was meeting its goals and it was recommended that the decree establishing the NCAB be extended (Dirksen et al., 1991).

For a survey of activities in the fields of research programming and advice we would refer to the reports issued by the Health Research Council (RGO) on stepping up AIDS research and the AIDS research programmes in 1988-1990 and 1991-1992 (RGO, 1987; PccAo, 1989; PccAo, in preparation). In addition the PccAo has drawn up an inventory of AIDS research in the Netherlands (PccAo, 1990).

Although not unique to AIDS, a striking feature is the fact that in the Netherlands, AIDS policy, AIDS care and especially AIDS control are a joint effort by all the relevant parties: the government, the scientific community, the health care system, social services, public information service, those concerned and their legal representatives. In many cases it was the representative organizations that took a lead in initiating HIV/AIDS prevention activities, although by international standards the Dutch authorities soon took its lead from the work being done in the private sector (Shilts, 1987; Coppoolse, 1988; Tillemans, 1988; Schnabel, 1988). What is unique internationally is the far-reaching cooperation up to the highest level with representative organizations. Whereas in the United States and many European countries, AIDS has ushered in the setting up and recognition of interest groups and led to the establishment of a large number of community-based organizations and AIDS service organizations, in the Netherlands there already existed a dialogue between community-based organizations and the government and it was generally possible to build on existing facilities. Despite a number of major tensions, e.g. during the debate in 1983 about safeguarding the nation's blood supply, there is nevertheless a broadly collective, jointly determined strategy (Coppoolse, 1988; Schnabel, 1988).

Internationally, the Dutch reaction to AIDS stands out for the value attached to self-determination, privacy and the individual responsibility of the citizen and the absence, with a few individual exceptions, of the initially feared public backlash (Curran, 1989; Wayling, 1990; Bayer, 1991). As far as the legal framework of AIDS policy is concerned, this has translated itself into the marked importance attached to the preservation of individual civil rights. The scope of individual civil rights has played a decisive role in the conflict between individual interests and the interests of third parties, such as caregivers, employers, insurers or the public health system, and in the heated and fundamental debate concerning HIV testing. The implications for HIV-testing policy and the legal framework for such testing are discussed in sections 4.6-4.6.8.

The special nature of the disease called for a separate response.

Relevant factors included the fatal and untreatable nature of AIDS, the transmission of HIV by means of sexual intercourse and the concentration of HIV-infected persons among socially vulnerable groups: gay men and drug users. In contrast to the measures to combat other communicable diseases, the only prevention strategy for HIV and AIDS consisted of public information and education and the promotion of safe behaviour. The implications this had for the planning and implementation of HIV/AIDS prevention are discussed in sections 4.7-4.7.4. Within the health care system, AIDS raised questions of a psychosocial, psychiatric and somatic nature. Knowledge and expertise had to be built up over a brief space of time on the often complex, specialized care required and on the far reaching treatment and support of both for the person with HIV and the caregiver. Within the health care system this led to a large number of initiatives in the provision of care. These initiatives are discussed in terms of an integrated approach towards the psychosocial, psychiatric and somatic problems of AIDS patients in sections 4.8-4.8.3. We also examine initiatives on the part of people with AIDS and their representative organizations with respect to the planning and organization of care.

4.6.1 Characteristics of AIDS policy

Schnabel (1989b) cites the following characteristics of Dutch AIDS policy: the aim of normalization; relying on the effectiveness of an AIDS control policy based on personal responsibility; an emphasis on targeted prevention; and, wherever possible, fitting the care of people with AIDS into ordinary health care. Schnabel describes Dutch AIDS policy as first and foremost Dutch in nature and secondarily of relevance to AIDS: "The entire policy is geared to the 'normalization' of HIV and AIDS as a serious and difficult but ultimately not exceptional problem." In addition Schnabel notes that the policy is based on "preserving the social integration of identified patients wherever possible and limiting the risk of further spread by staying in contact with the core groups". Brandt (1987) and Paalman (1986) note in this respect the history of efforts to combat sexually transmitted diseases. Control, let alone coercion, has had little effect: even where a vaccine or antiviral therapy has been available for an STD, coercive measures have not brought the epidemic under control.

4.7 HIV-testing and conflicting interests

Dutch AIDS policy has been formulated against the background of developments in the field of individual civil rights. The ability to identify HIV-infected persons by means of an HIV-antibody test in 1985 created additional possibilities for HIV/AIDS prevention. The screening of donor blood for HIV meant that the safety of the nation's blood supply could be assured. In addition all sorts of possibilities arose for other applications of HIV-testing, such as routine screening in the course of medical treatment, screening when third parties are specifically at risk, public health screening and screening for insurance and other financial purposes (Markenstein and Goethart, 1989).

E. Roscam Abbing (1988) distinguishes a large number of situations in which HIV-testing might be considered and has summarized the interests that need to be protected or which could be harmed. He concludes that a clear judgement as to the desirability of testing can only be made after considering the pros and cons on a case-by-case basis and, where there is doubt, regards the pressure on the individual in a legal and psychological sense as the decisive factor[8].

4.7.1 Respect for individual civil rights

Since the Second World War increasing emphasis has been placed internationally on individual civil rights (Somerville and Orkin, 1989). With respect to the right of self-determination Markenstein and Goethart (1989) point to the Universal Declaration of Human Rights (UN, 1948), the International Covenant on Civil and Political Rights (UN, 1966) and the European Convention for the Protection of Human Rights and Fundamental Freedoms (Council of Europe, 1950). These treaties provide the international context within which each country is able at national level to determine civil rights with respect to the protection of privacy. In the Netherlands this resulted in the related and to some extent overlapping Articles 10 and 11 of the Constitution. These two articles, GW 10 and GW 11, were included in the Constitution in 1983 and came into force in 1988. Together the two articles are concerned with the personal sphere of life in the broadest sense of the word. GW 10 has particular significance for the protection of personal data. GW 11 focuses on

[8] The benefits of HIV testing may include: (1) enlarging insight into the epidemiology of HIV; (2) providing starting points for prevention and the planning of care provision, (3) enlarging the responsibilities at individual level for responsible behaviour; (4) maximizing the possibilities for care providers to protect themselves against HIV infection. Disadvantages are (1) the possibility of severe psychological/emotional and social consequences if a person tests positive; (2) the inability to link up a positive test result to necessary treatment; (3) the fact that the test does not provide absolute certainty because it only provides an indication at a given moment. He regards screening under pressure or coercion as disadvantageous for HIVAIDS prevention as it can lead to the evasion of prevention campaigns (E. Roscam Abbing, 1988).

another key element in the personal sphere of life, namely the integrity of the human body.

In order to put GW 10 and GW 11 into practice further legislation was required. Of particular relevance for the debate concerning AIDS are the Data Protection Act (WPR) and the Medical Treatment Agreement Bill (WGBO) of 1990. The GW 10 and GW 11 provide the basis for the requirement for consent, which provides the individual with protection from interference with his or her personal sphere of life, as well as the following rights: the right to information; the right to remain spared from undesired information; the right to confidentiality; the right to the protection of privacy with the respect to the registration of personal data; and the right of protection of privacy with respect to body material (Markenstein and Goethart, 1989).

Apart from GW 10 and GW 11 two other articles of the Constitution are of relevance for the debate, namely GW 1, which enshrines the principle of equality and the prohibition on discrimination, and GW 22, under which the government is obliged to take measures to promote public health (social fundamental right to health care). Activities concerning the Equal Treatment Act arise from GW 1, while legislation and administrative provisions in relation to access to and the financing of health care arise under GW 22. Of relevance for the debate concerning AIDS is the difference that individual civil rights are enforceable and are in principle fully operative, while that is not the case with respect to social civil rights such as GW 22.

Also relevant is the fact that limitations on individual civil rights are possible only with the greatest restraint, in exceptional situations and on the basis of statutory provisions. In the case of the right of self-determination, situations are conceivable in which the right of self-determination of others is interfered with, discrimination is possible and/or general interests and obligations come into conflict with individual interests and obligations[9].

---

[9] In this respect Leenen (1988) has formulated the exception principle, namely the requirement that the exception is governed by the same norm on which the exception is based. In line with Leenen the following criteria may be laid down with which statutory exception provisions to constitutional rights must comply:

- The relevance criterion: the reasons for the exception must be relevant and adequate.
- The motivation principle: the need for exception provisions must be properly grounded.
- The proportionality principle: a reasonable balance must be struck between the end and means.
- The subsidiarity criterion: it must be the only means of achieving the interest in question.

It should also be ensured that no less radical alternatives are available for achieving the same goal (Markenstein and Goethart, 1989; Te Braake, 1989; NCAB, 1989; Roscam Abbing, 1989).

4.7.2 *Predominantly non-mandatory screening policy*

Against the background of the legal framework outlined above, State Secretary Dees formulated a predominantly non-mandatory screening policy in his Policy Document on AIDS Policy. Apart from routine screening of donor blood, semen, tissue and organs, he considered that screening in a general sense would not contribute towards preventing the transmission of HIV. He also took the view that the lack of treatment facilities and the fact that HIV was not transmissable in social situations militated against a policy of greater screening. With respect to testing as part of medical treatment the State Secretary followed the recommendations of the Health Council: the hygienic measures already being used to counter the transmission of Hepatitis B (GR, 1987) provide adequate protection against infection with HIV. Considerable importance is attached to screening in connection with epidemiological studies, but this can only be done if the requirement of consent and the obligation to provide information have been complied with. Here too the protection of the private sphere of life applies with undiminished force[10].

4.7.3 *Large-scale seroprevalence screening*

Proposals for research into the distribution of HIV among the Dutch population by means of anonymous serological screening of blood collected for other purposes, whereby a working method was proposed that would ensure the data could not be traced back to the individuals concerned, gave rise to a fundamental debate. The Permanent Committee on AIDS of the Health Council (1989) and the NCAB (1989) issued divided reports on this proposal for screening and a discussion arose concerning the legal framework, ethical acceptability and necessity and importance of such research for AIDS control. The debate examined not just the screening itself but also the wider context of the problem. Topics examined included interference by third parties (including government) in the private life of citizens, the use of medical and other data for non-medical purposes and the possibility of conducting epidemiological and other patient or client-related screening (Huisman, 1988a; Lumey et at., 1989; Roscam Abbing, 1989; Vedder and Van der Burg, 1989; Van der Burg et al., Te Braake, 1989; Van den Boom et al., 1990).

Legally, the debate centered on the question as to whether the screening proposal entailed an infringement of individual civil rights.

---

10 Screening at the person's own request and upon medical indication are two other, obviously possible situations.

H. Roscam Abbing (1989), Markenstein and Goethart (1990) and Gevers (1989ab) consider this to be the case and conclude that the proposal is inadmissable without further legislation to provide a specific foundation for such screening. Akveld and Hermans (1989), by contrast, take the view that anonymous screening may be conducted without the need for special legislation. A difference of opinion arose concerning the question as to whether a right of objection would suffice, whereby each participant would be able to indicate whether his or her body material could be used for screening or whether the procedures should be based on a requirement of consent in the strict sense, whereby each participant is explicitly asked to provide consent.

In February 1990 State Secretary Simons decided not to concur with such screening, because he considered it would make only a limited contribution to prevention and care and was not of overriding importance in terms of public health. At the same time, the State Secretary emphasized that he attached major importance to epidemiological studies. In line with a recommendation issued by the Health Council the State Secretary supports selective epidemiological screening on a voluntary basis among "frontline group and situations", such as outpatient clinics for STDs (TK, 1990a; GR, 1990a). In relation to the statutory framework, the divergent views concerning the import and interpretation of individual civil rights led the government to propose a provision for anonymous scientific research in the WGBO. Under this provision, anonymous medical research is permitted on substances previously separated from the body in so far as the persons from whom those substances derived had no objection (TK, 1990c).

4.7.4 Screening in connection with financial interests

A second fundamental debate that attracted widespread interest arose when it became known that HIV-testing was being conducted in connection with medical examinations for appointments, life insurance or supplementary employment disability insurance. Employers and insurers have financial interests that conflict with the individual interests of the applicant. Legally, such testing is of a highly coercive nature, in that the person being tested is under an obligation of compliance or acceptance and, in the case of insurance, an obligation to inform the insurers so that the latter can determine the insurance risk. This debate too has not been conducted in isolation but has been examined in relation to such divergent topics as medical selection for access to welfare facilities, the dividing line between basic provision accessible to all and "luxury" facilities that are not vital for the functioning of society, the use of medical data outside health care and protecting the applicant's legal position. The central question in this respect for the government is whether self-regulation will suffice or whether statutory provisions are required[11] (Bergkamp and Van Wersch, 1989; Markenstein and Goethart, 1989; Te Braake, 1988; Gevers, 1988; NCAB, 1990bc).

4.7.5 *Employment medicals*

With respect to AIDS and employment medicals the Government takes the view that an HIV test should not form an integral element because it is unclear what implications seropositivity has for the ability to perform a job, HIV is not transmissable in normal work circumstances and there is presumably a low seroprevalence among the general population. The following guidelines have been laid down: (1) the determination of long-term risks may not form part of an employment medical, (2) an HIV test is rejected as part of an employment medical, and (3) an employment medical shall also qualify the applicant for inclusion in the pension fund (TK, 1990b).

Willems (1989) notes in a reconstruction of the debate surrounding employment medicals that there are major differences in medical examination practice and the position of the examining doctor and concludes that the rights and obligations of examinees are not commensurate with the financial interests of employers. Lourijsen et al. (1989) conclude that in 1987 the administration of employment medicals did not correspond with the ideas on the subject of the government, the Association for Health Law and the Joint Industrial Labour Council. With respect to HIV-testing it turned out that 2% (N = 102) of the general practitioners surveyed routinely tested for HIV in an employment medical and 23% occasionally. Of the 149 company doctors surveyed 5% occasionally tested for HIV.

At present the government takes the view of waiting to see whether self-regulation will suffice with respect to the problem of employment medicals.

4.7.6 *Insurance medicals*

In the Netherlands the debate about the insurance issue has focused on the use of HIV-testing for life insurance and supplementary employment disability insurance. Insurers take the view that HIV and AIDS cannot be insured against since the short life expectancy would

---

11 There are no general statutory provisions concerning the legal protection of job applicants or applicants for insurance.

necessitate a prohibitively high premium. In addition insurers are making allowance for substantial AIDS-related losses on existing insurance policies. Insurers also refer to the phenomenon of "risk selection", under which insurers who fail to screen out certain risks tend to attract high-risk applicants in that very category, with adverse consequences for the insurer's financial position (De Raadt, 1988).

Following consultations between the Netherlands Association of Life Insurers and the Royal Dutch Medical Association (KNMG) it was agreed in 1988 that applications in excess of NLG 200,000 should in general be subject to a compulsory HIV test. In a memorandum in the same year the Minister of Justice laid down that such tests should be conducted in accordance with the conditions of medical research. The testing is for example subject to medical professional secrecy, the registration of medical data is subject to the Data Protection Act and discrimination is prohibited. He further took the view that testing did not necessarily involve an unacceptable invasion of the examinee's private life, unlike questions concerning and research into matters of no relevance for the insurance, such as sexual identity. With respect to the social consequences of an HIV test the Minister observed that life insurance is be regarded as a "luxury", i.e. not something that is vital to the functioning in society (TK, 1987b).

The memorandum aroused fierce debate concerning both the NLG 200,000 guideline and the designation of life insurance as a luxury provision. In practice it was evident that HIV tests were also being conducted on medical indication for cover of less than NLG 200,000. Opinion differed on the ability to reach an objective medical indication. The National Commission for AIDS Control (NCAB) and experts in the field of health law referred to an unacceptable balance between the pros and cons for the insurance applicant (NCAB, 1990c; Willems, 1989; Bergkamp and Van Wersch, 1989).

On account of these problems, and prompted by the increasing possibilities for predictive medicine in a general sense, State Secretary Simons undertook in 1990 to strengthen the legal position of insurance applicants. In balancing the priorities the Minister wishes to take account of the importance of an effectively operating insurance industry, of the principle that social facilities should remain accessible to all, of individual civil rights and of the fact that participation in scientific research should not be indirectly deterred.

Despite these consultations between the parties concerned the insurance issue has not yet been resolved. The NCAB (1990b), KNMG (1991) and the Health Council (1991) regard HIV-testing as acceptable only in excess of a certain insured sum. Below that limit they do not regard an HIV test as legitimate. In this respect they are not thinking of a set limit, such as NLG 200,000, but of a variable sum, corresponding with the "real needs limit" of the examinee, depending on social circumstances. The NCAB (1990c) regards this issue as one of the major problems that will have to be resolved in order to counter the negative social impact of an HIV infection.

4.7.7 *Early intervention and clinical trials for therapies*

The case for HIV-testing could be viewed in a totally different light if an effective treatment for HIV infection were to be discovered. First steps in this direction are already evident as regards early intervention, with individuals in the pre-AIDS stage being administered therapies in order to counter or postpone the symptoms due to AIDS.

Medically speaking there are still numerous ambiguities and uncertainties surrounding early intervention, but in view of the rapid developments in biomedical research early intervention is expected to be a real option in the near future. Apart from an increase in the demand for and burden of care this can lead to an increase in the number of requests for tests. In the case of effective drugs that also extend life expectancy and/or drugs that enhance the quality of life, the NCAB (1990d) points to the necessity of avoiding possible negative social consequences of testing, for example by means of legislation on the insurance issue. In addition the NCAB takes the view that early intervention requires expertise in the field of medical treatment, counselling, information activities and psychosocial programmes. For the present the NCAB and the Health Council see no reason to change the present testing policy, under which individuals take the initiative to seek testing.

Roscam Abbing (1990) and Markenstein (1990) examine the medical law aspects of drugs research, the availability of effective medication and the principles for testing policy in the event of an adequate anti-AIDS therapy. In the absence of a therapy offering a genuine prospect of cure, they see no reason to depart from the present policy on testing. But even if an adequate remedy for AIDS were to be discovered, there would be no grounds on the basis of health law to introduce compulsory testing or a policy to promote testing on grounds other than the individual interests of a potential seropositive. As far as drugs research is concerned Roscam Abbing concludes that in the case of AIDS there is no legal justification for withholding the general availability of a drug shown to be efficacious in the experimental phase until that drug has been registered. Instead she argues that such drugs should be made widely available under strict national and international rules and agreements designed to protect the rights of patients and to monitor distribution.

4.7.8 *Impact of AIDS*

Consideration has not been given at any point to legislation specially directed towards AIDS or legislation that would curtail individual civil rights on the grounds of AIDS. Where the extra protection of individual rights has been at issue, e.g. in relation to medical examinations for prospective employees or the insurance question, the main emphasis has been on self-regulation. The only statutory regulation directly related to the AIDS debate - but not confined to AIDS - is the provision in the Medical Treatment Agreement Bill concerning anonymous scientific research on body material. It is possible that the insurance issue and developments concerning the availability of drugs still in the experimental stage will give rise to the need for additional legislation.

Contrary as feared in the US, Dutch policy would appear to be exemplary rather than exceptional (Bayer, 1991). Looking to the future it is probable that the debate surrounding AIDS will have an impact on the way in which STDs are tackled, now that it appears legally clear that epidemiological screening for contact tracing and partner notification is impermissible without prior consent, and the government must be exceptionally cautious about interfering in the private life of citizens. In addition it is probable that the debate about the insurance issue will broaden out into a discussion about access to social provision for people with congenital disorders and chronic diseases.

4.8 *Prevention and information*

4.8.1 *AIDS control and classic STD control*

Extensive experience has been gained in the Netherlands with the control of infectious diseases (Huisman, 1998b, Coutinho, 1989). The framework for doing so is provided by the Infectious Diseases (Control and Detection) Act, under which infectious diseases are classified into three groups according to the threat they pose to public health:

- A. as soon as the existence of such a disease is suspected the case must be notified to the Chief Medical Inspectorate (GHI), after which measures must be taken to prevent the further spread of the disease (e.g. polio or tuberculosis);
- B. the diseases must be notified within 24 hours of diagnosis (e.g. cholera and Hepatitis B);
- C. diseases are notified only in order to determine the epidemiological course of the disease which, in contrast to category A

and B diseases, can take place anonymously. Sexually transmitted diseases such as gonorrhoea and syphilis fall into category C.

On medical, social and political grounds it has been decided against including AIDS in any of the above categories for the purposes of AIDS control. Instead there is a system of anonymous registration of people with AIDS on a voluntary basis. HIV-infected persons are not registered.

The detection and treatment of infected persons, blocking the transmission route and protecting the exposed population are strategies for combating infectious diseases. In the light of the existing treatment possibilities, the emphasis in STD control in the 1970s lay on secondary prevention, early diagnosis and treatment. In the case of AIDS control, the only available strategy consists of primary prevention by means of information and the avoidance of behaviour involving a risk of HIV infection. In developing that strategy, AIDS control thereby introduced a new approach towards the control of sexually transmitted diseases on a large scale by making greater use of methods and techniques forming part of the new discipline of Health Information and Education (Van den Boom et al., 1991a).

4.8.2 HIV/AIDS information and education

The first information campaign directed towards men who have sex with men was started at an early stage of the AIDS epidemic in the Netherlands. The immediate reason for doing so was provided by the problem of safeguarding the nation's blood supply, which gave rise to the "blood debate" of 1983 in which, at the initiative of Buro GVO Amsterdam, the Chief Medical Inspectorate of Health (GHI), the blood banks, the GG & GD Amsterdam and the GGD Rotterdam, the gay movement and the National Association of Haemophiliac Patients (NVHP) all participated. The proposal to reject gay men as blood donors was rejected by the gay movement as unacceptable and discriminatory. The final result of these consultations was that men who have sex with men were informed about the new disease and asked to withdraw voluntarily as blood donors. Following a period of ad hoc cooperation between the various parties concerned it was decided in 1984 to adopt a more structural approach. This resulted in the establishment of the National AIDS Coordination Team (LCA) which, in 1987, was replaced in line with the Policy Document on AIDS Policy by the National Commission for AIDS Control (NCAB). Within the NCAB the various interest groups played a less prominent part and the national character of the AIDS problem was given greater emphasis (Coppoolse, 1988).

4.8.3 *Information and education activities*

At the start of the epidemic the prevention activities were primarily directed towards men who have sex with men and later also to IDUs. The actual implementation of these activities was largely left to organizations concerned with these target groups, such as the Ancillary Services Department (SAD), the NIVH-COC, the Schorer Foundation and the Federation of Junkie Unions. Apart from providing information for their own target group these organizations also came up with initiatives aimed at a broader public, such as the production by the SAD of the HIV/AIDS manual for general practitioners.

Since 1987 the WVC, NCAB and STD Foundation have organized multi-media prevention and information activities aimed at the general public, such as the " Flower with Bee" campaign (1987), "AIDS and Work" (1988), "Safe Sex on Holiday" (1988) and the "Excuses Campaign" (1989-1990). These poster campaigns were supported by leaflets, TV and cinema spots, advertisements in daily newspapers and weekly magazines, education programmes in schools and condom-distribution campaigns.

The information was designed in the first place to promote knowledge of HIV/AIDS and transmission routes, thereby encouraging a change in behaviour.

Figure 4.1 sets out a policy model developed by the Buro GVO Amsterdam, showing the various phases of the preventive strategy devised for each risk group during the period 1983-1988.

AIDS information and education is at present undergoing a number of shifts in emphasis. Group-specific information is becoming increasingly small-scale and outreach in nature and is concentrating to a greater extent on hard-to-reach and/or potentially high-risk behaviour such as marginalized youth, foreign commercial sex workers and specific groups of gay men. The campaigns for the general public are more concerned than previously with maintaining the level of knowledge about AIDS and the transmission of HIV and the preservation of public support as well as public involvement in the AIDS issue. Examples include the 1990 and 1991 campaigns aimed at promoting understanding of people with AIDS and the campaign "Are we taking AIDS seriously enough?".

4.8.4 *Need and importance of prevention*

Looking to the future there can be no doubt about the need and importance of primary prevention in order to avoid the transmission of HIV: information and the promotion of safer behaviour remain the only instruments for countering HIV infection. This means that the knowledge of AIDS and the changes in behaviour so far brought about need to be preserved and that measures to this end need to be taken for groups among whom this has been achieved only partially, if at all. There is a particular need for information to be provided to young people who are on the point of becoming sexually active. A number of questions and uncertainties surround the content and organization of HIV/AIDS prevention. In substantive terms, data from research into the determinants of risk behaviour and sexual life-styles will need to be incorporated into the information and education and efforts will need to be made to devise more systematic prevention programmes (Kok and Widdershoven, 1989; Kok and Sandfort, 1990). Greater attention is also being devoted to a long-term perspective for HIV/AIDS prevention. This might include an examination of the most effective strategies for consolidating changes in behaviour and analysis as to which prevention strategy, using which medium and on what scale, is the most effective for specific target groups (Coyle et al., 1991). The relationship between AIDS control and STD control may also come in for consideration, with attention to the desirability of integrating the two. As a logical extension this might include examination of the way in which a joint STD/AIDS control strategy might be organized and how STD control might benefit from the experience and expertise gained with primary prevention in the field of AIDS control. We shall be returning to these points in Chapter 9.

4.9 *Impact on the care system*

Special attention has been devoted to AIDS care since the start of the epidemic. AIDS differed from other diseases in that it was unclear what scale the epidemic would assume, what manifestations of the disease would occur, what treatment facilities would be required, how much of a burden would be imposed on the health system and what the associated costs would be. Problems were also foreseen in the treatment and care of AIDS patients on account of the emotional stresses of providing terminal care for young people, the fear that the virus might be transmitted, and possible negative consequences resulting from prejudice towards homosexuality, drug use and prostitution.

AIDS led to a large number of new initiatives in the field of care. Examples include programmes to improve the expertise of care providers, the introduction of new treatment facilities, the appointment of AIDS specialists, consultants and nursing staff, the setting up of AIDS wards in various hospitals and, more recently, the establishment of the National AIDS Therapy and Evaluation Centre (NATEC). Chapter 5 dealing with the baseline economic analysis examines the demands made by people with HIV and AIDS on care facilities. A number of initiatives in the field of care and support for people with AIDS and HIV are examined below.

4.9.1 Regional hospital centres

Given the lack of experience in treating AIDS patients the Health Council (1987) recommended that to begin with there should be a system of regional centralization of care in a limited number of well equipped hospitals providing high quality research, care and treatment. These hospitals would also be charged with passing on the know-how they had built up to others, so that effective care for HIV-infected persons could in due course also be provided elsewhere.

In 1990 this led to the provisional designation of 11 hospitals as regional centres. The criteria for such designation included experience with care for HIV-infected persons, the availability of good quality treatment facilities and a willingness to cooperate in research[12].

For the present, inpatient care for AIDS patients and HIV-infected persons is largely confined to the Regional Hospital Centres. The complexity of the disease and the pace of change in medical technology make it difficult to transfer knowledge to caregivers who do not have extensive contact with this patient group in daily practice (Weigel, 1991; personal communication). In addition the care of HIV-infected persons and AIDS patients is often highly labour-intensive in terms of medical treatment, nursing care and psychosocial support.

4.9.2 Psychosocial care and support

The limited ability to treat AIDS, and the fatal course of the disease, mean that allowance needs to be made at the outset of the epidemic for the fact that there will be a substantial requirement for care to

---

[12] The following hospitals were provisionally designated as regional centres: the teaching hospitals of Groningen, Nijmegen, Utrecht, Leiden, Rotterdam and Maastricht, Medical Spectrum Twente, Leyenburg Hospital The Hague, St. Elisabeth Hospital in Tilburg, Onze Lieve Vrouwe Gasthuis and Slotervaart Hospital in Amsterdam. The Academic Medical Centre serves a national reference function. Three other hospitals (Free University, Prinsengracht and Lucas Hospital) have been designated for the Amsterdam region. These do not act as regional centres but do form part of a structural cooperative arrangement between the Amsterdam Hospitals.

cope with the psychological and psychosocial problems associated with the disease. Examples include the psychiatric and psychosocial problems faced by the HIV-infected person, relatives and friends; the problems associated with the HIV-antibody test; coming to terms with a positive test result; the unpredictability of the course taken by the disease; and mourning (Bakker and Schrameijer, 1987; Mulder, 1990; Sno et al., 1990; Lunter et al., 1991; Van den Boom, 1991; Van den Boom et al., 1991b). This has been reflected in AIDS care policy by the explicit attention devoted to psychosocial care, as elaborated in the Framework Plan for Psychosocial Care for AIDS Patients (NCAB, 1988), which sets out differing strategies in terms of functions, care providers and outreach organizations.

Among other things the plan devotes special attention to the importance attached to pre- and post-test counselling. In this respect Roscam Abbing (1990), the Health Council (1990b) and the NCAB (1990d) point to the importance of good patient information when testing is requested for the purposes of early intervention. Since there is still major uncertainty about the effects of treatment, the point at which treatment can commence and the long-term side-effects, the patient must be given the opportunity of weighing up all the pros and cons in close consultation with the physician.

4.9.3 The influence of patients and patients' associations

People with AIDS are by and large well informed and articulate patients who have launched a large number of initiatives through their patients' associations. Apart from the HIV Association there is in the Netherlands also a division of ACT-UP, an international association of AIDS activists.

In itself it is a familiar enough phenomenon for patients in the terminal stage of an illness to grasp at any straw to lengthen or preserve life. In the case of AIDS, however, there has been a notably large number of initiatives organized by people with AIDS themselves and their representative associations and they have also had a marked impact on the content and organization of care. Defert (1989) even typifies the person with AIDS "as a new social reformer". Van den Boom et al. (1991a) refer in the Dutch context to the contribution they have made towards the extensive provision of information on therapies and the marked attention to patients rights as results that cannot be divorced from the efforts and actions of people with AIDS. The establishment of care facilities within the regular health care system, in which alternative and not always fully tested therapies are offered, is indissolubly bound up with the activities of the "Fight for Life" association.

Van den Boom et al. also note that AIDS activists have had a striking impact on clinical trials[13]. Among other things people with AIDS objected that it was taking too long for new drugs to be tested in trials and that alternative drugs such as Compound Q and KEMRON were not being included in trials. Other objections were that the research into new drugs was taking too long, that it was taking too long for results to be published and that the registration of drugs was far too slow a process. It became clear that good medical practice and patients' interests in having access to the most effective medication were at variance with one another. In practice this placed clinical trials under considerable pressure, leading among other things to the premature termination of studies since patients in the control group began taking the active drug or dropped out of the trial (Volberding et al., 1990). Roscam Abbing (1990) maintains that in this respect there are by definition conflicting interests of scientific research, industry, insurance, government and patients. She concludes that in the case of AIDS, considerations of fairness and equal accessibility to treatment militate in favour of the widespread availability outside trials and before registration of drugs that have been shown to have any degree of efficacy. Strict conditions would, however, need to be laid down for the monitoring and evaluation of availability. Among other things these conditions would relate to early registration, dosage, indication and the findings from follow-up research.

The campaign surrounding and interest in clinical trials to do with AIDS have resulted in shortened procedures, broader criteria for participation, the acceleration of trials by conducting various stages simultaneously, the speedier publication of results and faster registration. Merigan (1990) is convinced that these changes will not remain confined to AIDS but will in due course come to serve as new standard procedures for clinical trials.

4.10 Summary

This chapter has examined social developments in the field of sexuality, gay emancipation, hard-drug use and commercial sex work and the changes in these areas due to AIDS. The public reaction to AIDS has also been examined.

In the field of sexuality the consequences of sexual liberalization

---

[13] Scientific research into the effectiveness of new drugs often takes years. New drugs are only tried on people after extensive laboratory research and trials with animals. This final, human-testing part of the research consists of three stages: stage 1 - safety; stage 2 - effectiveness; stage 3 - dosage and comparison with other drugs. A drug can only be registered and made available to large groups of patients if the trials indicate that it is safe, effective and has no side-effects.

and constants and trends in attitudes towards sexuality and sexual behaviour have been examined. The advent of AIDS is described against the background of and in interaction with this sociosexological context. Relevant areas of concern from sexological research for projections of the spread of HIV among the heterosexual population are also examined. The social consequences of AIDS for gay men are described against the background of gay emancipation, tolerance towards and discrimination against gay men and the initiatives and impact of organizations of gay men in prevention and the care of people with AIDS. The AIDS and drugs problem is set in the context of the rise of hard-drug addiction, Dutch policy on drug dependence, the life-styles of hard-drug users and the coordination of AIDS and drugs policies. With respect to AIDS and commercial sex work, developments are noted in the sex industry and in prostitution policy.

The "Dutch reaction" to AIDS is outlined in terms of the debate concerning the application of HIV-testing and the decisive role that respect for individual civil rights has played in that context. The formulation of the testing policy and the discussions concerning large-scale seroprevalence screening and HIV-testing for employment medicals and applications for life insurance are reconstructed against the background of the Dutch legal framework. These discussions are used to outline the legal framework for long-range studies. In the field of HIV/AIDS prevention special attention has been devoted to the structure, organization and implementation of the prevention policy, with special emphasis on a staged, systematic and targeted approach. The description of the care provided for people with AIDS examines initiatives in somatic and psychosocial care and attention is devoted to changes brought about in AIDS care and especially clinical trials by initiatives on the part of people with AIDS and patient associations.

References

Akveld, J.E.M., H.E.G.M. Hermans
Rapport Anonieme screening op HIV infecties; juridische aspecten
EUR, Rotterdam, 1989

Atteveld, J.M.A. van
Het Nederlandse drugsbeleid in vergelijking met andere Westeuropese landen: liberaal?
Tijdschrift voor Alcohol, Drugs en andere Psychotrope stoffen, 14 (1988), 1, 3-11

Bakker, M., F. Schrameijer
Aids: psychosociale problemen en daarop gerichte hulpverlening; een literatuurstudie
NcGv, Utrecht, 1987, NcGv-reeks 109

Bayer, R.
Public Health Policy and the AIDS epidemic; an end to HIV exceptionalism?
New England Journal of Medicine, 324 (1991), 21, 1500-1504

Belderbos, F., J. Visser (red.)
Beroep: Prostituée
Stichting Welzijns Publicaties, Utrecht, 1987

Berg, A.H. van den, M. Blom (m.m.v. S. Altink)
Heroïneprostitutie
SUA/Mr. de Graafstichting, Amsterdam, 1987

Bergkamp, P., P.J.M. van Wersch
Het testen op AIDS bij het afsluiten van verzekeringen
In: H.D.C. Roscam Abbing, F.C.B. van Wijmen (red.), *Wetgeving gezondheidszorg in perspectief*, Kluwer, Deventer, 1989, serie gezondheidsrecht 22, 97-108

Bieleman, B., J.J. Bosma, K. Swierstra
Cocaïne: van mythe tot probleem
Tijdschrift voor Alcohol, Drugs en andere Psychotrope stoffen, 16 (1990), 1, 11-16

Bijkerk, H.
Epidemiologie
In: E. Stolz, D. Suurmond (red.), *Seksueel overdraagbare aandoeningen*, Stafleu, Alphen aan de Rijn, 1982

Bisset, C., G. Jones, J. Davidson, B. Cummins, S. Burns, J.M. Inglis, R.P. Brettle

Mobility of injection drug users and Transmission of HIV
Lancet, juli 1, 1989, 44

Blom, M., O. Janssen
Molukse heroïnegebruikers in Nederland; een typologie van levensstijlen van Molukse heroïnegebruikers
Groningen, Criminologisch Instituut, 1987

Bolt, A.
Jeugd en seksualiteit in Nederland; een vergelijking tussen enquètemateriaal uit 1968 en 1981
Tijdschrift voor Seksuologie, 13 (1989), 266-275

Boom, F.M.L.G van den, J.C. Jager, L.H. Lumey, E.J. Ruitenberg
Het wetenschappelijk AIDS-onderzoek: Randvoorwaarden van de programmering
In: I. Ravenschlag, M. de Wachter, H. Zwart (red.), *Aids: instellingen, individu en samenleving*, Ambo, Baarn, 1990, 155-179

Boom, F. van den
AIDS in de familie; een persoonlijke reflectie
Maandblad Geestelijke volksgezondheid, 46 (1991), 1, 3-17

Boom, F. van den, P. Schnabel, D. Reinking
AIDS als bedreiging en uitdaging voor de homobeweging
Tijdschrift voor Gezondheid en Politiek, 1991a, september, 2-5

Boom, F. van den, T. Gremmen, H. Roozenburg
AIDS: leven rond de dood; nabestaanden over ziekte, dood en rouw
NcGv, Utrecht, 1991b, NcGv-reeks 91-16

Boutellier, J.C.J.
Enkele cijfers over prostitutie
Justitiële Verkenningen, 13 (1987), 1, 36-44

Braake, Th.A.M. te
Grenzen aan risicoselectie; over de rol van de HIV-test bij verzekerings- en aanstellingskeuringen
Tijdschrift voor Gezondheidsrecht, 1988, 402-412

Braake, Th.A.M. te
Het gebruik van medische mogelijkheden voor andere doeleinden
In: H.D.C. Roscam Abbing, F.C.B. van Wijmen (red.), *Wetgeving gezondheidszorg in perspectief*, Kluwer, Deventer, 1989, serie gezondheidsrecht 22, 97-108

Brandt, A.M.
No Magic Bullet; A Social History of Venereal Diseases in the United States

since 1880
Oxford University Press, New York/Oxford, 1987

Buning, E.
De GG & GD en het drugprobleem in cijfers deel IV
GG & GD Amsterdam, Amsterdam, 1990

Burg, W. van der, A.H. Vedder, A.K. Huibers
Anoniem bevolkingsonderzoek naar de verspreiding van HIV-infectie; ethische overwegingen
Medisch Contact, 44 (1989), 1, 7-9

Cobelens, F.G.J., P.C. Schrader, Th.A. Sluijs
Acute dood na druggebruik in Amsterdam
GG & GD Amsterdam, Amsterdam, 1990

Cohen, P.
Drugs as a social construct
Elinkwijk, Utrecht, 1990, dissertation

Coppoolse, P.A.
AIDS, preventie en besluitvorming
Vereniging Humanitas afdeling Rotterdam, Rotterdam, 1988, publikatie nr. 4

Coutinho, R.A.
Van pokken, syfilis en AIDS; geschiedenis van de infectieziektenbestrijding door de eeuwen heen
Drukkerij Bij, Amsterdam, 1989, inaugurele rede

Coyle, S.L., R.F. Boruch, C.F. Turner (eds.)
Evaluating AIDS prevention programs; expanded edition
National Academy Press, Washington DC, 1991

Curran, J.
A Global Survey of AIDS Legislation
Presentatie *V International Conference on AIDS*, Montreal, 1989

Defert, D.
A new social reformer. The patient
In: D. Ostrow (ed.), *Behavioral aspects of AIDS*, Plenum Publishing Corporation, 1989, 1-6

Dercksen, A., E. van der Veen
Centrum Anti-Discriminatie Homoseksualiteit: Meldingen van meldpunten 1989
Utrecht, Interfacultaire werkgroep Homostudies / CAdH, 1990

Dirksen, A.G., H.P. Griffioen, R.M. Lapré, A. Meijerman, H.J. Troelstra
Evaluatie-onderzoek Nationale Commissie Aids Bestrijding
KPMG, Utrecht, 1991

Dobbeling, M., P. Koenders
Het topje van de ijsberg; inventarisatie van tien jaar discriminatie op grond van homoseksualiteit en leefvorm
RUU, Homostudies, 1984, publicatiereeks Homostudies 3

Driessen, F.M.H.M.
Methadonverstrekking in Nederland
Bureau Driessen, Sociaal Wetenschappelijk Onderzoek en Advies, Rijswijk/Utrecht, 1990

Driessen, A., L. van de Velden, F. van den Boom, J. Derks
Steun van De Regenboog; vrijwillige hulpverlening aan verslaafden met AIDS
NcGv, Utrecht, 1991, NcGv-reeks 91-12

Es, J.C. van, C.W. Kramers, G.W. de Weert van Oene, R.F. Schreuder, R.A. te Velde (red.)
Leefomstandigheden Leefwijzen en Gezondheid; een aanzet voor scenario's
STG, Rijswijk, 1990

Frenken, J.
Seksuele liberalisering en post-liberale seksualiteit
In: E. Ketting, J. de Jong Gierveld, I. Weeda, J. Frenken, P. Schnabel, *Samen-leven in onzekerheid; de invloed van enkele sociale ontwikkelingen op intieme relaties*, NISSO, Zeist, 1984a, 43-67

Frenken, J.
Strafbare seksualiteit; opvattingen en aanpak van politie, justitie en hulpverlening
Van Loghum Slaterus, Deventer, 1984b

Frenken, J.
Seksuele moeilijkheden in Nederland; een overzicht
Maandblad Geestelijke volksgezondheid, 42 (1987), 1, 3-18

Gagnon, J.H.
Sexuality across the Life Course in the United States
In: C.F. Turner, H.G. Miller, L.E. Moses (eds.), *AIDS; sexual behavior and intravenous drug use*, National Academy Press, Washington D.C., 1989, 500-537

Gelder, P.J. van, J.H. Sijtsma
Horse, coke en kansen: sociale risico's en kansen onder Surinaamse en Marokkaanse harddruggebruikers in Amsterdam: I Surinaamse harddruggebruikers

UvA, Instituut voor Sociale Geografie, 1988a

Gelder, P.J. van, J.H. Sijtsma
Horse, coke en kansen: sociale risico's en kansen onder Surinaamse en Marokkaanse harddruggebruikers in Amsterdam: II Marokkaanse harddruggebruikers
UvA, Instituut voor Sociale Geografie, 1988b

Gemert, F. van
Mazen en netwerken; de invloed van beleid op de drugshandel in twee straten in de Amsterdamse binnenstad
UvA, Instituut voor Sociale Geografie, 1988

Gevers, J.K.M.
Medische keuringen
Nederlands Tijdschrift voor Geneeskunde, 132 (1988), 22, 1018-1021

Gevers, J.K.M.
Het gebruik van afgenomen lichaamsmateriaal in epidemiologisch onderzoek
Nederlands Tijdschrift voor Geneeskunde, 133 (1989a), 4, 173-175

Gevers, J.K.M.
AIDS en mensenrechten: Het onderzoek op HIV-infectie
NJCM, 14 (1989b), 2, 133-143

Griensven, G.J.P. van
Epidemiology and prevention of HIV infection among homosexual men
GG & GD Amsterdam / UvA, 1989, dissertation

Groenendijk, H.
Twintig jaar homosexualiteit in het MGv; 1966-1986
Maandblad Geestelijke volksgezondheid, 42 (1987), 9, 923-949

Haan, H.A. de, J.A.R. van den Hoek, H.J.A. van Haastrecht, C.W. van der Meer, R.A. Coutinho
Relatieve lage HIV-prevalentie onder druggebruikers in Den Haag ondanks riskant spuitgedrag
Nederlands Tijdschrift voor Geneeskunde, 135 (1991), 6, 218-221

Haverkamp, G.
Carrière- en scènevorming onder autochtone heroïnegebruikers
Tijdschrift voor Criminologie, 1984, 2, 136-148

Health Council (GR)
AIDS-problematiek in Nederland; richtlijnen voor groepsonderzoek en adviezen voor preventie
GR, The Hague, 1986, no. 1986/22

Health Council (GR)
De zorg voor patiënten met AIDS en andere ziekteverschijnselen als gevolg van infectie met het humaan-immunodeficiëntievirus
GR, The Hague, 1987, no. 26

Health Council (GR)
Onderzoek naar de verspreiding van HIV-infectie in Nederland
GR, The Hague, 1989, no. 1989/08

Health Council (GR)
Verspreiding van het AIDS-virus in Nederland: methoden van onderzoek
GR, The Hague, 1990a

Health Council (GR)
Vroegtijdige medische interventie bij met HIV geïnfecteerde personen
GR, The Hague, 1990b

Health Council (GR)
De HIV-test en levensverzekeringen; advies uitgebracht door de Beraadsgroep Gezondheidsethiek en Gezondheidsrecht van de Gezondheidsraad
GR, The Hague, 1991, nr. 1991/04

Hoek, J.A.R. van den, R.A. Coutinho, H.J.A. van Haastrecht, A.W. van Zadelhoff, J. Goudsmit
Prevalence and risk factors of HIV infection among drug users and drug-using prostitutes in Amsterdam
In: A. van den Hoek, *Epidemiology of HIV Infection among drug users in Amsterdam*, Rodopi, Amsterdam, 1990, dissertation, 29-34

Hoek, J.A.R. van den
personal communication, 1991

Hoogma, M.
Een politieke tragikomedie
Intermediair, 26 (1990), 27, 15, 17, 19

Huisman, J.
Anoniem serologisch bevolkingsonderzoek op het vóórkomen van HIV-infektie: een noodzaak!
Tijdschrift voor Sociale Gezondheidszorg, 66 (1988a), 301-302

Huisman, J.
De strijd tegen besmettelijke ziekten: nog steeds een uitdaging
Erasmus Universiteit, Rotterdam, 1988b, inaugurele rede

Hulsman, L.H.C.
Het Nederlandse heroïnebeleid in internationaal perspectief
Tijdschrift voor Criminologie, 1984, 2, 76-97

Jacobs, C., R. Bijl
GGZ in getallen 1991
NcGv, Utrecht, 1991, NcGv 91-14

Janssen, O., K. Swierstra (m.m.v. P. Barneveld)
Heroïnegebruikers in Nederland; een typologie van levensstijlen
RUG, Kriminologisch Instituut, 1982

Johnson, A.M., J. Wadsworth, P. Elliot, L. Prior, P. Wallace, S. Blower, N.L. Webb, G.I. Heald, D.L. Miller, M.W. Adler, R.M. Anderson
A pilot study of sexual lifestyles in a random sample of the population of Great Britain
AIDS, 1989, 3, 135-141

Ketting, E., Ph. van Praag
Abortus Provocatus Wet en Praktijk; een internationaal vergelijkende analyse van de abortuspraktijk zoals die na wetswijziging in tien westerse landen is ontstaan
NISSO, Zeist, 1983

Kok, G.J., G.A.M van Widdershoven
De noodzaak van een betere AIDS-voorlichting
Tijdschrift voor Seksuologie, 13 (1989), 30-42

Kok, G.J., Th. Sandfort
AIDS preventie, voorlichting en gedragsverandering
1990, in druk

Koninklijke Nederlandsche Maatschappij tot bevordering der Geneeskunst (KNMG),
commissie Medische Ethiek
Risicokeuringen in Medisch Perspectief
KNMG, Utrecht, 1991

Kooy, G.A.
Seksualiteit, huwelijk en gezin in Nederland; ontwikkelingen en vooruitzichten
Van Loghum Slaterus, Deventer, 1975

Kooy, G.A. (sam.)
Sex in Nederland; het meest recente onderzoek naar mening en houding van de Nederlandse bevolking
Utrecht/Antwerpen, Spectrum paperback, 1983

Korf, D.J.
Heroïnetoerisme II; resultaten van een veldonderzoek onder 382 buitenlandse dagelijkse opiaatgebruikers in Amsterdam
UvA, Instituut voor Sociale Geografie, 1987

Laeyendecker, L.
Waardenverandering: de cultuur als probleem
In: L. Halma, F. Heunks (red.): *De toekomst van de traditie; vier visies op een onderzoek naar waarden en normen*, Tilburg, University Press, 1988, 6-30

Leenen, H.J.J.
Handboek Gezondheidsrecht
Samsom, Alphen a/d Rijn, 1988

Lourijsen, E.C.M.P., H. Hoolboom, W.L.A.M. de Kort
De medische aanstellingskeuring; een inventarisatie van de mate waarin en de wijze waarop Nederlandse bedrijven en artsen medischeaanstellingskeuringen (laten) verrichten
Directoraat Generaal van de Arbeid, NIPG/TNO, 1989, S 53-1

Lumey, H.L., H. Houweling, J.C. Jager
Noodzaak en mogelijkheden van prevalentie onderzoek naar HIV-infectie in Nederland
Nederlands Tijdschrift voor Geneeskunde, 133 (1989), 923-927

Lunter, C.H., H.N. Sno, F.M.L.G. van den Boom
HIV patiënten op een polikliniek psychiatrie
Nederlands Tijdschrift voor Geneeskunde, 1991, geaccepteerd

Markenstein, L.F., R. Goethart
Gezondheidsrechtelijke aspecten van AIDS; testen op HIV antistoffen
Rijksuniversiteit Limburg, Gezondheidsrecht, 1989

Markenstein, L.F.
Gezondheidsrechtelijke aspecten van aids; implicaties van toenemende interventiemogelijkheden bij HIV-infectie voor het (beleid inzake) testen op HIV-antistoffen
Rijksuniversiteit Limburg, Gezondheidsrecht, 1990, nr. 11-d

Merigan, T.C.
You can teach an old dog new tricks; How AIDS trials are pioneering new strategies
New England Journal of Medicine, 323 (1990), 19, 1341-1343

Middendorp, C.P.
Culturele veranderingen in Nederland, 1965 - 1970
Intermediair, 10 (1974), 11, 1,3,5,7,9

Middendorp, C.P.
Verdere culturele veranderingen in Nederland?: De periode 1970 - 1974
Intermediair, 11 (1975), 19, 1,3,5,15

Ministry of Culture, Recreation and Social Work (CRM)
Advies voor de wettelijke bestrijding van discriminatie wegens homofilie
CRM, Rijswijk, 1981

Mooij, A.
De ziektes van de revolutie; geslachtsziekten in Nederland vanaf de jaren zestig
In: G. Hekma, B. van Stolk, B. van Heerikhuizen, B. Kruithof (sam.), *Het verlies van de onschuld; seksualiteit in Nederland*, Amsterdams Sociologische Tijdschrift / Wolters Noordhof Groningen, 1990, 121-150

Mulder, C.L.
De invloed van psychosociale variabelen op het beloop van HIV-infectie: een overzicht
Gedrag en Gezondheid, 18 (1990), 4/5, 157-166

Werkgroep AIDS en Prostitutie van de Nationale commissie AIDS-bestrijding
Notitie 'AIDS en Prostitutie'
NCAB, Amsterdam, 1988

Nationale Commissie AIDS-bestrijding (NCAB)
- *Raamplan AIDS en de psychosociale zorg*
  NCAB, Amsterdam, 1988
- *Advies over grootschalig HIV-seroprevalentie onderzoek op anonieme basis*
  NCAB, Amsterdam, 1989
- *Het AIDS- en drugbeleid in Nederland: de stand van zaken*
  NCAB, Amsterdam, 1990a
- *AIDS en particuliere verzekeringen*
  NCAB, Amsterdam, 1990b
- *Buiten spel; over toegankelijkheidsproblematiek bij (kans op) HIV-infectie en AIDS*
  NCAB, Amsterdam, 1990c
- *Vroegtijdige interventie bij personen met een HIV-infectie; maatschappelijke gevolgen, en gevolgen voor het voorlichtings-, zorg- en testbeleid*
  NCAB, Amsterdam, 1990d
- *Interne evaluatie 1987-1991*
  NCAB, Amsterdam, 1991

NCAB/SOA-stichting
AIDS en prostitutie 1990
NCAB/SOA-stichting, Amsterdam/Utrecht, 1990

Nederlands centrum Geestelijke volksgezondheid (NcGv)
Gids Geestelijke gezondheidszorg 1990-1991
Bohn Stafleu Van Loghum bv, Houten, 1990

Nederlands Instituut voor Alcohol en Drugs (NIAD)
Spuitomruiladressen in Nederland
NIAD, Utrecht, 1990

Nederlandse Vereniging Consultatiebureaus Alcohol en Drugs (NVC)
LADIS 1988, jaarstatistieken uit het landelijke alcohol en drugs informatiesysteem
NVC, Utrecht, 1990

NZR, sectie GGZ i.s.m. Stichting Informatiecentrum voor de Gezondheidszorg (SIG)
- *Patiëntenregister intramurale geestelijke gezondheidszorg (PIGG), landelijke tabellen psychiatrie, Algemeen Psychiatrische Ziekenhuizen, 1988*
  NZR / SIG, Utrecht, 1990a
- *Patiëntenregister intramurale geestelijke gezondheidszorg (PIGG), landelijke tabellen psychiatrie, Klinieken voor Verslavingsziekten 1988*
  NZR / SIG, Utrecht, 1990b

Paalman, M.
AIDS: welke lessen kunnen uit de SOA-bestrijding getrokken worden?
SOA-bulletin, 7 (1986), 1, 4-6

Piot, P., M. Laga
Prostitutes: a high risk group for HIV-infection
Sozial- und Präventivmedizin, 33 (1988), 336-339

Programma coördinatie commissie AIDS-onderzoek (PccAo)
Inventarisatie AIDS onderzoek in Nederland
PccAo, The Hague, 1990

Raad voor Gezondheidsonderzoek (RGO)
Advies stimulering AIDS-onderzoek
RGO, The Hague, 1987

Raad voor Gezondheidsonderzoek (RGO), Programma coördinatie commissie AIDS-onderzoek (PccAo)
- *Programma AIDS-onderzoek 1988- 1990*
  RGO, The Hague, 1989
- *Programma AIDS-onderzoek 1991- 1992*
  RGO, The Hague, in preparation

Raadt H.K. de
AIDS en verzekerbaarheid
Rede tijdens symposium *'AIDS een nieuwe verantwoordelijkheid voor*

gezondheidszorg en onderwijs', studiedag georganiseerd door stichting Leffelaar, 11-10-1988, Amsterdam

Rijk, K. de, F. van den Boom
Psychosociale hulpverlening AIDS; vijf jaar hulpverlening door de Schorerstichting
NcGv, Utrecht, 1989, NcGv-reeks 89-6

Roscam Abbing, E.W.
Testbeleid, AIDS-bestrijding en belangenverdediging; een analysekader
Medisch Contact, 43 (1988), 16, 487-491

Roscam Abbing, H.D.C.
Medische (persoons)gegevens, lichaamsmateriaal en wetenschappelijk onderzoek
Tijdschrift voor Gezondheidsrecht, 1989, 362-369

Roscam Abbing, H.D.C.
AIDS in het gezondheidsrecht: Behandelingsperspectief
In: J.K.M. Gevers, S.M.S.M. van de Goor, J.F.L. Roording, H.D.C. Roscam Abbing, *AIDS in het recht*, Ars Aequi Libri, Nijmegen, 1990, 14[illegible]-156

Schmidt, G.
The influence of AIDS on sexuality
In: Maria Paalman (red.), *Promoting safer Sex: prevention of Sexual Transmission of AIDS and other STD*; proceedings of an International Workshop, May 1989, The Netherlands, organized by The Dutch Foundation for Sexually Transmitted Diseases (STD Foundation), Swets en Zeitlinger, Amsterdam / Lisse, 1990, 39-47

Schnabel, P.
Seksualiteit, sociologisch gezien
In: J. Frenken, *Seksuologie; een interdisciplinaire benadering*, Van Loghum Slaterus, 1980, 13-36

Schnabel, P.
De gezondheidszorg: van immuniteit tot publiek domein
In: A.M.J. Kreukels, J.B.D. Simons (red.), *Publiek domein; de veranderende balans tussen staat en samenleving*, Boom, Meppel Amsterdam, 1988, jaarboek Beleid en Maatschappij 1987/1988, 172-201

Schnabel, P.
Een veranderende kijk op seksualiteit
Tijdschrift voor Seksuologie, 13 (1989a), 208-218

Schnabel, P.
De diepten van een epidemie; over de maatschappelijke gevolgen van AIDS
In: A. Noordhoff-de Vries, *AIDS; een nieuwe verantwoordelijkheid voor*

gezondheidszorg en onderwijs, Swets en Zeitlinger, Amsterdam/Lisse, 1989b, 15-33

Schnabel, P.
Het verlies van de seksuele onschuld
In: Gert Hekma, Bram van Stolk, Bart van Heerikhuizen, Bernard Kruithof (red.), *Het verlies van de onschuld; seksualiteit in Nederland*, Amsterdams Sociologisch Tijdschrift / Wolters Noordhoff, Groningen, 1990, 11-50

Selwyn, P.A., D. Hartel, W. Wasserman, E. Drucker
Impact of the AIDS epidemic on Morbidity and Mortality among Intravenous Drug Users in a New York City Methadone Maintenance Program
American Journal of Public Health, 79 (1989), 10, 1358- 1363

Shilts, R.
And the band played on: politics, people and the AIDS epidemic
Penguin-pockets, London, 1988

Skidmore, C.A., J.R. Robertson, A.A. Robertson, R.A. Elton
After the epidemic: follow up study of HIV seroprevalence and changing pattern of drug use
British Medical Journal, 300 (1990), 219-223

Sno, H.N., J.G. Storosum, J.A. Swinkels
AIDS en Psychiatrie
Jaarboek voor Psychiatrie en Psychiatrie 1990, in druk

Sociaal en Cultureel Planbureau (SCP)
Sociaal en cultureel rapport 1988
SCP, Rijswijk, 1988

Sommerville, M.A., A.J. Orkin
Human Rights, discrimination and AIDS: concepts and issues
AIDS, 1989, 3 (suppl. 1), S283- 287

Stemvers, F.A.
Meisjes van plezier; de geschiedenis van de prostitutie
Fibula-Van Dishoeck, Weesp, 1985

Straver, C.J., A. van Stolk
De kans op verbeiding van AIDS onder de Nederlandse bevolking
Maandblad Geestelijke volksgezondheid, 43 (1988), 4, 379-394

Swierstra, K.
Drugcarrieres; van crimineel tot conventioneel
Stichting drukkerij Regenboog, Groningen, 1990, dissertation

Tielman, R.
Homoseksualiteit in Nederland
Boom, Amsterdam/Meppel, 1982, dissertation

Tillemans, G.
AIDS, beleid en organisaties; beschrijving en analyse van de beleidsvorming rondom AIDS en het ontstaan van een organisatienetwerk daarbij
KUN, politicologie en bestuurskunde, 1988, doctoraalscriptie

Turner, C.F., H.G. Miller, L.E. Moses
AIDS; Sexual Behavior and Intravenous Drug Use
National Academy Press, Washington D.C., 1989

Tweede Kamer der Staten Generaal (TK)
- Nota inzake het AIDS-beleid
  Tweede Kamer der Staten Generaal, 1987-1988, 19218, nrs. 8-9 (TK, 1987a)
- Juridische aspecten van verzekering in geval van AIDS-risico
  Tweede Kamer der Staten Generaal, 1987-1988, 19218, nr. 10 (TK, 1987b)
- Notitie over het Nederlandse beleid inzake het testen op antistoffen tegen het zogenaamde human immunodeficiency virus (HIV)
  Tweede Kamer der Staten Generaal, 1988-1989, 19218, nr. 35 (TK, 1989)
- Regeringsstandpunt inzake onderzoek naar de verspreiding van HIV-infectie in Nederland
  Tweede Kamer der Staten Generaal, 1989-1990, 19218, nr. 39 (TK, 1990a)
- Kabinetsstandpunt met betrekking tot de medische keuring bij aanstelling
  Tweede Kamer der Staten Generaal, 1989-1990, 19218, nr. 40 (TK, 1990b)
- Juridische aspecten, verbonden aan het gebruik van lichaamsmateriaal voor medisch wetenschappelijk anoniem onderzoek
  Tweede Kamer der Staten Generaal, 1989-1990, 19218, nr. 43 (TK, 1990c)

Vedder, A.H., W. van der Burg
AIDS en Ethiek; een verkenning van ethische en rechtsfilosofische vragen rond HIV-infectie en AIDS
RUU, Centrum voor Bio-Ethiek en Gezondheidsrecht, 1989

Verweij, G.C.G.
Het gebruik van de anticonceptie-pil stijgt nog steeds
Maandbericht Gezondheid, 1989, 7, 14-19

Volberding, P.A., S.W. Lagakos, M.A. Koch
Zidovidine in asymptomatic human immunodeficiency virus infection: a controlled trial in persons with fewer than 500 CD-4 positive per cubic milimeter
New England Journal of Medicine, 322 (1990), 941-949

Vogels, T., R. van der Vliet
Jeugd en seks; gedrag en gezondheidsrisico's bij scholieren
SDU, The Hague, uitgeverij Koninginnegracht, 1990

Wayling, S. (ed.)
Current status of HIV/AIDS prevention and control policies in the European region: 1990 update
WHO, Regional Office for Europe / Global Program on AIDS, Copenhagen, 1990

Weigel, H.M.
personal communication, 1991

Wigersma, L.
Huisartsgeneeskundig handelen bij klachten over de geslachtsorganen en de seksualiteit
MEDITekst, Lelystad, 1990, dissertation

Wijngaart, G.F. van de
Competing perspectives on drug use: the Dutch experience
RUU, 1990, dissertation

Willems, W.
De AIDS test bij aanstellingskeuringen en verzekeringen; een deelstudie van het project 'De strijd rond de Aidstest'
Centrum voor Onderzoek van Maatschappelijke Tegenstellingen, RUL, 1989

Zessen, G.J. van, Th. Sandfort
Het onderzoek naar seksualiteit in Nederland
In: G.J. van Zessen, Th. Sandfort (red.), *Seksualiteit in Nederland; seksueel gedrag, risico en preventie van AIDS*, Swets & Zeitlinger, Amsterdam/Lisse, 1991, 11-33

Zessen, G.J. van, C. Straver
De mogelijke verspreiding van HIV onder de Nederlandse bevolking
In: G.J. van Zessen, Th. Sandfort (red.), *Seksualiteit in Nederland; seksueel gedrag, risico en preventie van AIDS*, Swets & Zeitlinger, Amsterdam/Lisse, 1991, 205-224

Zwart, M.W. de
Alcohol, tabak en drugs in cijfers
NIAD, afdeling Onderzoek, 1989

5 Baseline analysis of the economic impact of HIV/AIDS 1982-1991

5.1 Introduction

In addition to its effects on the patient and those close to him or her, AIDS also has societal consequences, which to some extent can be expressed in economic terms. The first publications on the economic impact of AIDS, produced in the United States, report costs for the treatment and care of AIDS patients varying between $75,000 and $100,000 per person per year (Hardy et al., 1986; Pascal, 1987). More recent publications quote considerably lower cost estimates, ranging from $25,000 to $40,000 (Hay et al., 1988; Bloom and Carliner, 1988; Hellinger, 1988).

Cost estimates focus primarily on hospital costs (Andrulis 1990; Bez, 1989; Borleffs et al., 1990). In addition, mention is always made of the importance of determining indirect costs, such as lost (productive) years of life, loss of quality of life and sickness absence from work. A number of authors express the economic impact of AIDS by making comparisons with other illnesses (Over, 1989; Scitovsky and Rice 1987; Jager et al., 1990, Leidl et al., in preparation). Description of the economic impact of AIDS is important for proper planning of the level of care facilities needed. It is also important to gain an insight into the associated financial consequences (Schreuder, 1990). In an EEC context, this is taking place in the "Concerted Action on the Statistical Analysis and Mathematical Modelling of AIDS" (Jager and Ruitenberg (eds.), 1988; in preparation; RIVM/Bilthoven, 1988) and the "Study on Economic Aspects of AIDS and HIV infection" (Schwefel et al. (eds.), 1990; Drummond and Davies (eds.), 1990). Our methodology is in line with that used in these projects. The inventory of the costs of AIDS/HIV in the Netherlands is based to a large extent on a cost survey carried out for 1988 (Wiggers and Bergsma, 1990ab).

5.2 Classification

In the economics of health care, two classifications are widely used for expressing the financial/economic consequences of AIDS - direct versus indirect costs, and patient-related versus general programme costs (Johnson, 1988; Bilheimer, 1989ab; Bloom and Glied, 1989; Drummond and Davies, 1988; Rovira, 1990; Rutten, 1989; Jager and Postma, 1989).

Direct costs of the epidemic arise from the treatment of AIDS patients and HIV-infected persons, research, public information programmes and prevention. These are costs which can be related directly to sickness or infection. *Indirect* costs arise because goods cannot be produced as a result of HIV or AIDS-related premature death or illness. The illness leads to indirect costs associated with sickness absence; death can be expressed in terms of potential years of life lost (PYLL).

Patient-related costs are directly associated with the individual in the AIDS or pre-AIDS stage. They are the costs associated with treatment and care in a hospital or home care situation, but may also include indirect costs resulting from sickness absence or premature death. Non-patient-related or *general programme costs* are linked to research, prevention, public information and the maintenance of certain services for the benefit of the entire population, such as HIV-testing facilities.

The best way of combining the results of epidemiological surveys with studies into the economic consequences of AIDS is to express these in terms of *patient-related* and *general programme costs*. We can directly link these patient-related costs to the incidence and prevalence of HIV and AIDS, expressed in the disease stages in the Centers for Disease Control (CDC) classification.

In computing the costs of AIDS, we have decided not to use a monetary value for the PYLL to express production loss; not only can objections of an ethical nature be raised against such a model, but there is also a general lack of clarity concerning the expression of production loss in financial terms.[1]

In calculating the economic impact of AIDS we have laid the stress on the costs of AIDS incurred within the health care system. This choice means that certain economic consequences are left out of this part of the baseline analysis, such as the consequences for private insurance where there is no acceptance obligation - e.g. life insurance. Costs which are borne by the patient him or herself have also been left out of consideration.

This chapter catalogues the economic impact of AIDS on the basis of the categories "direct versus indirect costs" and "general programme costs versus patient-related costs". The emphasis here is on the direct costs. The cost categories are dealt with for each health care sector separately, and at the end of the discussion of each sector we formulate the assumptions for scenario analysis.

---

1 It is sufficient here to refer to several methods; the 'willingness to pay' the 'human capital' and the 'friction cost method' (Hay, 1989; Van Haselen, 1987; Drummond et al, 1988)

5.3 *Patient-related impact*

5.3.1 *Hospital*

Three studies are available in the Netherlands which look at the scale of hospital care and costs resulting from the inpatient and outpatient care and treatment of patients with HIV or AIDS. One study was carried out jointly by the Teaching Hospital attached to the University of Amsterdam (AZUA) and the Netherlands Institute for Preventive Medicine (NIPG) (Wiggers and Bijlsma 1989; Bijlsma, 1990). The second study was carried out by the University Hospital Utrecht (AZU) and the National Institute for Health and Environmental Protection (RIVM) (Borleffs and Jager, 1989; Dijkgraaf et al, 1989; Jager et al., 1989). Finally, a study was carried out by the Slotervaart Hospital (SZ) and KMPG Klynveld Management Consultants (KPMG, 1989abc; Gosselink and Vandermeulen, 1989; Danner et al., 1989). Table 5.1 gives an estimate of the average costs (per observation year in a given stage) emerging from these studies.

Table 5.1 **Hospital costs and hospitalization days (between brackets) in NLG per observation year (1988 cost levels); after Postma et al., accepted.**

	AZUA/NIPG		AZU/RIVM		SZ/KPMG	
CDC II and III	-	(9.1)[1]	4,700	(1.1)	8,500	(13.9)
CDC IV	-	(58.4)[2]	47.400	(51.1)	35,900	(52.5)
All stages	42,500	(37.4)	18,400	(23.1)	30.100	(17.4)

1. Figure relates to pre-AIDS stage
2. Figure relates to AIDS

As far as possible, the costs have been differentiated into CDC IV and CDC II and III (Centers for Disease Control, 1986; 1987a) and are expressed as costs per *observation year*. All amounts are expressed in 1988 guilders.

The average costs in the AZUA/NIPG study are put at NLG 42,500. In the AZU/RIVM study, this figure is NLG 18,400 for the entire population, NLG 4,700 for patients in the CDC III and II stages, and NLG 47,400 for patients in CDC category IV. Average costs in the SZ/KPMG study amount to NLG 30,100, with NLG 8,500 in the pre CDC IV stages and NLG 35,900 for CDC IV patients. For patients in category CDC IV, the number of hospitalization days in the studies is 51.1 (AZU/RIVM) and 52.5 (SZ/KPMG). In the pre-CDC IV stages, this number is 1.1 and 13.9 days respectively. In the AZUA/NIPG study, the opposition AIDS versus pre-AIDS was adopted (Centers for Disease Control, 1987b). Here, the number of hospitalization days per observation year amounts to 58.4 in the AIDS stage and 9.1 in the pre-AIDS stage.

Data on the total duration of the disease, i.e. from the first contact after HIV infection up to the point of death, are only available for 127 patients in the AZUA/NIPG study. Patients are admitted to hospital on average more than three times. The average number of hospitalization days is 77, which for 3.3 admissions works out at an average hospital stay per admission of 23.3 days. The costs amount to NLG 87,000 per patient.

Table 5.1 shows that the average costs per observation year vary between NLG 18,400 and NLG 42,500, while the costs for patients in category CDC IV range from NLG 35,900 to 47,400. The spread in the number of hospitalization days per observation year for patients in the CDC IV stage is small: 51.1 - 52.5 days. In addition, a recent analysis from the AZU/RIVM study for the period July 1989 to January 1991 shows a significant fall to 27.3 hospitalization days per observation year (Dijkgraaf et al., 1991). Since it is not yet known what effect this fall will have on the costs of hospital care, we have expressed it for the present *only* in terms of hospitalization days.

Several factors may be responsible for the differences in costs and production figures (Scitovsky and Over, 1988). These may include the *operationalization of the costs and cost types*, for example in terms of cost prices (SZ/KPMG) or tariffs (AZUA/NIPG), or a mixture of the two (AZU/RIVM); differences in the *period* and *location* covered by the study; possible differences in medical technology and treatment *protocols*; differences in the *size* and *composition* of the patient population; and whether or not *follow-up measurements* were carried out. Differences e.g. occur between patient groups; the costs per observation year in 52 for gay/bisexual men and injecting drug users in the CDC IV stadium are estimated at NLG 34,800 and NLG 8,800 respectively, with the number of hospitalization days being 48 and 9 respectively (Postma et al., in preparation). The latter findings differ from what might be expected on the basis of other available literature (Arno, 1986; Hiatt et al., 1990; Epstein et al., 1990).

Table 5.2 **Hospital costs and days in hospital per person year for AIDS in US $[1,2]**

Reference	Cost level	Hospitalization days	Costs
US[3]			
Hellinger (1988)	1986	23	29,100
Hellinger (1990)	1989	38	38,400
Hay et al. (1988)	1986	19	25,300
Andrulis et al. (1987)	1986	59	38,300
Lafferty et al. (1988)	1986	47	32,700
Europe			
AZUA/NIPG	1988	58	
AZU/RIVM	1988	51	19,800
SZ/KPMG	1988	53	15,000
Koock-Walewski (1989)	1986	130	23,500
AZUA/NIPG[4]	1988	99	
Australia[3]			
Whyte et al. (1987)	1986	58	26,400

1 The figures for AZU/RIVM and SZ/KPMG apply to CDC IV
2 Conversions between different currencies are based on purchasing power indexes (Organisation for Economic Cooperation and Development, 1989); $1 is equivalent to NLG 2.40
3 Taken from Scitovsky and Over (1988)
4 Subgroup of patients who died during the observation period

Table 5.2 places the results of the Dutch studies in an international perspective. The Table gives estimates of the number of hospitalization days needed by people with AIDS, and shows the hospital costs per observation year. Studies carried out in the US show noticeably higher cost estimates than those in the Netherlands, while the estimates of the number of hospitalization days needed are usually lower. This is due to the high all-in cost of a day's hospitalization in the US, i.e. the costs of a day in hospital including overheads, medication and treatment. Hellinger (1990) puts this cost at $1,000, as compared to a figure of NLG 928 as used by the AZU/RIVM, and NLG 684 in the SZ/KPMG study. Few European studies are known which are comparable in design with the Dutch study. The (West) German study carried out by Koock-Walewski covers the period 1.1.1985 to 30.6.1987 and contains only data on only a small number of patients who were monitored during the entire period of illness until death. For comparison with the need for hospitalization days in the Netherlands, data have been included here on the subgroup "deceased patients" from the AZUA/NIPG study.

The above cost estimates for Dutch hospitals include the costs of psychiatric consultations. Not every hospital in the Netherlands has a psychiatric consultancy department, so that differences in the extent and costs of the care provided are possible. Sno et al. (1990), in a study involving 97 people with HIV infection or AIDS at the Academic Medical Centre (AMC) in the period 1983-1989, observed a total of 116 psychiatric or psychological disorders or problems. In 1988 and 1989, psychiatric consultation was requested for 41 and 43 HIV-infected persons respectively. Of the total of 355 and 321 patients, respectively, who were admitted during these two years because of HIV or HIV-related problems, this amounts to a consultation percentage in 1988 of 11.5%, and of 13.4% in 1989. Lunter et al. (1991) report that of the 600 HIV-infected persons who had been in contact with the AMC up to May 1990, approximately 5% had been treated at the psychiatric outpatients clinic.

5.3.1.1 Assumptions for scenario analysis

In expressing the consequences of AIDS for hospitals and linking this to epidemiological developments, we have taken as a basis the three studies in Table 5.1. The estimates for the CDC IV and pre-CDC IV stages have also been adopted in the scenarios for the AIDS and pre-AIDS stages, respectively.

5.3.2 Nursing homes

In 1987, two nursing homes in Amsterdam began offering care to people with AIDS, and in 1988 they reserved a total of four beds for this purpose (Wiggers and Bergsma, 1990ab). Since that time, other nursing homes have also equipped themselves to offer nursing care to people with AIDS: as at April 1989, 16 AIDS patients were admitted to nursing homes in Amsterdam, three in the Hague and two in Rotterdam. On the assumption of a need for admission to a nursing home among 10% of AIDS patients in the terminal phase, a bed occupancy rate of 95% and a length of stay of 60 days, the Dutch National Commission for AIDS Control (NCAB) calculated a need for seven beds in 1990 (NCAB, 1989).

According to the guidelines published by the Central Council on Health Care Charges (COTG), nursing home fees in 1988 were NLG 220 per day. Per AIDS bed in a nursing home this means an annual total in fees of NLG 80,300 per bed. The ancillary expenses are estimated at NLG 48,000 per bed for AIDS patients (NCAB, 1989).

5.3.2.1 *Assumptions for scenario analysis*

People with AIDS do not appear to make extensive use of nursing care. We have based our scenarios on the NCAB estimates of a demand for care by 10% of people with AIDS and a duration of nursing care of 60 days. It should be borne in mind here, however, that this type of care provision for people with AIDS has only recently got underway, and that an increase in the requirement is not unlikely (Weigel, personal report, 1991). This would mean that the estimates of the use of nursing-home beds in our scenarios could be too low. We have expressed the costs in accordance with the COTG guideline for 1988, excluding ancillary costs.

5.3.3 *Regular district nursing*

Research among relatives of 52 deceased AIDS patients shows that the help of the district nursing was sought in 18 cases (Van den Boom et al., 1991). No data are available from this study regarding the duration of the care. The National Home Nursing Association estimates that approximately 200 people with AIDS received care from the district nursing service in 1990. In addition, the province of South Holland keeps records on 12 patients, which show that the average time span between diagnosis of AIDS and the first contact with the district nursing service was approximately one year, and the average period of care around three months (National Home Nursing Association, 1988; 1989; Mostert, personal report, 1990).

The costs of nursing, including overheads, are put at NLG 90 per hour (Wiggers and Bergsma, 1990ab); this estimate would seem to be rather high (Mannaerts, personal report).

5.3.3.1 *Assumptions for scenario analysis*

We have assumed a need for district nursing care among 35% of AIDS patients. We have estimated the duration of care at three months and have assumed an intensity of 5 hours' care per week. All in all, this comes to a total of 60 hours' care among 35% of AIDS patients. We have assumed a cost of NLG 90 per contact hour.

5.3.4 *Regular home help*

The Central Council for Home Help Services estimates that 27,500 contact hours were devoted to people with AIDS in 1988, with a further 14,800 hours being spent on support, consultation, administration, etc. The AIDS Health Care Project Survey showed that in September 1990, 9 hours' home help were provided per patient per week (National Home Nursing Association, 1991); this compares with a figure of 7 hours for 1989 (Laverman, 1989; personal report). The study among surviving relatives of people with AIDS shows that the home help service was involved with 38% of people with AIDS (Van den Boom et al., 1991). No information is available on the duration of the help provided. Wiggers and Bergsma (1990a) assume an hourly rate of NLG 35 excluding overheads. This hourly rate is multiplied by a factor of 1.5 to give the costs including overheads, such as consultation hours etc.

5.3.4.1 Assumptions for scenario analysis

We have assumed the same duration of care for home help as for district nursing. For 9 hours' care per week, this comes to 108 hours of home help for 38% of AIDS patients. The cost calculations include overheads.

5.3.5 Intensive home care

The National Council for Public Health defined home care in 1989 as "the totality of care, nursing, treatment and assistance given to the person in need of care in the domestic setting, which is carried out through "self-help" initiatives, an informal support network, voluntary work and/or (supplementary) professional care, and which is designed specifically to enable the person in need of care to remain in the domestic setting."

One of the objectives of government health care policy is to increase the role of home care (Commission for the Structure and Financing of Health Care, 1987; Ministry of Welfare, Health and Cultural Affairs, 1989). The experiments carried out with intensive home care are in line with this objective. Intensive home care is intended for patients whose medical condition indicates admission to hospital or nursing home, but for whom there are no medical objections to nursing at home. It is a condition for intensive home care that the duration of care must be short. Intensive care is provided for 6 weeks, with the possibility of extension by a further 6 weeks, by the general practitioner, district nursing service, home help service, social services department, informal support network and voluntary service. Within the framework of the Regulation on Experiments in Home Nursing, intensive home care projects have been initiated in Amsterdam, Groningen and the provinces of West Brabant and Zeeuws

Flanders. An average of NLG 200 per day of care may be borne by the additional care subsidy. The costs per patient over the whole period of home care, i.e. including periods of regular home care, must not exceed NLG 350 per day. A subsidy ruling governing intensive home care for the whole of the Netherlands came into effect in May 1990 (Ministry of Welfare, Health and Cultural Affairs, 1991).

AIDS was one of the diagnosis categories selected in the final report of the Experiments in Home Nursing (Miltenburg, 1989; Miltenburg et al., 1990; Ramakers et al., 1990). The 1,996 users of intensive home care included 37 AIDS patients, who received care for an average of 22 days, although 86% received intensive home care for less than one week. AIDS patients received 56 hours' "extra" home care per week, of which 44 hours were intensive home care.

5.3.5.1 Assumptions for scenario analysis

Until recently, intensive home care was an experimental service with a small number of participating AIDS patients. How much use AIDS patients will make of the service in the coming years will depend on initiatives taken by regions where there is as yet no intensive home care system, and also on the possibilities for substitution. We look at a number of substitution options in the care scenarios (Chapter 8). The reference scenario assumes intensive home care for 5% of AIDS patients for 22 days. For the costs per day we will use NLG 200 per day.

5.3.6 General practitioners

A survey carried out amongst all general practitioners in the Netherlands by the Ancillary Services Foundation (SAD) showed that 88.7% of GPs had held HIV or AIDS-related consultations in the year up to July 1989; the figure for practices in the West of the Netherlands was 92.8%, where 25% of the practices had at least one AIDS patient. The project "Advancement of Expertise and Support of General Practitioners" reported on the practical support given to 4 heavily-loaded Amsterdam general practices (Hochheimer et al., 1988; Wigersma et al., in print; SAD 1989a, 1989b, 1990).

The results showed that the number of consultations and visits in connection with HIV-related problems was approximately 6 per patient per year for seropositive pre-AIDS patients and 10 for AIDS patients. In the 6 months preceding the last measurement, 80% of the seropositive patients and 87% of the AIDS patients consulted their general practitioner. The average length of each consultation or visit was 12 minutes for HIV-infected persons and 27 minutes for AIDS patients. Of the total of 1327 consultations and visits given to seropositive patients and AIDS patients during these 6 months, 49% lasted less than 20 minutes and 51% were longer than this. Only 14% of the visits lasted less than 20 minutes. For each consultation lasting less than a quarter of an hour, a fee of NLG 28 is charged, while a double rate is charged for consultations lasting longer than 20 minutes.

Wiggers and Bergsma (1990ab) estimate that there were around 31,000 consultations in 1988, assuming 6,184 general practitioners each giving 5 consultations per year for AIDS-related problems. The latter estimate also includes consultations for men and women with no HIV infection, including requests for an HIV antibody test by heterosexuals without a demonstrable AIDS risk. This would seem to be a high estimate in view of the recent publication showing 2.6 AIDS consultations per general practitioner per year (Moons and Peters 1990). On the basis of the SAD study, showing 282 AIDS patients in 1988 and a maximum of 1500 persons who were aware of their seropositive status, it is possible to estimate the number of patient-related consultations in 1988 (Wiggers and Bergsma, 1990ab; Health Council, 1990); such an estimate would give a figure of around 12,000 consultations.

5.3.6.1 Assumptions for scenario analysis

We draw a distinction in the scenario analysis between patient-related and general programme costs (i.e. non-patient-related costs). For the patient-related costs we have assumed 10 consultations for AIDS patients and 6 consultations for persons in the pre-AIDS stage. In establishing the non-patient-related costs of the general practitioner, we have assumed that in 2 out of 3 consultations the patient is not infected with HIV and that each general practitioner has 2.6 AIDS consultations. This produces in a total for general programme costs of NLG 112,000 (Moons and Peters 1990; Wiggers and Bergsma 1990ab).

5.3.7 Psychosocial support: Regional Institutes for Ambulant Mental Health Care (RIAGG), Social Work (AMW), the Schorer Foundation

The RIAGGs and the AMW are regarded as cornerstones of the policy on psychosocial support in relation to HIV (National Commission for AIDS Control (NCAB), 1988). It is not possible to estimate the demand for care from RIAGGs and the social services, although the impression is that RIAGGs have so far not been involved to any large extent in providing support in HIV-related problems.

The psychosocial care provided in relation to AIDS has until now been concentrated within the Department of Psychosocial Support for AIDS (APHA) of the Schorer Foundation, a national foundation providing help and service with problems related to homosexuality. In the period from May 1986 to April 1989 278 people with AIDS and HIV, and those close to them made use of one or more of the services of the APHA. The APHA's budget in 1989 was more than one million guilders (De Rijk and Van den Boom, 1989). Apart from the provision of care, prevention and information activities and the training of buddies were also financed from this budget.

5.3.7.1 Buddy help

So-called buddy projects have been operating in the Netherlands since 1984 in order to meet the needs of people with AIDS for material and moral support. Buddies are trained volunteers who offer practical and emotional help and support to people with AIDS. Among the organizations involved in the organization of buddy projects in the Netherlands are the basic health care institutions, the primary health care organizations and category-specific organizations such as the Schorer Foundation, the Central Education Commission and drug aid agencies. Five projects, including the large-scale buddy projects set up by the Schorer Foundation and the Rainbow Foundation in Amsterdam, are restricted to gay men and injecting drug users. For 1990, the subsidy applied for in respect of buddy projects was NLG 900,000 (Van den Boom and de Rijk, 1989; Driessen et al., 1991).

Up to 1.1.91 there were 25 operational buddy projects in the Netherlands, in which 520 buddies had been active with 500 clients. Half of these buddies were involved in the project set up by the Schorer Foundation. It is estimated that 25% of people with AIDS made use of the buddy help service in 1990. 80% of the client population are gay men. Up to now, buddies have assisted an average of 3 clients; this calculation includes buddies who are still active, which means that the average number of clients per buddy will increase further. The time invested by buddies has been fixed at a minimum of 8 hours per week, and buddies are active for an average 110 weeks (De Rijk et al., in preparation).

On the basis of the above findings an approximation can be made of the total number of hours of buddy help provided. In calculating the annual figures, we have restricted ourselves to gay men; the number of hours of buddy help given to this category in 1990 was 64,000.

5.3.7.2 Assumptions for scenario analysis

We express the psychosocial care provided by RIAGGs, the AMW and the Schorer Foundation as memorandum items in the scenarios, because no data are available to enable an accurate estimate to be given in terms of patient-related costs. For buddies, we have taken as our basis the key figures listed above, and will restrict ourselves in the scenarios to buddy help given to homosexual men.

5.3.8 Use of medicines: AZT

In mid-1987 azidothymidine (AZT) became available in the Netherlands for the treatment of people with AIDS and seropositives. In 1990, 10,020 units of AZT, each of 10,000 mg, were placed with pharmacists, and 1,213 units at hospitals (Wellcome Pharmaceuticals bv, personal report, 1990); hospitals have thus distributed barely 10% of all AZT. The costs of using AZT and other medicines in hospitals are included in the hospital costs stated in section 5.2.1 (see also Scitovsky et al., 1990); information on the use of medicines consumed outside the hospital environment is only available for AZT.

AZT is not prescribed in fixed doses, doses vary between 500 and 1500 mg per day. The purchase price of AZT is NLG 33 per 1,000 mg (10 x 100 mg), excluding VAT.

5.3.8.1 Assumptions for scenario analysis

We have assumed an AZT dosage of 1,000 mg per day for a period of one year. In the scenarios it is assumed that 10% of the costs of AZT have been included in the hospital costs. The VAT-exclusive price has been used as a basis for calculating costs.

Table 5.3 **Estimates of the economic impact of AIDS per person year (the figures between brackets refer to persons in the pre-AIDS stage, per person year, who are aware of their sero-positive status); 1988 cost level, in NLG.**

Category	Estimate	References
Hospital costs		
SZ/KPMG	35,900 (8,500)	1, 4
AZU/RIVM	47,400 (4,700)	2, 4
hospitalization days		
SZ/KPMG	52.5 (13.9)	1, 4
AZU/RIVM	27.3 (1.1)	2, 4
Nursing home		
costs	660	5, 6
length of stay (days)	3.0	5, 6
District nursing		
costs	945	6, 7, 8
contact hours	10.5	7, 8
Home help		
costs	1076	6, 8, 9
contact hours	20.5	8, 9
Intensive home care		
costs	110	10
length of care (days)	0.55	10
AZT use at home		
costs	5422	11
General practitioner		
costs	490 (210)	12, 6
consultations	10 (6)	12
Buddy help		
hours (for gay men)	98	8,13

1 KPMG (1989abc); Danner et al. (1989); Gosselink and Vandermeulen (1989). 2 Borleffs and Jager (1988); Dijkgraaf et al. (1989); Jager et al. (1990); Borleffs et al. (1990); Dijkgraaf et al. (1991). 3 Wiggers and Bijlsma (1989); Bijlsma (1990). 4 Postma et al. (accepted). 5 NCAB (1989). 6 Wiggers and Bergsma (1990ab). 7 Mostert, personal report (1990). 8 Van den Boom et al., 1991. 9 National Home Nursing Association (1991). 10 Miltenburg et al. (1990); Ramakers et al. (1990). 11 Wellcome Pharmaceuticals bv, personal report (1990). 12 SAD (1989ab; 1990). 13 De Rijk et al. (in preparation).

5.3.9 Survey of patient-related costs

Table 5.3 gives a summary of the assumptions we have used in calculating the patient-related economic impact of AIDS. We have expressed the demand for care, and the associated costs, per person year per disease stage. Put another way, we have assumed that a person is in the pre-AIDS or AIDS stage for a full year. We have put the average survival period of people with AIDS at two years. The amounts between brackets relate to an HIV-infected person in the pre-AIDS stage who is aware of his or her serostatus. The information above concerning the use and costs of care in fact relates only to persons who (whether or not in connection with HIV/AIDS-related complaints) have been in contact with the health care services and are therefore *aware* that they are seropositive.

5.3.10 1990 cost comparison

In Table 5.4, the patient-related costs of HIV/AIDS for the year 1990 are compared with relevant statements costs and production in the health care sector as published by the Financial Statement on Health Care (FOZ) 1991 (Ministry of Welfare, Health and Cultural Affairs, 1991). In making this comparison, it has been assumed that 25% of the prevalence in the pre-AIDS stage are *aware* that they are seropositive. The total of patient-related costs for HIV/AIDS in 1990 is estimated at NLG 51.2 million. Wiggers and Bergsma (1990ab) estimate the patient-related costs for 1998 at almost NLG 20 million.

The hospital bed need for HIV/AIDS in 1990 was 84 on the basis of Dijkgraaf et al. (1991), and 227 days if we take KPMG (1989abc) as a basis. A bed occupancy of 75% has been assumed. Taking the total number of beds in the Netherlands as a whole (66,000) this means that the bed requirement for HIV/AIDS amounts to between 0.13 and 0.34%. On the basis of the SZ/KPMG and AZU/RIVM studies, the costs of HIV/AIDS amount to 0.28 and 0.30%, respectively, of the total hospital costs.

Of 51,000 recognized beds in nursing homes, of which 27,000 are for non-psychogeriatric patients, 6 beds are needed for AIDS patients; this is equivalent to 0.01% of the total number of beds, or 0.02% of the non-psychogeriatric beds. At a daily rate of NLG 220, this brings the total costs to NLG 520,000.

The home care costs created by HIV/AIDS amount to NLG 2.3 million, which represents 0.05% of the home care cost items selected in this study. The use of AZT (assuming that 90% of the AZT is distributed outside hospitals) amounts to (4.2*100)/(0.90*4.100 =) 0.11% of the total medicine use in the Netherlands. Finally, the Table shows that buddy help was given during 1450 complete working weeks in 1990.

Table 5.4 **The need for care and the costs (in millions NLG; 1988 cost level) resulting from AIDS and HIV[1] per category in 1990 (1988 cost levels). Comparison with totals for all illnesses (taken from the Financial Statement on Health Care 1991), for the year 1989 (cost in millions NLG).**

	HIV/AIDS	Total
Beds		
hospital	84 - 227	66,000
nursing home	6	27,000[2]
Costs		
hospital	41.0 - 44.1	14,900[3]
nursing home	0.5	3,900
Out-of-hospital		
hours of district nursing	8,190	
hours of home help	15,990	
intensive home care (days)	429	
GP consultations	16,904	
Out-of-hospital costs		
district nursing	0.7	900[4]
home help	0.8	1,700
intensive home care	0.1	21
general practitioner	0.7	1,800
Costs of medicine use	4.2[5]	4,100
Total costs	51.2[6]	27,400
Buddy help for gay men		
number of hours		58,000

1 Based on 25% *aware* of seropositivity
2 Only includes beds for somatic patients; excludes beds for psychogeriatrics
3 Inclusive of medical specialists, dental specialists and ambulance transport
4 Inclusive of vaccination programme costs
5 Relates only to AZT, excluding in-hospital use
6 Based on hospital costs at NLG 44.1 million

5.4 *Programme costs*

In addition to patient-related costs, there are also programme costs. These costs cannot be attributed to a person in one of the stages of the disease, but relate to the costs of research, prevention and information, training and services provided for the entire population. Wiggers and Bergsma (1990ab) estimate the programme costs in 1988 at NLG 56 million. What follows is based mainly on their cost estimate.

5.4.1 *Research*

The AIDS Research Programme Coordination Committee (PccAo) of the Health Research Council (RGO) estimates the costs of implementing the complete AIDS research stimulation programme at NLG 11.5 million in 1990, and NLG 13.5 million in 1991 and 1992. These costs are borne by the Ministry of Welfare, Health and Cultural Affairs and by the Prevention Fund. Wiggers and Bergsma (1990ab) estimate the costs of research in 1988 at NLG 14.2 million. This sum includes the costs borne by the Ministry of Welfare, Health and Cultural Affairs (including the costs of AIDS research within the RIVM), costs borne by the Prevention Fund and expenditure on research under the aegis of the EEC.

5.4.2 *Prevention*

Wiggers and Bergsma (1990ab) subdivide prevention measures into public information, including Health Information and Training, testing of sperm and organ banks, needle-exchange schemes, the testing of blood donors and deactivation, and preventive measures by dentists and in hospitals. The total costs of prevention in 1988 were estimated at more than NLG 31 million, of which almost 50% was taken up by preventive measures by dentists. The costs of testing for HIV antibodies and deactivation by heat treatment in blood banks are estimated by Wiggers and Bergsma at NLG 12.7 million.

5.4.3 *Tests*

Wiggers and Bergsma (1990ab) estimate the number of HIV ELISA tests in 1988 at between 803,190 and 920,000. The upper limit was determined on the basis of the number of tests sold, while the lower limit is a conservative estimate of the number of persons tested. 703,500 tests were carried out in 1988 in blood banks, 26,375 tests in connection with life assurance policies and 6,172 tests through the general practitioner, or at alternative test sites operated by the Municipal Medical Departments (GGD) and the Ancillary Services Foundation (SAD). A generous margin of 1% was added to this number of tests to allow for the number of tests which had to be repeated. Exact figures are available for the Western Blot confirmation tests for 1988, when 6,330 tests were carried out.

Wiggers and Bergsma (1990ab) estimate the costs of ELISA tests in 1988 at a minimum of NLG 9.2 million, with NLG 7.7 million going on the blood bank tests and the costs of the Western Blot tests accounting for NLG 1.2 million. The Municipal Health Departments charge a privately insured individual NLG 25-30 for a test; these are the costs of the ELISA test or a Western Blot confirmation test, including a repeat where necessary. For a test through the general practitioner, the normal consultation fee of NLG 28 is charged.

The costs of Pre- and Post-Test Counselling (PPTC) are estimated by Wiggers and Bergsma on the basis of the fee for a consultation. For 1988 this means a minimum for PPTC of NLG 249,000. The NCAB (1990) considers that good PPTC involves consultation costs of NLG 74. On this basis, the costs of PPTC in 1988 would be a minimum of NLG 891,000, which would bring the costs of the ELISA tests to NLG 9.8 million. We have based the scenarios on the NCAB standard for PPTC; the costs of the ELISA and Western Blot tests together then amount to NLG 11 million.

5.4.4 Summary of programme costs

We estimate the total programme costs at NLG 47 million, which excludes a figure of NLG 15 million for preventive measures by dentists, but includes NLG 100,000 for preventive measures by general practitioners and NLG 11 million for tests. For the remaining items, we have adopted the figures given by Wiggers and Bergsma (1990ab) of NLG 14.2 million for research, NLG 16 million for prevention and NLG 6 million for other general programme costs.

Our justification for stating the costs of prevention by dentists separately is as follows. Dentists have incurred costs for measures designed to prevent transmission of HIV, and these costs have been passed on to third parties. Although the same safety measures apply in principle in hospitals, Wiggers and Bergsma (1990ab) do not include any costs for hospitals because the existing precautionary measures against the transmission of viruses such as Hepatitis B are already considered adequate (Health Council 1986); AIDS is therefore not considered to involve any additional costs. A different argument is possible here, however: dentists can also be considered to take precautionary measures against Hepatitis B, which would mean that this cost item is incorrectly attributed solely to AIDS. All in all, however, stating this cost item separately appears justified.

5.4.4.1 Assumptions for scenario analysis

Due to the difficulty of linking costs of this type to epidemiological models, we have adopted a constant figure of NLG 47 million in the scenarios for the programme costs for HIV/AIDS for the period 1990-2000. In the reference scenario, this figure functions as a reference point for the study of patient-related costs which are, by contrast, linked directly to epidemiological models.

5.5 Commentary

This chapter contains an overview of the patient-related and general programme costs of AIDS in the Netherlands. The reconstruction leads to an estimate of the total costs of AIDS in the Netherlands of at least NLG 98 million. Comparison with the results obtained by Wiggers and Bergsma shows that this represents a sharp increase, resulting from a rise in the number of AIDS patients and the associated patient-related costs.

Table 5.3 enables an estimate to be made of the costs per HIV-infected person and/or AIDS patient. This leads to the following results per person year per AIDS patient.

- The costs of inpatient and outpatient care amount to NLG 35,900 (SZ/KPMG) or NLG 47,400 (AZU/RIVM);
- We estimate the out-of hospital costs at NLG 8,700, of which NLG 700 can be attributed to costs in the nursing home.

For HIV-infected persons, taken here to be persons in the pre-AIDS stage (aware *and* unaware of their serostatus), we have estimated these amounts at NLG 50 for out-of-hospital care and NLG 2,100 (SZ/KPMG) and NLG 1,200 (AZU/RIVM) for in-hospital treatment. It is clear that for persons in the pre-AIDS stage, the costs of out-of-hospital treatment will be higher than stated here. However, the only information we have available concerns costs related to general practitioner visits.

These findings imply a total average cost for HIV/AIDS per patient over the entire period of infection up to death of NLG 126,000 (AZU/RIVM) or NLG 112,900 (SZ/KPMG). These figures are based on an average survival period of two years following diagnosis of AIDS, and an average of 11 years for the pre-AIDS stage.

The English-language literature contains estimates per person year which vary from $25,000 to $100,000 (Hay et al., 1988; Bloom and Carliner, 1988, Hellinger, 1988; see also Table 5.2). The Dutch estimate per person year is rather lower, for which a number of reasons can be cited. In addition to the composition of the case mix (stage of the disease, distribution across core groups), it is important to bear in mind that the causal factors of the costs vary from country to country. For example, the costs of a hospital admission are created to a large extent by the "hotel costs" (the costs of simply residing in the institution) and the nursing costs (the costs associated with care). The salary levels of nursing staff are an important factor here.

The care of people with AIDS in the Netherlands does not cover its costs. Ancillary costs arise because the costs of care and treatment in hospital are higher than the amount which the hospital receives through application of the Function-oriented Budgeting System developed by the Central Council on Health Care Charges. The SZ/KPMG study puts these ancillary costs at 80%. It is important to bear in mind here that these ancillary costs cannot be assumed to be constant over time, and the study results would gain a great deal of credibility if the same methodology was applied to one or more other disease categories.

5.6 *Summary*

In working out the baseline analysis of the economic impact of the HIV/AIDS epidemic, we have opted for a subdivision of the costs into two categories:

- direct versus indirect costs
- patient-related versus general programme costs

The emphasis in this chapter is on the direct patient-related costs. This choice results from the fact that these costs can be readily linked to the epidemiological models presented in Chapter 2. The indirect costs (including Potential Years of Life Lost) were discussed in Chapter 3. In addition to a reconstruction of the costs of AIDS, an indication is given for each cost category of which values or basic principles have been adopted in scenario analysis.

The estimated patient-related costs for HIV/AIDS for the year 1990 come to NLG 51.2 million, while the total costs of out-of-hospital care amount to NLG 2.9 million. The quantity of AZT distributed outside the hospital is estimated to have a value of NLG 4.2 million. The largest part of the costs - NLG 44.1 million - is borne by the hospitals (see figure 5.1).

Figure 5.1 Patient-related costs of HIV/AIDS per category (in millions NLG; 1988 cost level). The hospital costs are based on Borleffs et al. (1990).

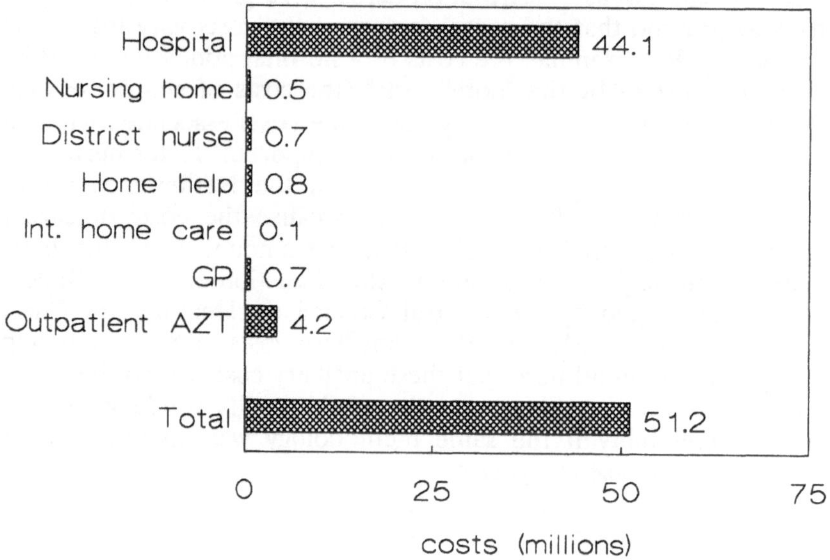

Figure 5.1 is based on the results of several studies into the use of care and the costs of HIV/AIDS. The results of these studies show some variation, even after conversion to the same dimensions. This may be explained by a number of factors, including design of the study, operationalization of the term "costs" and characteristics of the patient population.

The costs of general prevention and information programmes, HIV-antibody tests and research, are estimated at NLG 47 million (1988 cost levels). These amounts excludes the preventive measures taken by dentists and in hospitals. Apart from nominal growth, it will be assumed in the scenario analysis that these costs remain constant up to the year 2000.

References

Andrulis, D.P.
The US hospital AIDS survey: structure and substance
In: D. Schwefel, R. Leidl, J. Rovira, M.F. Drummond (eds.), *Economic Aspects of AIDS and HIV Infection*, Springer-Verlag, Berlin, 1990

Andrulis D.P., V.S. Beers, J.D. Bentley, L.S. Gage
The provision and financing of medical care for AIDS patients in US public and private teaching hospitals
JAMA, 258 (1987), 1343-1346

Arno, P.S.
The Nonprofit Sector's Response to the AIDS Epidemic: Community-based Services in San Francisco
American Journal of Public Health, 76 (1986), 11, 1325-1330

Bez, G.
La prise en charge des malades infectes par le V.I.H.: utilisation des structures hospitaliers et coût
Cah. Socio. Démo. Méd., 29 (1989), 2, 107-135

Bilheimer, L.
Data gaps in modeling AIDS Service Utilization and Costs
Presentatie op *V International Conference on AIDS*, Montreal, 1989a (ThHO3)

Bilheimer, L.
AIDS cost modelling in the US: a pragmatic approach
Health Policy, (1989b), 11, 147-168

Bloom, D.E., G. Carliner
The economic impact of AIDS in the United States
Science, 239 (1988), 604-610

Bloom, D.E., S. Glied
The evolution of AIDS economic research
Health Policy, (1989), 11, 187-196

Boom, F.M.L.G. van den, T. Gremmen, H. Roozenburg
AIDS: leven rond de dood; Nabestaanden over ziekte, dood en rouw
NcGv, Utrecht, 1991, NcGv-reeks 91-16

Borleffs, J.C.C., J.C. Jager
Registratie en kostenschatting van klinische en poliklinische werkzaamheden voor patiënten met HIV-infectie
Nederlands Tijdschrift voor Geneeskunde, 133 (1989), 15, 767-772

Borleffs, J.C.C., J.C. Jager, M.J.J.C. Poos, M.G.W. Dijkgraaf, R.M.A. Geels, H. Vrehen, A.J.P. Schrijvers
Hospital cost for patients with HIV infection in a University hospital in The Netherlands
Health Policy, (1990), 16, 43-54

Bijlsma, P.R.E.
The Costs of Hospital Care of AIDS Patients at the Teaching Hospital of the University of Amsterdam
In: D. Schwefel, R. Leidl, J. Rovira, M.F. Drummond (eds.), *Economic Aspects of AIDS and HIV Infection*, Springer-Verlag, Berlijn, 1990

Centers for Disease Control (CDC)
Classification of HTLV-III/LAV infections
Annals of Internal Medicine, (1986), 105, 234-237

Centers for Disease Control (CDC)
Classification system for HIV infection in children under 13 years of age
MMWR, (1987a), 36, 225-236

Centers for Disease Control (CDC)
Revision of the CDC surveillance case definition for Acquired Immunodeficiency Syndrome
MMWR, (1987b), 36 (suppl 1S), 1-15

Commissie Structuur en Financiering Gezondheidszorg
Bereidheid tot verandering
The Hague, 1987

Danner, S.A., P.L. Meenhorst, W. Pauw, P. Reiss
Diagnostiek en behandeling van patiënten met een HIV infectie
Bohn, Scheltema & Holkema, 1989

Dijkgraaf, M.G.W., J.Th.L. Jong, M.J.J.C. Poos, J.C.C. Borleffs, J.C. Jager
A relational database for monitoring hospital activities, costs of care and quality of life related to treatment of HIV infection and AIDS
In: J.C. Jager, E.J. Ruitenberg (eds.), *AIDS impact assessment; modelling and scenario-analysis*, RIVM/Bilthoven, in voorbereiding

Dijkgraaf, M.G.W., J.C.C. Borleffs, M.J.J.C. Poos, J.C. Jager, A.J.P. Schrijvers
Monitoring hospital resource use and cost: a three-and-a-half year follow-up
Presentatie op *VII International conference on AIDS*, Florence, 1991 (MD112)

Driessen A., L. van de Velden, F. van den Boom, J. Derks
Steun van de Regenboog; Vrijwillige hulpverlening aan verslaafden met AIDS

NcGv, Utrecht, 1991, NcGv-reeks 91-12

Drummond, M.F., G.L. Stoddart, W.G. Torrance
Methods for the economic evaluation of health care programmes
Oxford University Press, Oxford, 1987

Drummond, M.F., L.M. Davies (eds.)
AIDS: The challenge for economic analysis
Health Services Management Centre, World Health Organisation, University of Birmingham, 1990

Drummond, M.F., L.M. Davies
Treating AIDS: the economic issues
Health Policy, (1988), 10, 1-19

Epstein, A.M., M.A. Stern, J.S. Weismann
Do the poor cost more? A multihospital study of patients' socioeconomic status and use of hospital resources
New England Journal of Medicine, (1990), 16, 1122-1128

Gosselink, A., L.R.J. Vandermeulen
Dummy rapportage over de uitkomsten van de landelijke toepasbaarheid van de uitkomsten van het meerkosten onderzoek AIDS-hulpverlening
Nationaal Ziekenhuisinstituut, Utrecht, 1989

Hardy, A.M., K. Rauch, D. Echenberg, W.M. Morgan, J.W. Curran
The economic impact of the first 10.000 cases of Acquired Immunodeficiency Syndrome in the United States
JAMA, 1986, 209-211

Haseler, H.W.J.
Produktieverlies als gevolg van verkeersongevallen
Stichting het Nederlands Economisch Instituut, Rotterdam, 1987

Hay, J.W., D.H. Osmond, M.A. Jacobson
Projecting the medical costs of AIDS and ARC in the United States
Journal of Acquired Immune Defidiency Syndromes, 1 (1988), 5, 466-485

Health Council (GR)
AIDS-problematiek in Nederland; richtlijnen voor groepsonderzoek en adviezen voor preventie
GR, The Hague, 1986, no. 1986/22

Health Council (GR)
Vroege medische interventies bij personen die met AIDS-virus zijn geïnfecteerd
GR, The Hague, 1987, no. 1987/16

Hellinger, F.
Forecasting the personal medical care costs of AIDS from 1988 through 1991
Public Health Reports, 103 (1988), 3, 309-319

Hellinger, F.
Updated forecasts of the medical care costs of treating persons with AIDS, 1990-1994
Presentatie op *VI International Conference on AIDS*, San Francisco, 1990(FD122)

Hochheimer, E.H., A.H. Heijnen, L. Wigersma (eds.)
HIV-wijzer voor de huisarts
Stichting Aanvullende Dienstverlening, Amsterdam, 1988

Hiatt, R.A., C.P. Quesenberry Jr, J.V. Selby, B.H. Fireman, A. Knight
The cost of acquired immunodefiency syndrome in northern California. The experience of a large prepaid health plan
Arch. Intern. Med., 150 (1990), 4, 833-838

Jager, J.C., E.J. Ruitenberg (eds.)
Statistical Analysis and Mathematical Modelling of AIDS
Oxford University Press, Oxford, 1988

Jager, J.C., E.J. Ruitenberg (eds.)
AIDS impact assessment: modelling and scenario-analysis
RIVM/Bilthoven, in voorbereiding

Jager, J.C., M.J. Postma
De AIDS-epidemie: prognoses en economische gevolgen
In: H. Vuijsje, R. Coutinho (red.), *Dilemma's rondom AIDS*, Swets & Zeitlinger, Amsterdam/Lisse, 1989

Jager, J.C., M.J. Postma, F.M.L.G. van den Boom, D.P. Reinking, J.J.C. Borleffs, S.H. Heisterkamp, J.A.M. van Druten, E.J. Ruitenberg
Epidemiological Models and Socioeconomic Information: Methodological Aspects of AIDS/HIV Scenario Analysis
In: D. Schwefel, R. Leidl, J. Rovira, M.F. Drummond (eds.), *Economic Aspects of AIDS and HIV Infection*, Springer-Verlag, Berlijn, 1990

Jager, J.C., M.J. Postma, R. Leidl, B. Majnoni d'Intignano en A.E. Baert
AIDS impact scenarios: questions for the years to come
AIDS, 4 (1990), 11, 1166-1167

Johnson, A.M.
Economic aspects of care and prevention of HIV infection and AIDS
In: J.C. Jager, E.J. Ruitenberg (eds.), *Statistical Analysis and Mathematical Modelling of AIDS*, Oxford University Press, Oxford, 1988

Johnson, A.M.
Services for the management of HIV infection: problems for planners
In: D. Schwefel, R. Leidl, J. Rovira en M.F. Drummond (eds.), *Economic Aspects of AIDS and HIV Infection*, Springer-Verlag, Berlijn, 1990

Koock-Walewski, A.
Was kostet AIDS? - Eine Kosten - Leistungs - Analyse stationaerer Faelle
Schwer, Stuttgart, 1989

KPMG Klynveld Bosboom Hegener, Organisatie-adviseurs
Kosten en meerkosten van ziekenhuiszorg voor HIV-geïnfecteerden
KPMG, Utrecht, 1989a

KPMG Klynveld Bosboom Hegener, Organisatie-adviseurs
(Meer)kostenonderzoek AIDS-functie; Deelrapport 2, Medische en verpleegkundige protocollen
KPMG, Utrecht, 1989b

KPMG Klynveld Bosboom Hegener, Organisatie-adviseurs
(Meer)kosten AIDS-functie; Deelrapport 3, Kostenonderzoek en kostprijsbepaling
KPMG, Utrecht, 1989c

Lafferty, W.F., S.G. Hopkins, J. Honey, J.D. Harwell, P.C. Shoemaker, J.M. Kobayashi
Hospital charges for people with AIDS in Washington State: utilization of a statewide hospital discharge data base
American Journal of Public Health, (1988), 78, 949-952

Laverman, H.
Nota 'AIDS (HIV) in de thuiszorg' vanuit de gezinsverzorging gezien
Stichting Centrale Raad voor Gezinsverzorging, Driebergen, 1989

Laverman, H.
persoonlijke mededeling, 1991

Leidl, R., M.J. Postma, M.J.J.C. Poos, J.C. Jager, B. Majnoni d'Intignano, A.E. Baert
Construction of socioeconomic AIDS-scenarios based on routine surveillance data
In: J.C. Jager, E.J. Ruitenberg (eds.), *AIDS impact assessment; modelling and scenario analysis*, RIVM, Bilthoven, in voorbereiding

Lunter, C.H., H.N. Sno, F.M.L.G. van den Boom
HIV patiënten op een polikliniek psychiatrie
Nederlands Tijdschrift voor Geneeskunde, 1991, geaccepteerd

Mannaerts, H.M.
persoonlijke mededeling, 1991

Miltenburg, T.
Experimenten thuisverpleging; een tussentijdse evaluatie
Instituut voor Toegepaste Sociale Wetenschappen, Nijmegen, 1989

Miltenburg, T., C. Ramakers, J. Mensink, F. Tjadens
Experimenten thuisverpleging deel 1; eindrapport intensieve thuiszorg
Instituut voor Toegepaste Sociale Wetenschappen, Nijmegen, 1990

Ministry of Welfare, Health and Cultural Affairs(WVC)
Financieel Overzicht Zorg 1991
WVC, Rijswijk, 1991

Ministry of Welfare, Health and Cultural Affairs (WVC)
Doelgericht veranderen; Ontwerp-Kerndocument Gezondheidsbeleid voor de jaren 1990-1995
WVC, Rijswijk, 1989

Mostert, H.
persoonlijke mededeling, 1990

Nationale Commissie AIDS Bestrijding (NCAB)
- *Raamplan AIDS en de psychosociale zorg*
  NCAB, Amsterdam, 1988
- *Advies inzake zorgverlening aan AIDS-patiënten in verpleeghuizen*
  NCAB, Amsterdam, 1989
- *Vroegtijdige interventie bij personen met een HIV-infectie*
  NCAB, Amsterdam, 1990

Nationale Kruisvereniging (NKV)
Kruiswerk, thuis in gezondheid; meerjarenraming tot 1995, verantwoording vanaf 1983
NKV, Bunnik, 1988

Nationale Kruisvereniging (NKV)
Kruiswerk: voor zorg en voorzorg; meerjarenraming kruiswerk tot 1996, verantwoording vanaf 1984
NKV, Bunnik, 1989

Nationale Kruisvereninging (NKV)
Enquête Gezondheidszorgproject AIDS
NKV, Bunnik, 1991

Over, M.
A production function approach to estimating the aggregate macro-economic impact of AIDS on Central African economics
Presentatie op *V International Conference on AIDS*, Montreal, 1989 (THO15)

Pascal, A.
The costs of treating AIDS under Medicaid: 1986-1991
Rand Corporation, Santa Monica, 1987

Postma, M.J., M.G.W. Dijkgraaf, J.C.C. Borleffs, D.P.Reinking, F.M.L.G. van den Boom, J.C. Jager
Omvang en kosten van ziekenhuiszorg voor HIV-geïnfecteerden; een vergelijking en integratie van Nederlandse studies
Tijdschrift voor Sociale Gezondheidszorg, 1991, geaccepteerd

Ramakers, C., T. Miltenburg, J. Mensink, N. Welling, F. Tjadens, C. Tunissen
Experimenten thuisverpleging deel 2; eindrapport intensieve thuiszorg in de praktijk
Instituut voor Toegepaste Sociale Wetenschappen, Nijmegen, 1990

Rijk, K. de, F. van den Boom
Psychosociale hulpverlening AIDS; Vijf jaar hulpverlening door de Schorer-stichting
NcGv, Utrecht, 1989, NcGv-reeks 89-6

Rijk, K. de, F.M.L.G. van den Boom
Buddy-projecten in Nederland; een inventarisatie van knelpunten en mogelijke oplossingen
Maatschappelijk Gezondheidszorg, 18 (1990), 5, 32-36

Rijk, C. de, J. Drent, F. van den Boom
Buddy-zorg in perspectief; vrijwilligershulpverlening voor mensen met AIDS: meerwaarde en grenzen
NcGv, Utrecht, in voorbereiding

Rijksinstituut Instituut voor Volksgezondheid en Milieuhygiëne (RIVM)
Second workshop on Quantitative Analysis of AIDS
RIVM, Bilthoven, 1988

Rovira, J.
Economic aspects of AIDS
In: D. Schwefel, R. Leidl, J. Rovira, M.F. Drummond (eds.), *Economic Aspects of AIDS and HIV Infection*, Springer-Verlag, Berlijn, 1990

Rutten, F.F.H.
Kostenaspecten
In: J.D.F. Habbema, A.F. Casparie, J.H. Mulder, F.F.H. Rutten (red.),

Medische Technology Assessment en gezondheidsbeleid, Samsom Stafleu, Alphen aan de Rijn, 1989, Reeks gezondheidsbeleid - deel 4

Schreuder, R.F.
Scenarios as a tool to support health planning and management
In: D. Schwefel, R. Leidl, J. Rovira, M.F. Drummond (eds.), *Economic Aspects of AIDS and HIV Infection*, Springer-Verlag, Berlijn, 1990

Schwefel, D., R. Leidl, J. Rovira, M.F. Drummond (eds.)
Economic Aspects of AIDS and HIV Infection
Springer-Verlag, Berlijn, 1990

Scitovsky, A.A., M.W. Cline, D.I. Abrams
Effects of the Use of AZT on the Medical Care Costs of Persons with AIDS in the First 12 Months
Journal of the Acquired Immune Deficiency Syndromes, 3 (1990), 9, 904-912

Scitovsky, A.A., M. Over
AIDS: costs of care in the developed and the developing world
AIDS, (1988), 2(suppl 1), S71-S81

Scitovsky, A.A., D.P. Rice
Estimates of the Direct and Indirect costs of Acquired Immunodeficiency Syndrome in the United States, 1985, 1986 and 1991
Public Health Reports, 102 (1987), 5-17

Sno, H.N., J.G. Storosum, J.A. Swinkels
AIDS en psychiatrie
Jaarboek Psychiatrie 1990, geaccepteerd

Stichting Aanvullende Dienstverlening (SAD)
Voortgangsrapportage project deskundigheidsbevordering huisartsen
SAD, Amsterdam, juni 1989

Stichting Aanvullende Dienstverlening (SAD)
Tweede voortgangsrapportage project deskundigheidsbevordering huisartsen
SAD, Amsterdam, november 1989

Stichting Aanvullende Dienstverlening (SAD)
Derde voortgangsrapportage project deskundigheidsbevordering huisartsen
SAD, Amsterdam, mei 1990

Wellcome Pharmaceuticals bv
Persoonlijke mededeling, 1990

Whyte, B.M., D.B. Evans, E.J. Shreurs, D.A. Cooper
The costs of hospital-based medical care for patients with the acquired

immunodeficiency syndrome
Med J Aust, (1987), 147, 269-272

Wigersma, L., A.M. Heijnen, E.H. Hochheimer, H. Kloosterman
Learning about HIV in General Practice in The Netherlands
Britisch Medical Journal, in druk

Wiggers, C.C.M.C., E.W. Bergsma
De kosten van AIDS/HIV in Nederland in 1988: een inventarisatie
NIPG/TNO, Leiden, 1990a, TNO-rapport

Wiggers, C.C.M.C., E.W. Bergsma
De kosten van AIDS en HIV in Nederland in 1988
Economisch Statistische Berichten, juni, 1990b

Wiggers, C.C.M.C., P.R.E. Bijlsma
Kosten van ziekenhuisbehandeling van AIDS-patienten in het AZUA/-AMC in de periode 1982-1988
Tijdschrift voor Sociale Gezondheidszorg, 67 (1989), 7, 227-231

Part III Scenario analyses

6 Reference scenario: Impact of AIDS in 1995 and 2000

6.1 Introduction

Since the beginning of the AIDS epidemic prognoses have been put forward concerning the prevalence of HIV and the number of people with AIDS to be expected in the near future as a consequence. Many of these estimates are based on data from the AIDS records, combined with the application of mathematical modelling techniques. In the Netherlands, the data on AIDS are provided by the Chief Medical Officer of Health (GHI); on a European level, data can be obtained from the Quarterly Reports of the E.C. World Health Organisation's (WHO) Collaborating Centre on AIDS in Paris, while worldwide figures are available from the WHO in Geneva.[1]

Estimates in the Netherlands put the number of HIV-infected persons in 1987 at between 10,000 and 20,000 and forecast a cumulative total of more than 3,000 people with AIDS by 1990, for whom 136-300 beds would be needed (Houweling et al., 1987; Dutch Health Council, 1987). In fact, these forecasts proved to be too pessimistic: on 31.12.1990 the cumulative total of people with AIDS, corrected for the lagging-behind of the reports, was 1,652, with the number of HIV-infected persons being estimated at 7,500-9,000 and 9,000-12,000 respectively (Van de Water et al., 1990; Jager et al., 1990b). The estimate in Chapter 3 of this study is also of this order, i.e. a cumulative total of 6,000-7,000 HIV-infected persons at 1.9.1989.

Recent estimates have been based on a more refined back-calculation technique, more data were available on the incidence of AIDS, and the incubation period was better documented. In view of the lack of data on seroprevalence, (determinants of) risk-producing behaviour, and uncertainty concerning the doubling time (rate of

---

1 As regards forecasts of the development of AIDS which (also) relate to the Netherlands, reference can be made to publications by Chin et al. (1990), Downs et al. (1987, 1988), Jager et al. (1988, 1989, 1990ab), Heisterkamp et al. (1989), Bindels et al. (1990), Verbrugh (1990), Houweling et al. (1987, 1990) and Van de Water et al. (1990). A recent report is also available from a workshop organized by the Centers for Disease Control (CDC) in Atlanta, USA, which gives the results of forecasts on AIDS in the US up to 1993 (CDC, 1990).
In addition to the above publications, which are based primarily on AIDS diagnoses and the application of mathematical models, forecasts have also been made which are based on Farr's Law (Vandenbroucke 1990), seroprevalence data combined with estimates of the size of core groups (Cox et al., 1989), and calculations of the risk of spread of the epidemic based on the Basic Reproduction Rate (Bonneux and Houweling, 1989).

spread of the epidemic), epidemiological prognoses are not made for periods longer than three years ahead. Figure 6.1 shows the most recent estimate of AIDS incidence for the period 1991-1993, with the associated confidence intervals (Jager et al. 1990b).

Figure 6.1 **Reported and corrected AIDS incidence per half-year (A = first half-year, B = second half-year), model modifications, extrapolations up to and including 1993 and limits of the 95% confidence interval. Calculations based on reports at 1.1.91.** (Source: GHI).

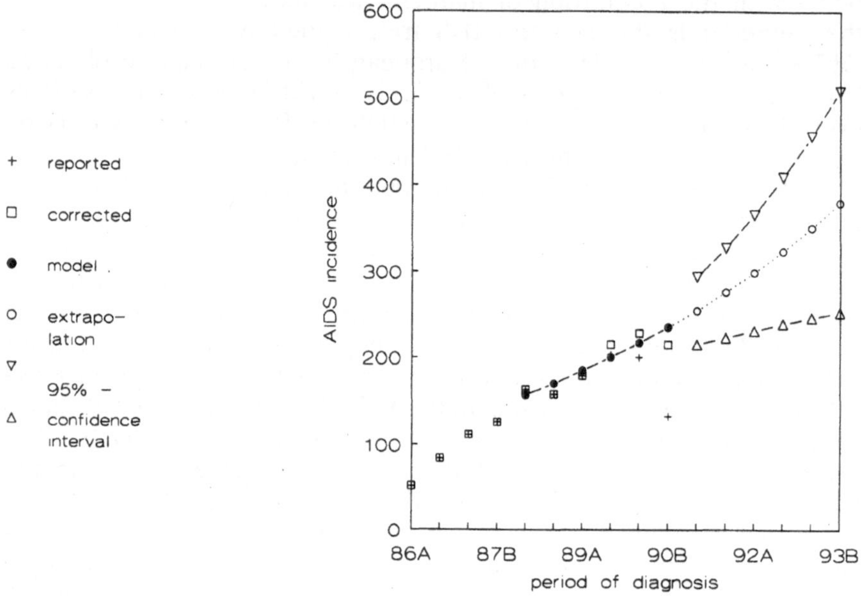

The reference scenario uses the same type of data and similar methods to those on which short-term extrapolations are based. Just as with these short-term extrapolations, therefore, we have had to contend with margins of uncertainty, which means that forecasts for the medium term are not justified. A medium-term perspective can be included in scenario analyses, however, because these involve *projections* of the consequences of AIDS up to the year 2000 rather than forecasts.

6.2 *Methods, data and underlying principles*

Chapter 2 introduced the reference scenario and the method of scenario analysis. The reference scenario relates to the period 1991-2000 and is based on the assumption that *no fundamental changes* take place with respect to the baseline analysis. In other words, the current epidemiological course continues unaltered, the fight against AIDS and the care of people with AIDS continue to be as effective over the next 10 years as at the end of the 1980s, and the social context of the epidemic is not fundamentally different in 2000 than in 1990. The baseline analyses in Chapters 3-5 describe the initial situations which form the basis of the reference scenario.

The reference scenario looks at the epidemiological course and its impact from an economic and socio-cultural perspective. Various parameters were identified for the purpose of the scenario analysis, and these form the basis for studying projected final situations of the epidemic and provide indicators which express the epidemiological course and its consequences. Table 2.1 in Chapter 2 contains these parameters and indicators.

The epidemiological studies in the reference scenario were carried out using statistical modelling techniques. The empirical basis of the epidemiological course in this chapter consists of notifications of AIDS corrected for reporting delays, and the estimated seroprevalence up to 1.1.1989, estimated with the help of back-calculation. We have taken account in the studies of the degree of progression towards AIDS and the possible spread of the epidemic, by linking data on the incubation period distribution and assumptions concerning the doubling time. This was discussed in detail in Chapter 2.

Projections of the impact of HIV/AIDS must take account of the fact that the incubation period is a long one. Some of the impact of AIDS for the health care sector in the coming decade are therefore attributable to developments which took place in the first decade of the HIV epidemic. As far as HIV/AIDS prevention is concerned, this means that the impact of the disease up to the year 2000 can only partially be averted through public information and the promotion of behavioural change.

In the elaboration of the reference scenario we express this by splitting the impact of AIDS into two components: (1) a reference scenario in which the impact of AIDS are projected on the basis of an unchanged continuation of the present trend in the doubling time, and (2) a subscenario, in which those consequences of AIDS are projected which can be attributed entirely to epidemiological developments in the first decade. Henceforth we shall refer to the scenario which follows path (1) as the *reference scenario* and the scenario based on (2) as the *subscenario.*

(1) is based on an epidemiological course in which we extrapolate the current trend in AIDS incidence forward to the year 2000. In mathematical modelling terms this amounts to a projection based on an assumed increasing doubling time, i.e. a slowdown in the growth of the incidence of AIDS. The assumptions made for the incubation period distribution are based on the compartmental model discussed in Chapter 2, adapted to take account of data from the San Francisco Clinic Cohort Study (Lifson et al., 1990), with 11 years as the average term of the progression to AIDS. It has also been assumed that 100% of HIV-infected persons ultimately develop AIDS. We have taken two years as the survival period following diagnosis of AIDS.

Given current insights, the reference scenario offers the best approximation of the impact of AIDS up to the year 2000. The subscenario is based on an approximation of the development in HIV infections up to 1.1.1989. The back-calculation method based on the quadratic exponential function, as set out in the Appendix to Chapter 2, was used in estimating the course of the HIV epidemic. The other assumptions are the same as those in the reference scenario.

The subscenario has a function at the level of target-setting, and comparison with the reference scenario gives an impression of the degree to which the AIDS crisis can be steered through public information and the promotion of behavioural change.

In order to obtain an *indication* of the maximum effect of primary prevention through public information and the promotion of behavioural change, the impact of the spread of HIV in the first decade must be separated out to leave the impact of the reference scenario: this is logical, since the HIV incidence shown by the subscenario can no longer be combated through an HIV/AIDS-prevention programme. It should be emphasized that the subscenario is a component of the reference scenario, and must not be seen as an alternative to it or a "best case" variant of it. It is assumed in the subscenario that no more HIV infection has occurred since 1.1.1989, whereas in fact Chapters 3 and 4 discuss in some detail HIV infections since this date. The subscenario thus gives too low an estimate of those consequences of the reference scenario which can no longer be influenced through public information and behavioural change. Accounting for the high degree of uncertainty concerning seroprevalence in the Netherlands means it is at the moment the most accurate way to express the unavoidable consequences of AIDS.

The impact associated with the epidemiological projections is expressed using indicators. To some extent these are consequences which are directly dependent on the incidence and prevalence of AIDS/HIV, such as the number of PYLL, the lethality and the patient-related economic impact. To some extent also, they are the consequences not directly linked to developments in the epidemics, such as the costs of testing and of HIV/AIDS-prevention programmes, and the socio-cultural consequences of AIDS. Table 6.1 summarizes the aspects which have been differentiated within the reference scenario. The left-hand column contains the elements of the reference scenario, while the right-hand column lists the sections of this Chapter where these elements are discussed.

Table 6.1 **Elements of the reference scenario: impact of AIDS in 1995 and 2000.**

Elements of reference scenario (and subscenario)	**Section**
Socio-epidemiological aspects	
- incidence and prevalence of AIDS/HIV	6.3
- PYLL/lethality	6.3
Consequences of AIDS	
- patient-related economic impact	6.4.1
- programme-level impact for general programmes	6.4.2
Social context	6.5

6.3 Reference scenario and subscenario: epidemiological aspects

Figure 6.2 shows the reported AIDS incidence, corrected for reporting delays, in the period 1982-1990, and two projections of the epidemiological course, up to 1995 and 2000 respectively. Figure 6.3 shows the estimates of AIDS prevalence.

It can be seen from Figure 6.2 that the incidence of AIDS rises from 635 in 1995 to 747 in the year 2000. On the basis of the HIV epidemic up to 1.1.1989, an AIDS incidence of 415 in 1995 appears unavoidable, while at least 230 AIDS patients can be expected in the year 2000. By way of comparison, the AIDS incidence in 1990, corrected for reporting delays, was 443. The subscenario shows that if no new HIV infections had occurred after the 1.1.1989, the AIDS incidence in 1985 would be 30% higher in 1995 and 66% higher in the year 2000, than in the reference scenario. This gives an *impression* of the HIV incidence which can *potentially* be averted through AIDS prevention.

Figure 6.2 **AIDS incidence per year in the reference scenario and the subscenario: reported and corrected for reporting delays (up to and including 1990), and extrapolated to the year 2000. Reference scenario: extrapolation of current trend in AIDS incidence; subscenario: course of the AIDS epidemic resulting from the HIV incidence up to 1.1.1989.**

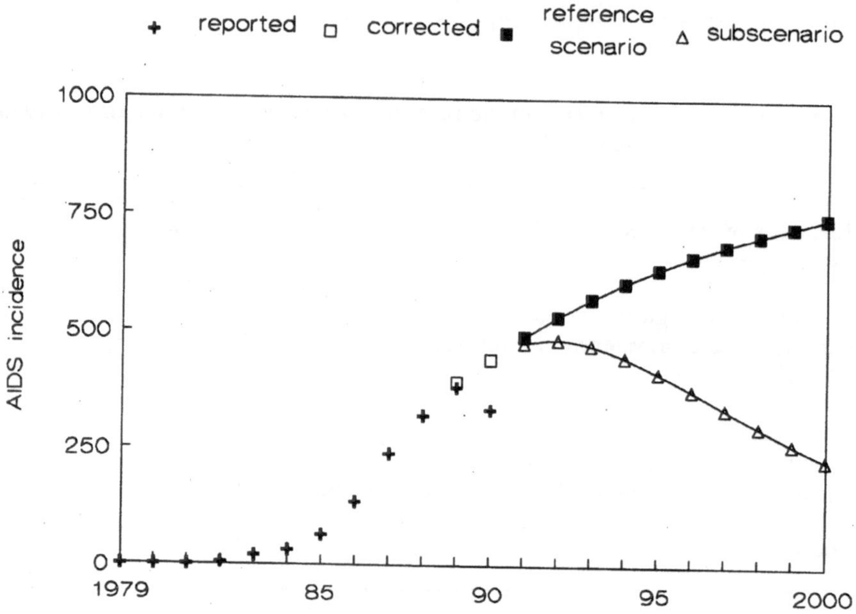

Table 6.2 contains a numerical summary of the epidemiological results of the reference scenario. The figures between brackets are the results of the subscenario. The table shows the incidence at 31 December and the prevalence at 30 June; the latter date was chosen because linking with cost studies is carried out on the basis of prevalence midway through the year. In addition to data on the HIV/AIDS epidemic, calculations of lethality and PYLL are also given.

It can be seen that for the period 1982-2000, with unchanged developments, a cumulative AIDS incidence of rather more than 8,000 must be expected. The subscenario shows that allowance must in any event be made for *more* than 5,459 people with AIDS. Expressed in terms of cumulative AIDS incidence over the period 1991-2000, this gives figures of 6,366, and *more* than 3,807 respectively. Compared with the cumulative AIDS incidence of 1,652 up to 1.1.1991, this means that the AIDS incidence in the period 1991-2000 will be almost four times as high as in the first decade of the epidemic. The subscenario shows that the cumulative AIDS incidence in the period 1991-2000 will in any event be twice as high as the cumulative AIDS incidence up to 1.1.1991.

The lethality figures show that, with an unchanged survival period, the cumulative total of people dying from AIDS will increase substantially over the next 10 years, from an estimated 560 up to 1989 (CBS, 1991) to more than 6,500 in the year 2000. The subscenario shows that by the year 2000 almost 5,000 persons will have died from AIDS.

Table 6.2 **Reference scenario: epidemiological aspects of AIDS/HIV in 1995 and 2000 (figures between brackets relate to subscenario: epidemiological aspects on the basis of the HIV epidemic up to 1.1.1989).**

	1995		2000	
AIDS incidence	635	(415)	747	(230)
AIDS prevalence	1,208	(892)	1,456	(528)
Cumulative AIDS incidence 1991-...	2,835	(2,299)	6,366	(3,807)
Cumulative AIDS incidence 1982-...	4,487	(3,951)	8,018	(5,459)
HIV prevalence	9,171	(3,884)	10,382	(1,920)
Cumulative HIV incidence 1979-...	12,506	(6,736)	16,998	(6,736)
Lethality	3,247	(3,088)	6,543	(4,966)
PYLL (per 1000 population)	1.27	(1.05)	1.53	(0.65)

Figure 6.3 and the prevalence figures in Table 6.2 enable an assessment to be made of the increase which, according to the reference scenario, can be expected in the demand for health care facilities up to the year 2000. At an assumed constant average survival period of two years, the AIDS prevalence amounts to 1208 in 1995 and 1456 in the year 2000. Of these two totals, almost 900 and more than 500, respectively, will be people with AIDS who became infected during the first decade of the epidemic. By way of comparison, on 1.1.1991 the estimated AIDS prevalence was 716. In other words, the reference scenario predicts twice as many people with AIDS in the year 2000 as in 1991.

Figure 6.3 **AIDS prevalence in the reference scenario and subscenario. Assumptions: survival period following diagnosis of AIDS is two years, otherwise identical to figure 6.2.**

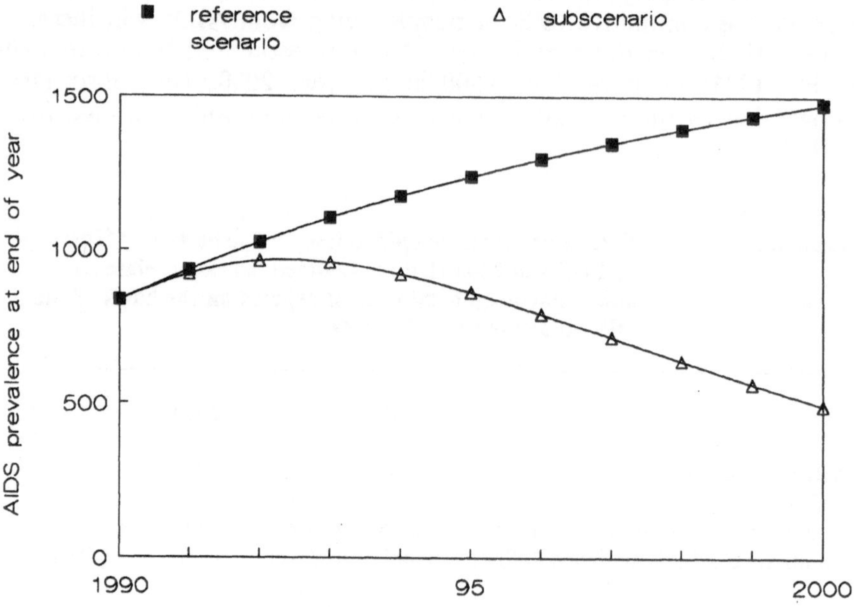

In Chapter 3 the PYLL for 1990 was fixed at 0.75 per 1000 inhabitants. In Table 6.2 the PYLL in the reference scenario is 1.53 in the year 2000, an increase of more than 100% compared to 1990. The PYLL figure gains extra significance when compared with other illnesses (Jager et al., 1990c). Figure 6.4 is an update of Jager et al. (1990c), and shows a comparison with the PYLL per 1000 inhabitants as a result of lung cancer, road traffic accidents, infectious diseases other than AIDS, and suicide. The PYLL for causes of death other than AIDS is based on linear extrapolation from the mortality statistics for the period 1980-1988 (Dutch Central Statistical Office), and is set against the PYLL resulting from AIDS in the reference scenario. Figure 6.4 shows that by 1990 the PYLL from AIDS has reached the PYLL level resulting from other infectious diseases, and that by 1995 the level begins to approach the extrapolated PYLL resulting from road traffic accidents and suicide.

Figure 6.4 **PYLL per 1000 inhabitants: observations and extrapolations. AIDS incidence according to the reference scenario.**

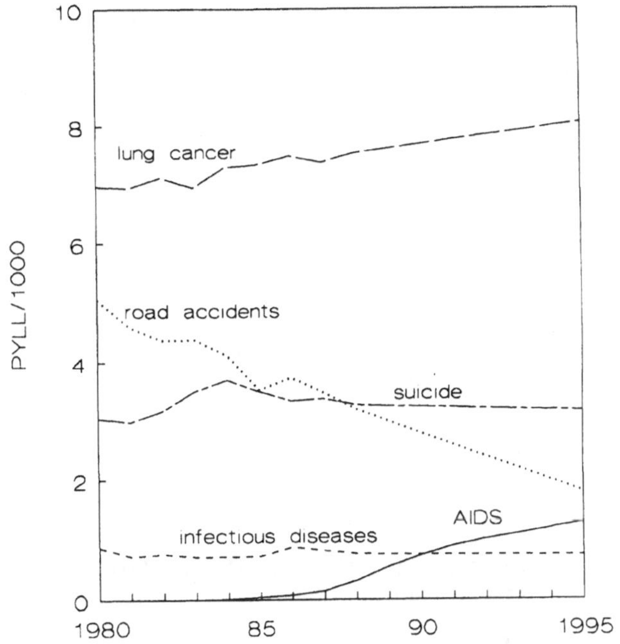

6.3.1 Incidence and prevalence of HIV in 1995 and 2000

The incidence of AIDS shown in the reference scenario is based on the postulated development of the HIV incidence. We have determined this development using the back-calculation method devised by Hay (1989) and the assumptions regarding the incubation period distribution which also form the basis of the subscenario projection.[2] Figure 6.5 shows a reconstruction of the HIV incidence from 1979 onwards for the reference scenario and the subscenario; Figure 6.6 shows the prevalence in the pre-AIDS stage.
The reconstruction of the number of HIV infections in the subscenario shows an increase in the incidence of AIDS up to and including 1985, followed by a sharp fall in 1987 and 1988. In the reference scenario projection, this rise and fall is even more marked. It can also be seen that the estimated HIV incidence in the reference scenario is almost 2000 in the period 1989-1990. The projected cumulative incidence for the period 1989-2000 would be around 12,000 - almost twice as many as in the period 1979-1988.

---

[2] Hay's working method is described in the Appendix to Chapter 2.

Figure 6.5 **Estimated HIV incidence in reference scenario and subscenario.**

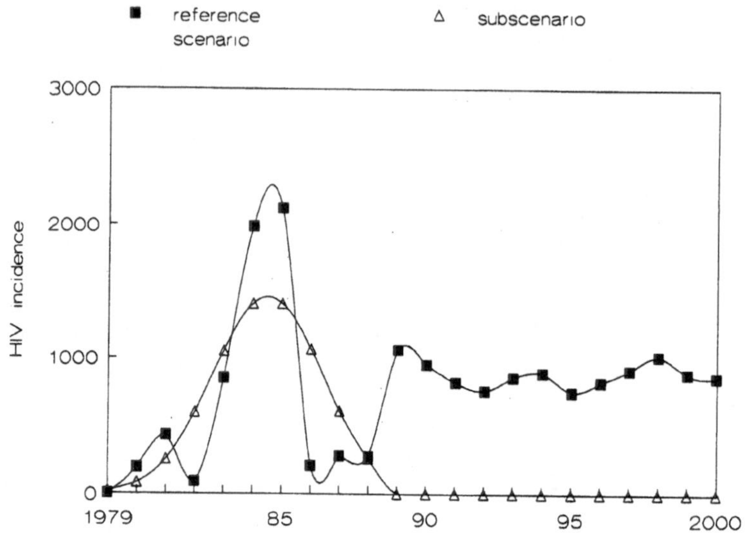

Figure 6.6 **Estimated prevalence in the pre-AIDS stage in reference scenario and subscenario.**

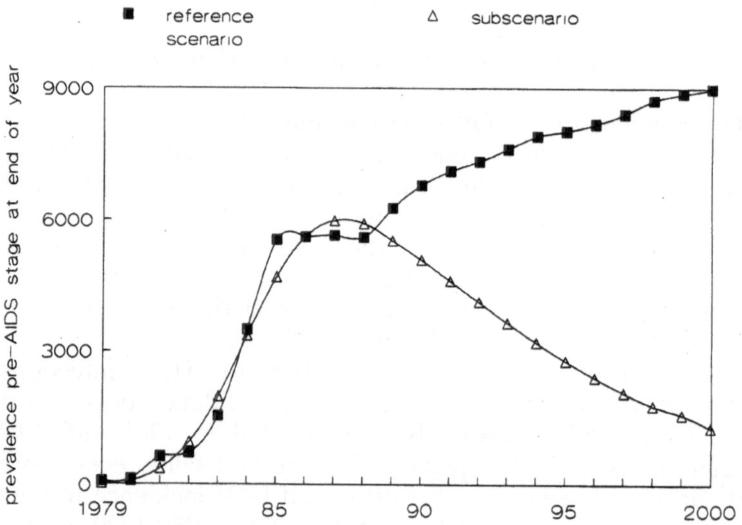

Figure 6.6 expresses the prevalence in the pre-AIDS stage. Adding the AIDS prevalence from Figure 6.3 gives the HIV prevalence. Table 6.2 shows the HIV prevalence estimates which result from this addition - more than 9,100 HIV-infected persons halfway 1995 and more than 10,000 halfway the year 2000.

The estimate of HIV incidence in the reference scenario can also be evaluated from the perspective of HIV/AIDS prevention. The expectation that there will be new HIV infections during the next ten years would seem to be realistic. The literature contains specific instructions for avoiding risk behaviour and relapse amongst men who have sex with men. The AIDS incidence projected in the reference scenario corresponds to an HIV incidence of 750-1000 per year in the period 1991-2000. This is the same as the 1986 level of incidence, and is considerably higher than the incidence in 1987-1988. An important question for the HIV/AIDS prevention effort is how much pressure this development in the HIV epidemic puts on the underlying principles of the reference scenario: is this level of HIV incidence possible with an unchanged effect of HIV/AIDS prevention and a concentration of HIV infections among gay men and IDUs? A further relevant question as a direct corollary to this concerns the degree to which the HIV incidence in the reference scenario justifies extra efforts to combat HIV. We shall return to the consequences for HIV/AIDS prevention in a strategic sense in the Commentary.

6.4 *Impact of HIV/AIDS in 1995 and 2000*

6.4.1 *Patient-related impact of HIV/AIDS*

Section 5.2 describes the patient-related economic impact of AIDS to date and formulates assumptions for the scenario analysis. Table 5.3 in Chapter 5 gives for each indicator the assumptions which we adopt here.

As regards the in-hospital costs, a number of assumptions proved to be possible. For calculations on the basis of prevalence we assumed a cost of NLG 35,900-47,400 per person year in the AIDS stage and NLG 4,700-8,500 in the pre-AIDS stage. These costings are based on hospitalization periods ranging from 51.1 to 52.5 days. Since recent analyses have shown that the number of hospitalization days has fallen to something over 27 (Dijkgraaf et al., 1991) we shall look in the reference scenario at a bed use of both 52.5 days (KPMG, 1989abc), and 27.3 per person year. No analysis has yet been carried out of the implications for hospital costs of the observed fall in bed use, and the cost calculations have therefore been based on a bed requirement of 51.1-52.5 days (Postma et al., accepted). A bed occupancy of 75% is assumed.

Table 6.3 **Patient-related economic impact of HIV/AIDS in 1995 and 2000. Reference scenario and subscenario (between brackets); 1988 cost level. Assumptions relating to persons in the pre-AIDS stage: in the subscenario 50% are *aware* of seropositivity in 1995, 75% in the year 2000; in the reference scenario, 25% are *aware* of seropositive status.**

Bed need				
Hospitals				
- 27.3 days/person-year AIDS[1]	128	(95)	154	(57)
- 52.5 days/person-year AIDS[2]	333	(247)	393	(154)
Nursing homes	10	(7)	12	(4)
A: Costs (NLG * 1,000,000)				
Hospitals				
- Borleffs et al. (1990)	66.6	(49.3)	79.5	(29.9)
- KPMG (1989abc)	60.3	(44.7)	71.2	(27.8)
Nursing homes	0.8	(0.6)	1.0	(0.4)
Out-of-hospital care need				
District nursing contact hours	12,700	(9,400)	15,300	(5,500)
Home help contact hours	24,764	(18,286)	29,800	(10,800)
General practitioner consultations	24,025	(17,896)	27,900	(11,500)
Days intensive home care	700	(500)	800	(300)
RIAGG/AMW	memorandum[3]		memorandum	
B: Costs (NLG * 1,000,000)				
District nursing	1.1	(0.8)	1.4	(0.5)
Home help	1.3	(1.0)	1.6	(0.6)
General practitioner	1.0	(0.8)	1.2	(0.5)
Intensive home care	0.1	(0.1)	0.2	(0.1)
AZT use at home	6.6	(4.8)	7.9	(2.9)
Total costs (A + B) (NLG * 1,000,000)[4]	77	(57)	93	(35)
Buddy help				
Requests	115	(75)	135	(40)
Hours	90,000	(68,000)	106,00	(40,000)
Drug-dependency outreach	memorandum		memorandum	
Care for next of kin/survivors	memorandum		memorandum	

1 Source: Dijkgraaf et al., 1991
2 Source: KPMG, 1989abc
3 Memorandum: No adequate indication found, either in hours or costs
4 Based on Borleffs et al., 1990

Table 6.3 shows the impact of AIDS for the care sectors described in Chapter 5 for the reference scenario and the subscenario. This is based on the assumption that it is possible to meet the need for care. All financial figures are based on the 1988 cost level.

It should be emphasized that, although Table 6.3 reflects a considerable proportion of the direct patient-related costs, it does not give a total picture. We are therefore dealing with a summary of the *minimum* patient-related consequences of AIDS. A number of cost items have been included as memorandum items: these are costs for which no adequate information is available. In addition, the summary does not show the financial indirect costs of HIV and AIDS.

Information on the use of care and the costs in the pre-AIDS stage is based on seropositives who are *aware* of their HIV infection. We have used the assumption from Chapter 5 in the reference scenario, namely that 25% of the HIV-infected persons are *aware* of their seropositivity (Health Council, 1990). In the subscenario it has been assumed that 50% of the HIV-infected persons in 1995, and 75% in the year 2000, are aware of their condition. This assumption is based on the idea that the percentage of people who are aware of their seropositive status will increase over time due to contacts with the support organizations resulting from HIV-related complaints, or due to use being made of alternative test locations. The calculated HIV-related costs are based on HIV prevalence estimates.

Table 6.3 shows that in the year 2000 (52.5 days per person-year, the hospital bed need for HIV/AIDS will be 393. Comparing this with the subscenario, we see that half the number of beds for AIDS patients are occupied by persons who became infected during the period 1991-2000.

According to the reference scenario, this represents a need for 0.60% of the average total of 66,000 recognized beds in 1989. In nursing homes, 10 beds are needed for HIV/AIDS in the year 2000, which is 0.05% of the average total of 27,000 recognized nursing home beds for somatic patients in 1989.

Table 6.3 shows the following care categories expressed in financial terms: hospitals, nursing homes, general practitioners, district nursing, home help, intensive home care, and use of AZT at home. The sum of these amounts gives a total for the reference scenario of NLG 77 million in 1995 and NLG 93 million in the year 2000. The results emerging from the subscenario suggest that more than NLG 57 million will have to be set aside for 1995, and over NLG 35 million for the year 2000. In other words, maximally effective HIV/AIDS prevention after 1.1.1989 will have succeeded in reducing the costs of care in the year 2000 to less than 40% of the projected figure of NLG

93 million if developments continue unchanged.

Wiggers and Bergsma (1990ab) have estimated the minimum direct patient-related costs in 1988 at just under NLG 19 million. Table 6.3 shows that in the reference scenario the costs in 2000 are almost five times higher than this. Moreover, looking at costs in the subscenario shows that the consequences of AIDS/HIV for the health care sector *only become fully apparent after some time*. The subscenario also shows that the costs of HIV/AIDS continue to be higher than in 1988 up to the year 2000. It hardly needs pointing out that the subscenario underestimates the minimum costs to be expected.

Figure 6.7 compares the direct patient-related costs of HIV and AIDS with trends described in the Financial Statement on Health Care 1991 (Ministry of Welfare, Health and Cultural Affairs, 1991) for the categories hospitals, nursing homes (including psychogeriatric homes), general practitioners, district nursing, home help, intensive home care and pharmaceutical help.

Figure 6.7 **Costs (in millions NLG) according to the reference scenario of hospital care, nursing home care, district nursing care, home help, intensive home care and general practitioner care and medication use for HIV/AIDS; a comparison with the Financial Statement on Health Care, FOZ (Ministry of Welfare, Health and Cultural Affairs, 1991).**

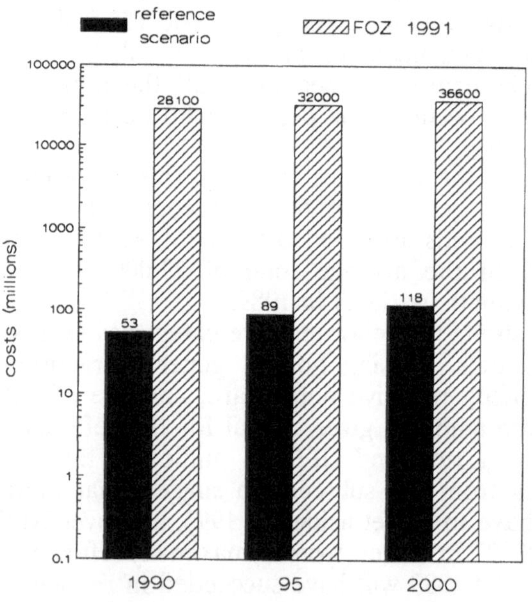

In the Financial Statement on Health Care we estimate the trend in terms of volume and cost level (the nominal growth) by extrapolation, based on the average annual growth per category over the period 1985-1989. This results in the following growth percentages: hospitals 1.5%; nursing homes 2.8%; district nursing 4.6%; home help 1.8%; general practitioners 5.0%. A figure of 5.0% has been taken for pharmaceutical help. This is lower than the growth percentage over the period 1985-1989, to allow for agreements on restriction of the growth (All Party Agreement). For intensive home care the 1990 volume was taken as a norm, and a nominal growth of 2 per cent applied.

In order to be able to compare the costs of HIV/AIDS with the Financial Statement on Health Care, a nominal growth figure for HIV/AIDS was also introduced, with 1988 being taken as the base year. This nominal growth was assumed to be 2 per cent, the average for the whole health care sector over the period 1985-1989. The costs of HIV/AIDS in the reference scenario amount to 0.28% of the cost estimate according to the Financial Statement on Health Care for 1995 (0.21% in the subscenario); for the year 2000 this percentage is 0.32% (0.12% in the subscenario). The cost categories selected make up almost 50% of the total health care costs in 1989 (Ministry of Welfare, Health and Cultural Affairs, 1991). We have based our estimates of hospital costs on Borleffs et al. (1990).

6.4.2 Non-patient-related impact of HIV/AIDS

In addition to patient-related consequences, AIDS also has consequences at programme level, such as the costs of prevention, research, policy and support and the costs of screening stocks of blood. These programme costs are only partially dependent on the epidemiological developments. With an unchanged policy, these costs will show little difference in 1995 and 2000 from their level in 1988. As in Chapter 5, therefore, we have adopted the following estimates of these costs: NLG 16 million for information and prevention; NLG 14 million for research; NLG 11 million for tests; NLG 6 million for miscellaneous costs. Adding these cost items together gives a total of NLG 47 million. In the case of prevention, the costs of preventive measures by dentists and in hospitals have not been included.

The estimate of programme costs must be considered as a minimum estimate. If developments continue unchanged, intensification of the needle exchange programme can be expected (Hartgers et al.,

1989; NCAB 1990).[3] A higher level of HIV prevalence will also mean that the number of conformation tests will be greater than to date. We shall return to the effects of early intervention on the costs of testing in Chapter 8.

6.4.3 Direct costs of HIV/AIDS

Figure 6.8 shows the direct costs of HIV/AIDS in 1990, 1995 and 2000. The costs in the reference scenario amount to NLG 124 million in 1995 and NLG 140 million in the year 2000, which represents an increase in the annual costs in the period 1990 to 2000 of more than NLG 40 million. In the subscenario, the costs amount to NLG 104 million in 1995 and in the year 2000 to NLG 82 million. The increase in the reference scenario is due entirely to developments in patient-related costs, which increase from 48% of total costs in 1990 to 67% in 2000.

Figure 6.8 can also be read from a target-setting perspective. It then becomes apparent that efforts in HIV/AIDS prevention, particularly in the period 1995 to 2000, can make a great difference to the costs. In 1995, the difference between the subscenario and the reference scenario is something over NLG 20 million, while by the year 2000 it has risen to NLG 60 million. Prevention efforts after 1990 could counter this rise in costs in the short and medium term. As regards the programme costs, Figure 6.8 suggests that the return on expenses for HIV/AIDS prevention in the *ideal* case could lead to a maximum return of NLG 60 million in the year 2000. A constant sum for HIV/AIDS prevention of NLG 16 million is assumed in the reference scenario, and a major question is to what extent this can produce a return of up to NLG 60 million in the year 2000. We shall return to this in the Commentary.

From a target-setting perspective, Figure 6.8 can also give rise to questions regarding the potential for reduction of patient-related costs. In this connection, we would refer to the limiting conditions for care, such as maintenance and, where possible, improvement of the current available treatment, and ensuring the provision of high quality care. In Chapter 8 we shall look in detail at the cost aspects of substitution of care.

---

[3] Extrapolation from current developments suggests a figure of 18 million needles in 1995 and 20 million in 2000, with half the needles being distributed within Amsterdam and half elsewhere.

Figure 6.8 **Patient-related and general programme costs: reference scenario and subscenario (1988 cost level; in millions NLG). Hospital costs are based on Borleffs et al. (1990).**

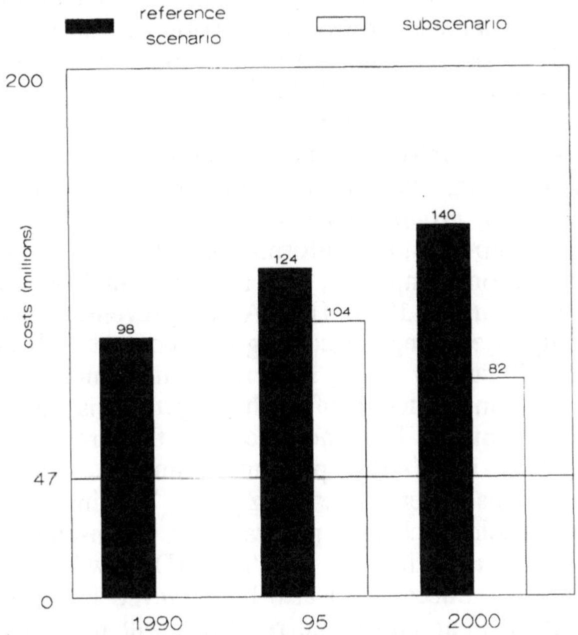

6.5 *The social context of the reference scenario*

Chapter 4 contains a description and analysis of the social context of the AIDS/HIV epidemic, and in the reference scenario this social context remains broadly unchanged. Expressed in terms of the parameters and indicators for scenario analysis, this amounts to the following:

The openness about (homo)sexuality which has arisen as a result of AIDS is permanent. The level of knowledge about AIDS and the transmission routes of HIV and other sexually transmitted diseases remains high. The need for protection during high-risk sexual behaviour is recognized. The incidence of sexually transmitted diseases (STDs), which fell in the mid-1980s and rose slightly at the end of that decade, remains below the level of the 1970s. Periodically repeated public information and prevention campaigns contribute to this and result in a growing realization that protection against sexually transmitted diseases is an essential element of sexual contact. This does not lead to large shifts in attitudes to sexuality.

Although the reassessment of the risks associated with unprotected anal sexual contact, in particular, has had some effect on the sexual behaviour itself, it is not possible to make absolute statements: on the one hand there are indications of behavioural change, particularly with respect to multiple partners, while on the other hand no large shifts have been found in sales of condoms, multiple partners or visits to commercial sex workers. Moreover, sexual behaviour is characterized by heterogeneity, which among other things includes (temporary) increases into risk behaviour.

In an unchanged situation, AIDS control in the year 2000 will be based on public information and the promotion of behavioural change. In addition, specific epidemiological monitoring will be carried out among groups which are susceptible to HIV and STD. The target group-oriented information strategy, combined with general information campaigns, will have attained a wider reach in the year 2000 than in 1990: HIV/AIDS prevention will have succeeded among other things in coming into contact with groups which are currently difficult to reach, such as ethnic minorities and foreign sex workers. The introduction of further regulations, such as abolition of the ban on brothels, have no effect on the prevention of HIV/-AIDS and STDs. HIV/AIDS prevention among hard-drug users is expected to increase over the coming years. The increasing effectiveness of the needle exchange programmes, counselling and bleach campaigns means that the risk profile of IDUs will be lower in the 2000 than in 1990. Success will also be achieved in the societal aims of AIDS control. Fear and panic reactions will not occur and there will be a degree of sympathy for people with HIV and AIDS, with no large-scale ostracism of those infected with HIV. In addition, the high level of tolerance towards to homosexuality in the Netherlands will continue unchanged.

The situation with respect to blood banks will be no less safe in the year 2000 than in 1985. The free movement of services and goods as a result of "Europe 1992" will have no effect on this or on any other aspects of the reference scenario. The increased movement of people has no consequences for the spread of HIV. The costs and organization of health care will also show no essential changes during the coming decade. The approach to the care of people with AIDS and HIV will continue to be characterized in the year 2000 by an integrated approach to the psychosocial, psychiatric and somatic problems of HIV infection and AIDS. Care will be provided in a coordinated way, and the planned and systematic dissemination of experience and expertise will contribute to the provision of high quality care.

Efforts in AIDS control and the care of people with AIDS cannot be seen separately from the safeguarding of individual civil rights. In conflicts surrounding the administration of the HIV-test and access to social facilities, individual civil rights relating to the protection of privacy and the integrity of the human body play a decisive role. A separate point of concern will be the new therapies which may be available in the year 2000. The rules of good medical practice in clinical trials, and the interest of people with AIDS in obtaining potentially helpful drugs as quickly as possible after their discovery, have led to changes in the procedures surrounding clinical trials, with active medicines being made available as early as possible to all patients who wish to be considered for them.

6.5 Commentary

The reference scenario shows that the expectations in the medium term are less sombre than the short-term prognoses put forward by Houweling et al. (1987), who estimated that the seroprevalence in 1987 would be as high as 10,000-20,000, and who did not rule out an AIDS incidence of almost 2000 in 1990. In the reference scenario we predict an AIDS incidence in the year 2000 of 747, and a cumulative total of HIV-infected persons of almost 17,000.

The reference scenario shows that such comparisons must not lead to optimism or complacency concerning the impact of AIDS up to the year 2000. Above all, the reference scenario makes clear that the impact of AIDS will only become *fully apparent* in the second decade of the epidemic. A doubling of the AIDS prevalence and a tripling of the patient-related costs compared to 1990 are likely. In addition, the reference scenario suggests that more than 6,500 persons will have died from AIDS by the year 2000.

The reference scenario also casts its shadow over the period beyond the year 2000, since a large part of the impact of the spread of HIV in the period 1991-2000 will only become apparent in the third decade of the AIDS epidemic. In this connection, the HIV incidence projected in the reference scenario for the period 1991-2000 is in fact greater than the estimated cumulative HIV incidence up to 1.1.1989.

There is a sizeable difference between the AIDS/HIV incidence in the reference scenario and that in the subscenario, and this difference increases over time. Directly in line with this, the reconstructed HIV incidence in the reference scenario shows that continued efforts in the area of public information and the promotion of behavioural change could enable thousands of HIV infections to be prevented. The reference scenario therefore leads to the conclusion that continued efforts in AIDS control are a necessary part of HIV/-AIDS prevention.

In the reference scenario the prevention efforts have been subsumed under the programme costs at 1988 levels. Similarly it has been assumed that HIV/AIDS prevention over the next ten years will remain as effective as in the past, and also that the present intensity of prevention efforts will have achieved as yet unattained targets by the year 2000. Kok (1991) refers in this connection to the phenomenon of "diminished returns" and states that, for an unchanged effect with respect to the baseline analysis, increased prevention efforts will be required. Section 6.3.3 refers to a financial return of up to NLG 60 million on prevention efforts in the medium term. Set against the present prevention budget of NLG 16 million, this means that a quadrupling of the prevention budget would still be financially viable. Obviously, the deaths and suffering which this will prevent are of much greater importance than the financial returns.

In the reference scenario the annual incidence of HIV in the period 1991-2000, with unchanged developments in the AIDS incidence, is estimated at between 750 and 1000. This is equal to the HIV incidence in 1986 in the subscenario, i.e. for the period in which the largest fall in HIV incidence was found in cohort studies. It is relevant in this connection to ask whether the reference scenario implicitly assumes a relapse into risk behaviour and/or a certain spread of HIV beyond the networks, core groups and geographical regions where the HIV epidemic began. It is also possible that, contrary to the description of the social context, there is a spread of HIV among ethnic minorities or an increase in HIV incidence as a result of the increasing mobility. If these developments were implicitly assumed in the reference scenario, this would lead to the projection of a future end-situation which conflicts with the assumptions of the reference scenario. If, on the other hand, the HIV incidence in the reference scenario is the result of unchanged developments, then the conclusion must be that AIDS control in the Netherlands is still far from achieving its goals. In this case, increased or more effective prevention efforts would seem to be indicated, rather than a continuation of the present level of the prevention effort.

From a societal perspective, a final situation is described in the reference scenario in which AIDS does not lead to radical changes in society. A great many underlying assumptions have been formulated in this connection, including the absence or fear and panic reactions, the safeguarding of individual civil rights, the fight against discrimination, the organization of high quality care and support, and the making available of new drugs at an early stage.

It has been implicitly assumed here that the present AIDS policy will continue, consisting essentially of an integrated approach to the biological, psychological and social consequences of AIDS. Apart from specific underlying principles in AIDS control which result from the Dutch socio-cultural and legal/ethical philosophy as characterized in Chapter 4, this also leads directly to activities such as seeking a solution to the insurance question and monitoring the guidelines covering use of the HIV-test during medicals for potential employees. It has been assumed that these matters will have been resolved by the year 2000. A change in the AIDS policy or the failure to find solutions to societal problems could have direct consequences for the epidemiological course, though this need not necessarily be the case. At any event, it leads to questions about the consequences for the maintenance of what can be termed "the public acceptance of the epidemic".

In this chapter we have elected not to compile a best-case and worst-case variant of the reference scenario. The projection of the consequences of AIDS in the subscenario is an over-optimistic approximation of a best-case variant: in contrast to what is assumed in the subscenario, there will indeed be a spread of HIV after 1.1.1989. The impact of AIDS will therefore, even in a best-case variant of the reference scenario, be *more widespread* than in the subscenario.

In theory, a projection of a worst-case variant could be based on an epidemiological course which in turn is based on the assumption of a constant doubling time of the AIDS incidence. In mathematical terms this amounts to extrapolation of the linear relationship between the logarithm of the AIDS incidence and time. Just as in the reference scenario, this projection could be based on AIDS incidence data from the last three years. This leads to a projection of the impact of AIDS based on constant growth in AIDS incidence as an alternative to the reference scenario, which is based on a decline in the growth of AIDS incidence.

Projections up to 1995, not presented in this chapter, show that such a variant leads to an explosive increase in the incidence of HIV and AIDS, with an AIDS incidence in 1995 of rather more than 1,000 and an HIV incidence of around 4,000 - almost a doubling and quadrupling, respectively, of the figures in the reference scenario. Extrapolation to the year 2000 would in effect amount to the projection of a doomsday scenario. Given the observed trend in AIDS incidence to date and the data from the baseline analyses in Chapters 3 and 4, this seems to us to be an over-pessimistic variant of the reference scenario.

In the construction of the reference scenario and the consideration of variants of this scenario, we are reminded yet again of the great uncertainty concerning the possible impact of AIDS. Scenario analyses may, for example, be hampered by a lack of data on seroprevalence, progression to AIDS and trends in the doubling time. By employing the most recent insights from the literature and consulting with experts, we have attempted to overcome as far as possible the lack of empirical data. Without supplementary data on essential points, we feel that a reference scenario other than that which we have compiled would be unjustifiably optimistic or pessimistic.

The above considerations do not rule out further reflection on how closely the reference scenario approaches reality. The short-term forecasts may offer counsel here; to date, short-term extrapolations have produced a pessimistic picture of developments in AIDS incidence, while in practice AIDS incidence is usually found at the lower limit of the confidence intervals. This has meant that forecasts have been adjusted downwards over the course of time. If the same phenomenon is active in the reference scenario, this would result in consequences of AIDS which are more widespread than in the subscenario, but less extensive than suggested in the reference scenario. However, the existing uncertainty means that developments are also possible which lead to a higher HIV/AIDS incidence than that suggested in the reference scenario. By way of illustration, we refer to - entirely possible - developments in the incubation period distribution. If the San Francisco Clinic Cohort Study were to show that the incubation period, rather than being an average of 11 years, lasts an average of 20 years, this would lead to a higher prevalence, and therefore possibly also incidence, of HIV.

A *qualitative* assessment and elaboration of the reference scenario is also possible by projecting intervening developments in the area of risk behaviour and prevention. Simulations are possible, differentiated according to core group, in which variation in introduced in the avoidance of risk behaviour, the effectiveness of prevention or the seroprevalence. Simulations are also possible in which a relapse into risk behaviour or the spread of HIV between core groups is analysed. These subjects are discussed in Chapter 7.

Changes in the impact of AIDS compared to the reference scenario are also possible as a result of developments in the area of care and medical technology. Examples here include the effects of an extension of the survival period following diagnosis of AIDS, the effects of early intervention or the substitutions of care. Each of these developments can lead to a different extent, composition or cost of care from that outlined in the reference scenario. We shall consider this in more detail in Chapter 8. As regards the social context, a reorientation of the AIDS control strategy or the organization of care could lead to changes with respect to the reference scenario. We shall look at these intervening developments in Chapter 9.

6.7 Summary

The reference scenario constructed in this chapter provides the best possible projection of the impact of the HIV/AIDS epidemic up to the year 2000. In the reference scenario we have assumed an unchanged continuation of the developments described in the baseline analyses in an epidemiological, socio-cultural and economic context. In the elaboration of the scenario we present the consequences of developments in the epidemic up to 1.1.1989 in a separate subscenario.

In terms of epidemiology, the reference scenario leads to an AIDS incidence of 6,366 in the period 1991-2000, and of almost 750 in the year 2000. The cumulative total of HIV-infected persons from 1979 onwards is estimated at almost 17,000, with an HIV prevalence in the year 2000 of more than 10,000. Of the 8,000 people with AIDS since 1982, 6,500 will have died by the year 2000. The subscenario shows what proportion of the consequences of the HIV/AIDS epidemic can no longer be avoided through public information and the promotion of behavioural change. The cumulative HIV incidence reconstructed for the subscenario, at 6,700 on 1.1.1989, leads to an AIDS incidence of 230 in the year 2000. Patient-related costs in the reference scenario amount to NLG 92.6 million in the year 2000, a fivefold increase over the costs in 1988. Comparison of HIV/AIDS cost categories with the Financial Statement on Health Care shows that care provided to people with AIDS accounts for 0.5% of the health care budget.

The non-patient-related costs of AIDS are only partly dependent on epidemiological developments. In the reference scenario we have fixed these costs at 1988 levels. Adding together all the costs produces a total of NLG 139 million in the year 2000. In 1990, patient-related costs account for 48% of the total; by the year 2000, this has risen to 67%. Comparison of the reference scenario with the subscenario shows that up to 60% of the patient-related costs relate to persons who became HIV-infected after 1.1.1989.

The social context in the reference scenario is largely unchanged from the baseline analysis. An indication is given of what this implies for the effectiveness of prevention, for sexual behaviour and for the public acceptance of the epidemic.

In the Commentary we look at the assumptions which lie at the basis of the reference scenario and the significance of the reference scenario for HIV/AIDS prevention and the social context of the AIDS epidemic. One of the conclusions drawn is that the impact of AIDS will only become fully apparent in the period 1991-2000, and that continued prevention efforts are advisable.

References

Bindels, P.J.E., J.T.L. Jong, M.J.J.C. Poos, A. Leentvaar-Kuijpers, R.A. Coutinho, J.C. Jager
Het epidemiologisch beloop van AIDS in Amsterdam, 1982 - 1988
Nederlands Tijdschrift voor Geneeskunde, 134 (1990), 390-394

Bonneux, L., H. Houweling
Is een epidemie van heteroseksueel overgedragen HIV-infectie mogelijk in Europa?
Nederlands Tijdschrift voor Geneeskunde, 133 (1989), 39, 1922-1926

Borleffs, J.C.C., J.C. Jager, M.J.J.C. Poos, M.G.W. Dijkgraaf, R.M.A. Geels, H. Vrehen, A.J.P. Schrijvers
Hospital costs for patients with HIV infection in a University Hospital in The Netherlands
Health Policy, 16 (1990), 43-54

Centers for Disease Control (CDC)
HIV prevalence Extimates and AIDS Case Projections for the United States: report based upon a workshop
MMWR, 39 (1990), no. RR-16

Centraal Bureau voor de Statistiek (CBS)
Vademecum Gezondheidsstatistiek
CBS, The Hague, 1991

Chin, J., P.A. Sato, J.M. Mann
Projections of HIV infections and AIDS cases to the year 2000; Update/Le Point
Bulletin of the World Health Organization, 68 (1990), 1, 1-11

Cox, D., R.M. Anderson, A.M. Johnson, M.J.R. Healy, V. Isham, A.D. Wilkie, N.E. Day, O.N. Gill, A. McCormick
Short term prediction of HIV-infection and AIDS in England and Wales; report of a working group
Her Majesty's Stationery Office, London, 1988

Downs, A.M., R.A. Ancella, J.C. Jager, J.B. Brunet
AIDS in Europe: Current trends and short-term predictions estimated from surveillance data, January 1981 - June 1986
AIDS, 1987, 1, 53-57

Downs, A.M., R.A. Ancella, J.C. Jager, S.H. Heisterkamp, J.A.M. van Druten, E.J. Ruitenberg, J-B. Brunet
The statistical estimation, from routine surveillance data, of past, present and future trends in AIDS incidence in Europe
In: J.C. Jager en E.J. Ruitenberg (eds.), *Statistical Analysis and Mathe-*

matical Modelling of AIDS, Oxford University Press, 1988, 1-16

Dijkgraaf, M.G.W., J.J.C. Borleffs, M.J.J.C. Poos, J.C. Jager, A.J.P. Schrijvers
Monitoring hospital resource use and cost: a three-and-a-half year follow up
Presentated at the *VII International Conference on AIDS*, Florence, 1991 (MD 112)

Geneeskundige Hoofdinspectie van de Volksgezondheid (GHI)
anonymous registration of AIDS-diagnoses
continuous registration

Hay, J.W.
Econometric issues in modelling the costs of AIDS
Health Policy, 11 (1989), 125-145

Health Council (GR)
De zorg voor patiënten met AIDS en andere ziekteverschijnselen als gevolg van infectie met het humaan-immunodeficiëntievirus
GR, The Hague, 1987

Health Council (GR)
Vroege medische interventies bij personen die met AIDS-virus zijn geïnfecteerd
GR, The Hague, 1990/16

Heisterkamp, S.H., J.C. Jager, A.M. Downs, J.A.M. van Druten, E.J. Ruitenberg
Predicting AIDS incidence: a statistical approach
Statistics in Medicine, 8 (1989), 963- 976

Hartgers, C., E.C. Buning, G.W. van Santen, A.D. Verster, R.A. Coutinho
The impact of the needle and syringe-exchange programme in Amsterdam on injecting risk behavior
AIDS, 3 (1989), 571-576

Houweling, H., J.C. Jager, R.A. Coutinho, H. Bijkerk, E.J. Ruitenberg
Epidemiologie van AIDS en HIV infecties in Nederland; huidige situatie en prognose voor de periode 1987-1990
Nederlands Tijdschrift voor Geneeskunde, 131 (1987), 19, 818-824

Houweling, H., J.C. Jager, R.A. Coutinho
Commentaar op 'Komt er een einde aan de AIDS-epidemie in Nederland? van H.A. Verburgh
Nederlands Tijdschrift voor Geneeskunde, 134 (1990), 667-668

Jager, J.C., S.H. Heisterkamp, E.J. Ruitenberg
De kwantitatieve analyse van de AIDS-epidemie

In: *Berichten uit het RIVM 1987*, Bilthoven, 1988, 218-221

Jager, J.C., M.J. Postma, F.M.L.G. van den Boom, D.P. Reinking, J.C.C. Borleffs, S.H. Heisterkamp, J.A.M. van Druten, E.J. Ruitenberg
Epidemiological models and socioeconomic information: methodological aspects of AIDS/HIV scenario analysis
In: D. Schwefel, R. Leidl, J. Rovira, M.F. Drummond (eds.), *Economic Aspects of AIDS and HIV infection*, Springer Verlag, Berlin, 1989, 262-281

Jager, J.C., M.J.J.C. Poos, M.J. Postma, H. Houweling, C.A. Postema, R.A. Coutinho
Short term scenarios on the socioeconomic impact of AIDS on society
Presentated at the *VI International Conference on AIDS*, San Francisco, 1990a (FD121)

Jager, J.C., M.J.J.C. Poos, H. Houweling, C.A. Postema, R.A. Coutinho
Prognose aangaande HIV-infectie en AIDS-epidemie in Nederland op basis van wiskundige analyse
Nederlands Tijdschrift voor Geneeskunde, 134 (1990b), 51, 2486-2491

Jager, J.C., M.J. Postma, R. Leidl, B. Majnoni d'Itignano, A.E. Baert
AIDS impact scenarios: questions for the years to come
AIDS, 4 (1990c), 11, 1166-1167

Kok, G.J.
persnal communication, 1991

KPMG Klynveld Bosboom Hegener, Organizational consultants
Kosten en meerkosten van ziekenhuiszorg voor HIV-geinfecteerden
KPMG, Utrecht, 1989a

KPMG Klynveld Bosboom Hegener, Organizational consultants
(Meer)kostenonderzoek AIDS-functie; interim report 2: Medische en verpleegkundige protocollen
KPMG, Utrecht, 1989b

KPMG Klynveld Bosboom Hegener, Organizational consultants
(Meer)kosten AIDS-functie; interim report 3: Kostenonderzoek en kostprijsbepaling
KPMG, Utrecht, 1989c

Lifson, A., N. Hessol, G.W. Rutherford, P. O'Malley, L. Barnhart, S. Buchbinder, L. Cannon, T. Bodecker, S. Holmberg, J. Harrison, L. Doll
Natural history of HIV-infection in a cohort of homosexual and bisexual men: Clinical and immunological outcome
Presentated at the *VI International Conference on AIDS*, San Francisco, 1990

Ministry of Welfare, Health and Cultural Affairs (WVC)
Financieel Overzicht Zorg 1991
WVC, Rijswijk, 1991

Nationale Commissie AIDS-bestrijding (NCAB)
Het AIDS en drugsbeleid in Nederland; de stand van zaken
NCAB, Amsterdam, 1990

Postma, M.J., M.G.W. Dijkgraaf, J.C.C. Borleffs, D.P. Reinking, F.M.L.G. van den Boom, J.C. Jager
Omvang en kosten van ziekenhuiszorg voor HIV-geïnfecteerden; een vergelijking en integratie van Nederlandse studies
Tijdschrift voor Sociale Gezondheidszorg, 1991, geaccepteerd

Vandenbroucke, J.P.
Het toekomstig beloop van de AIDS-epidemie in Nederland volgens de wet van Farr
Nederlands Tijdschrift voor Geneeskunde, 134 (1990), 51, 2479- 2482

Verbrugh, H.A.
Komt er een einde aan de AIDS-epidemie in Nederland?
Nederlands Tijdschrift voor Geneeskunde, 143 (1990), 666-667

Water, H.P.A. van de, C.C.M.C. Wiggers, C.C.J.H. Bijleveld, M. Berkane
Schatting van het aantal HIV-seropositieven in Nederland; implicaties voor het toekomstig verloop van de AIDS-epidemie
Nederlands Tijdschrift voor Geneeskunde, 134 (1990), 51, 2482- 2486

Wiggers, C.C.M.C., E.W. Bergsma
De kosten van AIDS/HIV in Nederland in 1988: een inventarisatie
NIPG/TNO, Leiden, 1990a

Wiggers, C.C.M.C., E.W. Bergsma
De kosten van AIDS en HIV in Nederland in 1988
Economisch Statistische Berichten, June 1990b

7 Risk behaviour and the spread of HIV

7.1 *Introduction*

There are wide international differences in the pattern of spread of HIV, and these justify differing expectations for the future. In the US, for example, an increase can be observed in STDs among ethnic minorities in the centres of large cities, and HIV has been found among young people (Holmes, 1989; Des Jarlais et al., 1991). Although it is not known whether the same developments are present in the Netherlands, the course of events in the US constitutes a warning: what is happening there can also happen here, adjustmed to fit the Dutch situation. For example, there may be developments which lead to a reduced effectiveness of prevention, or to the spread of HIV to sexual networks where rapid spread is possible, or to the creation of an independent epidemic within a relatively unpromiscuous population. It is therefore necessary to confront the present, cautiously optimistic prognoses with projections of intervening developments. These projections give an impression of the possible HIV incidence, and thus offer starting points for prevention and public information, because they give an insight into what effect must be produced by behavioural change in order to achieve control of the epidemic of HIV.

The condition for the spread of HIV is that potential risk contact must take place with an HIV-infected person. The concentration of HIV within a few groups in the Netherlands, and the indications for differences in HIV risk, suggest an approach differentiated on the basis of groups. Six behavioural scenarios have therefore been developed:

Scenario I	HIV/AIDS among men who have sex with men; reference scenario and subscenario;
Scenario II	HIV among men who have sex with other men; temporary versus permanent relapse;
Scenario III	HIV among IDUs; introduction & rapid spread versus plateauing in HIV infections;
Scenario IV	HIV among IDUs; spread by sexual contact and/or shared use of needles;
Scenario V	HIV among heterosexuals; independent epidemic of HIV infections.
Scenario VI	HIV among commercial sex workers and their clients.

Table 7.1 shows a summary for each behavioural scenario of the parameters studied, the indicators and the models used.

Table 7.1 **Parameters, indicators and models in behavioural scenarios I-VI.**

Scenario		Parameters	Indicators	Model[1]
I	HIV/AIDS among men who have sex with other men; reference scenario and subscenario	AIDS incidence	AIDS/HIV inc. AIDS/HIV prev.	MIDAS
II	HIV among males with homosexual partners; temporary vs. permanent relapse	risk behaviour no. of partners	HIV incidence HIV prevalence	MGM[2]
III	HIV among IDUs; saltatory increase ceiling in HIV infections	group size risk behaviour no. of partners	HIV incidence	-
IV	HIV among IDUs; spread via sexual contact and/or shared use of injection equipment	risk behaviour no. of partners	HIV incidence	MGM
V	HIV among heterosexuals; independent epidemic of HIV infections	risk behaviour no. of partners	HIV incidence	MGM
VI	HIV among prostitutes and their clients	risk behaviour no. of partners	HIV incidence	MGM

1 See Chapter 2 and appendices for an explanation of the models.
2 MGM = multi-group model.

Table 7.1 shows that in four of the six cases, namely Scenarios II, IV, V & VI, the effect of variation in risk behaviour and number of partners is studied on the basis of HIV incidence (and possibly prevalence) using the multi-group model (MGM).[1] Scenario I is constructed on the basis of the same collection of statistical methods as in the reference scenario (Chapter 6), applied individually to the group of men with male and female sexual partners. In Scenario III attention is also focused explicitly on the impact of a significant deviation from the group size from that in the baseline analysis

1 Following the terminology in the literature we use the term relapse in Scenario II. We are aware of the sensitivity around the term relapse, i.e. that for some people it is connected with concepts of blame. Therefore, we want to state explicitely that we use it in a strict neutral, non-moral sense.

(Chapter 4).

The central focus in this chapter will be on projections of the influence of behavioural change and the effectiveness of prevention on the incidence and spread of HIV. Linking these factors to the economic and socio-cultural impact of AIDS falls outside the scope of this chapter.

7.2 *Methods, data and underlying principles*

7.2.1 *Working method*

Projections of future developments in the HIV epidemic and the targets and effectiveness of the AIDS control programme are based largely on an approach in which data from epidemiological and socio-scientific research are used in conjunction with mathematical modelling. Examples of future projections of the epidemic of HIV infections include a report on England and Wales (Cox et al., 1988) and the working documents of the National Centre for Epidemiology and Population Health in Australia (Solomon et al., 1989; Solomon et al., 1990). One of the conclusions resulting from these studies is that projections are possible based on available data and models, though caution is needed in their interpretation. There is still a great deal of uncertainty on crucial points such as (1) the infectiousness, and the relationship between this and the progression to AIDS, the transmission of HIV and susceptibility to HIV infection; (2) the incubation period; (3) trends in HIV incidence in various risk groups and regions; (4) the avoidance of high-risk sexual behaviour and the shared use of injection equipment; (5) the effect of prevention and public information (Anderson, 1987, 1988a, 1990). Following a literature study, individual consultation and a workshop of experts, the conclusion is that it is still too early in the Netherlands to produce a coherent system of assumptions based entirely on empirical data and practical insights, with which scenario analysis using behavioural models would be possible: the data and insights available from research do not permit this. The simulations in this chapter are therefore based partly on assumptions.

The current stage of development of mathematical modelling also plays a role in this chapter. Modelling techniques are developing rapidly, with simple models becoming ever more complex, for example through the incorporation of variable infectiousness, effects of age on sexual behaviour, subdivision into different groups and regions, and differences in the duration of sexual relationships and number of partners (Withers, 1989; Fusaro et al., 1989; Castillo-Chavez, 1989; Lagergren, in preparation; Kaplan, 1989a; Kaplan and Lee, 1990). A start has also been made on the development of models which look at (sexual) behaviour and behavioural change as a result of prevention efforts. In such complex models it is important among other things to differentiate between one-off and permanent relapse (Aron and Wileyto, in preparation).

Bailey (1988, in preparation) takes the view that, from the perspective of policymakers and planners, and given the seriousness of the AIDS situation, it is not acceptable simply to wait for a definitive model and the definitive data. Moreover, conclusions which are relevant for policymakers can be derived from less complex models. Kaplan (1989b) supports Bailey by demonstrating that a simple model based on "random mixing" (arbitrary partner selection) leads in general to the same conclusion regarding the success of "safer sex" campaigns, as a model which is not based on random mixing.

On the basis of the developments in HIV incidence and the effects of risk behaviour described in Chapters 3 and 4, a specific number of projections has been chosen. The selection was inspired by questions relating to the extent, the rate of increase and decrease of HIV infections, possible transmission routes of the virus within and between differentiated groups, and the required effects of prevention.

The summary of results from epidemiological and socio-scientific research in Chapter 3 was determined partly by the possibilities for incorporating research data into mathematical models. For the projections in this chapter the following parameters are of particular importance: (1) infectiousness; (2) number of partners; (3) group size; (4) seroprevalence; (5) contacts between risk groups. The scenarios and projections in this chapter relate primarily to *risk behaviour*, *effectiveness of prevention* and the *transmission routes of HIV*. As a result of this, we have taken as our main variables in the projections the number of partners, the seroprevalence and the contacts between core groups. There is also variation in the transmission risk per contact type (anal and vaginal contact, shared use of injection equipment). The group sizes in the simulations correspond as far as possible to the estimates in Table 3.4 in Chapter 3. The estimates of the transmission risk are based on the international literature.[2]

---

[2] With respect to infectiousness, available studies relate mainly to transmission among gay men. Some studies focus on the estimate of the risk of transmission per partner, while others estimate the risk of HIV infection per sexual contact (DeGruttola et al., 1989; Holmberg et al., 1989; Jewell and Shiboski, 1990). Kaplan (1990), in modelling the findings from the San Francisco Mens' Health Study (Grant et al., 1987), concluded that the transmission risk per partner within this cohort, at an assumed seroprevalence of 50%, is 0.1. The estimated transmission risk per partner during receptive anal intercourse as found in the cohort study among gay men in Amsterdam, amounts to 0.04 (Van Griensven et al., 1990). The number of sexual partners in the latter study was approximately 14 per year. In applying mathematical models, the transmission risk is generally

7.2.2 *The multi-group model*

We have carried out the projections in this chapter on the basis of a multi-group model developed by the Catholic University of Nijmegen (KUN) and the National Institute of Public Health and Environmental Protection (RIVM) (Van Druten and Jager, 1991). For the mathematical basis and a complete description of the model, we refer to Chapter 2.

The model makes it possible to simulate the spread of HIV at different levels of risky sexual and injection behaviour, and with different numbers of persons and numbers of contacts within and between core groups. Six core groups are identified in the model: (1) men with a large number of multiple male partners; (2) other men with multiple male partners; (3) male injecting drug users; (4) female injecting drug users; (5) heterosexual males with multiple partners; (6) heterosexual females with multiple partners. Heterosexual contacts are not ruled out for groups (1) and (2). Two groups of men who have sex with men have been differentiated in order to take account in the simulations of heterogeneity in sexual behaviour.[3] The most important transmission routes of HIV are incorporated in this model, namely anal intercourse, shared use of injection equipment and vaginal intercourse. Group sizes can be incorporated into the model: these are assumed to remain constant, and not to change over the course of time as the result of inflow (new persons susceptible to risk of HIV) or outflow (death from AIDS). In order to avoid this leading to distortion of the results, our simulations relate to a period of

---

taken as an average value for the whole incubation period. In this connection, Roberts and Dangerfield (1990) developed a method which allows variable infectiousness to be incorporated. At an estimated ten partners per year and an incubation period averaging eight years, they estimated the following development in infectiousness: the transmission risk is 0.071 in the year following acute infection with HIV, 0 during the six-year period that HIV is present without symptoms, and 0.149 in the year prior to AIDS (Dangerfield and Roberts, 1989). In our simulations we have taken a transmission risk for homosexual anal intercourse which is of the same order as the above studies, namely 0.02. For heterosexual transmission, we have assumed a vaginal intercourse transmission risk of 0.0014 for each unprotected contact with an infected man. The transmission risk per contact with an infected woman has been assumed to be half as great. We have taken the transmission risk when sharing injection equipment to be 10 times as great as the risk of transmission during vaginal intercourse contact with an infected woman.

3 Anderson et al. (1986; 1989) found in this connection that persons with a large number of partners, in particular, are at greater risk of infection with HIV and make a greater contribution to the spread of HIV.

between three and five years.[4]

7.2.3 *The transmission matrix and the Yearly Effective Contact Rate*

Simulations using the multi-group model are based on a transmission matrix and a Yearly Effective Contact Rate (YECR) which is derived from this. Table 7.2 contains the transmission matrix which has been used thus far in simulations based on the model.

Table 7.2 **Transmission matrix. Transmission potential of HIV via anal intercourse, vaginal intercourse and shared use of injection equipment for: men with many multiple male partners (1), men with few male partners (2), female IDUs (3), male IDUs (4) males with multiple heterosexual partners (5) and females with multiple heterosexual partners (6).** Source; Van Druten and Jager, 1991.

	1	2	3	4	5	6
1	1.5	0.2	0.025	0.004	-	0.0035
2	0.05	0.5	0.016	0.001	-	0.0014
3	0.17	0.043	0.25	0.34	0.18	-
4	0.013	0.011	0.30	0.29	-	0.0087
5	-	-	0.0027	-	-	0.1
6	0.0014	0.0023	-	0.001	0.4	-

- = not applicable in the transmission matrix

Each of the three HIV transmission routes in this matrix is based on three matrices, so that in total there are nine matrices containing data on:

(i) the fraction of each group with contacts with persons from their own and other groups;

(ii) the number of new partners inside and outside the person's own group per year;

(iii) the transmission probability per partner.

[4] Models which allow for inflow and outflow, for example by incorporating age, lethality and progression to AIDS into the model, can be used for longer-term projections. Often, however, these are "single group" models, such as those developed by Griffiths and Williams (in preparation), De Haan and Dijkgraaf (in preparation) and Heisterkamp et al. (submitted).

As a result of the differentiation into groups and transmission routes, these matrices also contain empty cells. Shared use of injection equipment, for example, is only relevant for injecting drug users (groups 3 and 4). The transmission matrix summarises all transmission parameters which relate to the three transmission routes within and between Groups 1 to 6. The transmission matrix values were calculated by multiplying the proportions of persons with contacts within their own and other groups by the annual number of partners within each group and the risk of infection.[5]

The YECR can be derived directly from the transmission matrix. In the theory of communicable diseases this concept is defined as the number of new infections which is caused during a period of one year by a single infected person (in group j) in a completely receptive population (group i).[6] The $YECR_{ji}$ can be derived from the matrix by multiplying the matrix element by the size of group i divided by the size of group j. Expressed in a formula, this gives $YECR_{ji} = t_{ij} *N_i / N_j$.[7]

The empirical basis is crucial for the nature and coverage of mathematical models such as the multi-group model used here. The lack of detailed empirical information means that many parameters have not been validated (Van Druten and Jager, 1991). Socio-sexological research from the US, and initial results from Dutch research into the spread of HIV infections among gay men in Amsterdam, have been taken as a guide in earlier applications of the model. Mathematical models which are designed for the estimation or optimization of parameters also have been used. Note 1 contains a summary of these studies consulted. Where we have used the multi-group model, we have generally adopted the same coherent system of assumptions from the transmission matrix in Table 7.2 which has been used until now. This has the advantage of making comparisons possible between our simulations and simulations carried out earlier. Where our baseline analysis suggests different values for certain

---

5 An example may make the method of calculation clear. The value of 0.05 for the matrix elements in row 2, column 1, relates to the potential for transmission of HIV infections from men in Group 1 to men in Group 2 (element t_{21} in the matrix). Anal intercourse is the only relevant transmission route here. The proportion of men in Group 2 with contacts in Group 1 is 0.1, while the number of new partners per year for men in Group 2 is 25 and the assumed transmission risk per partner is 0.02. Multiplying these three figures together produces the value of 0.05 for this matrix element.

6 The $YECR_{ji}$ relates to direct transmission. In transmission from person A to C via person B, one infection is allocated to A, even though A is also the original source of infection for C.

7 In the case of transmission within the group, the YECR is obviously equal to the value of the matrix element, since N_i then equals N_j.

parameters, we have justified this for each simulation. Partial validation of the parameters from the model then takes place, although an exhaustive validation of parameters, or a structured sensitivity analysis, both of which are necessary for research into the quantitative analysis of the AIDS epidemic, are not an explicit objective of this study.

7.3 HIV/AIDS among men who have sex with men

7.3.1 Scenario I: HIV/AIDS among men who have sex with men; reference scenario and subscenario

As at 1.1.1991, 80% of people with AIDS in the Netherlands were men with multiple male partners, which translates into 1223 of the total of 1531 people with AIDS (Chief Medical Officier for Health, GHI).

Figure 7.1 **AIDS incidence among men with multiple male partners up to 2000: reconstruction and extrapolations for scenario I. Based on reported and corrected AIDS incidence at 1.1.1990. Extrapolations according to methods and assumptions from reference scenario and subscenario.**

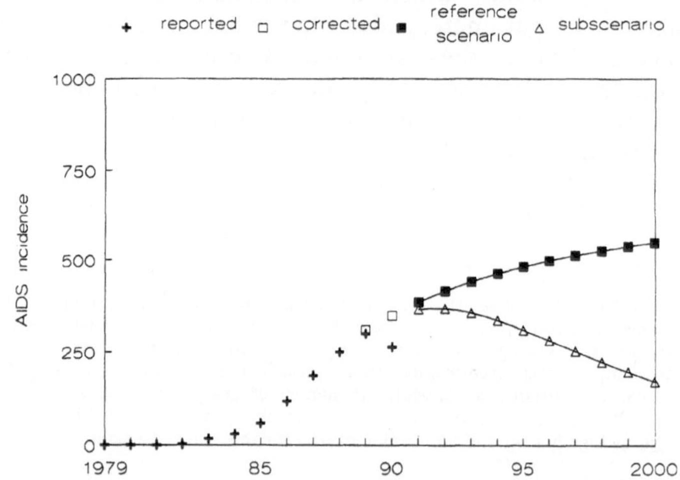

Using the methodology and assumptions in the reference scenario (Chapter 6), the course of the AIDS epidemic and the epidemic of HIV in this core group was reconstructed and projections carried out. The results of this scenario are shown in Figures 7.1 and 7.2, which show the AIDS and HIV incidence, respectively, up to the year 2000 for the reference scenario and subscenario. Figures 7.3a and b show the results of the projections expressed in terms of AIDS and HIV prevalence figures.

It can be seen from Figure 7.2 that the estimated cumulative incidence of HIV is 5,124 at 1.1.1989. According to the reference scenario, the projected HIV incidence in the period 1989-2000 is almost 7,500 for men who have sex with men. On 1.1.1991 the projected prevalence in the pre-AIDS stage is 5,000 in the reference scenario, and 4,000 in the subscenario.

Figure 7.2 **Estimated HIV incidence among men with multiple male partners up to 2000: reconstruction and extrapolation for scenario I. Methods and assumptions analgous to reference scenario and subscenario.**

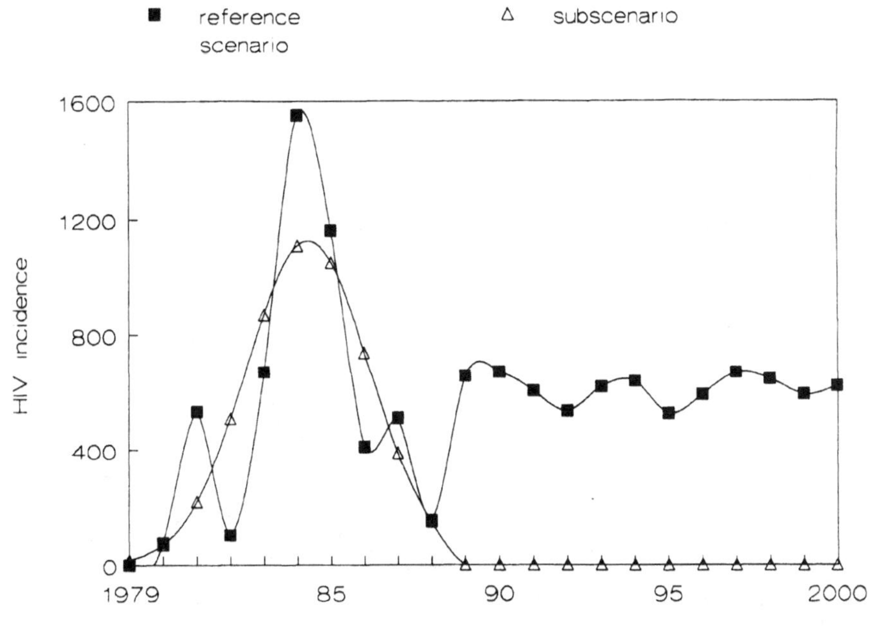

Figure 7.3 **Prevalence in AIDS and pre-AIDS stages among men with multiple male partners up to 2000: reconstruction and extrapolations for scenario I. Derived from Figures 7.1 and 7.2 and methods and assumptions from reference scenario and subscenario. 7.3a: AIDS prevalence; 7.3b: prevalance in the pre-AIDS stage.**

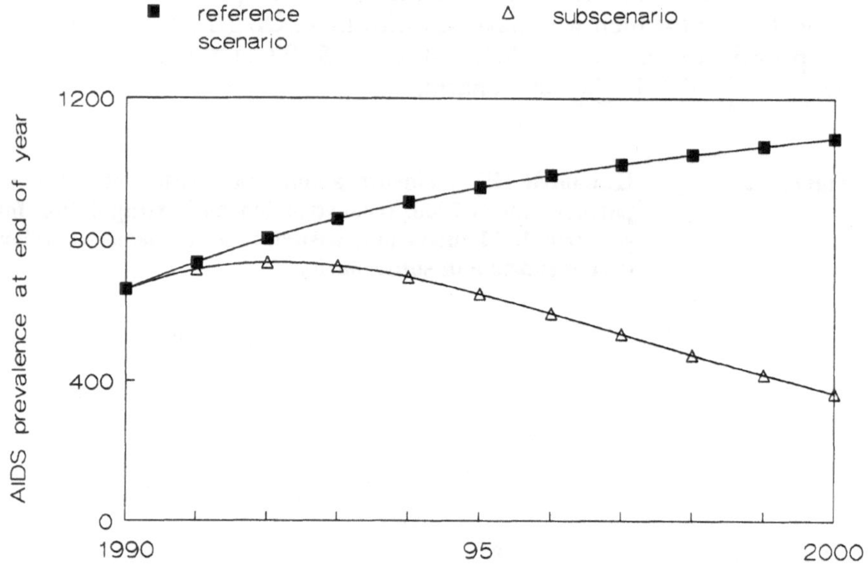

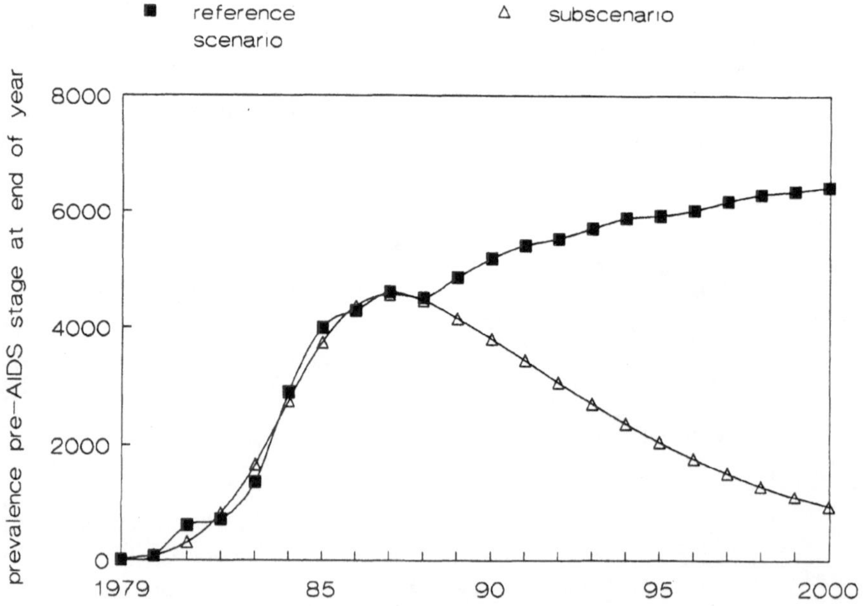

7.3.2 *Scenario II: HIV among men who have sex with men; temporary versus permanent relapse*

7.3.2.1 *Introduction*

The following questions are important when projecting the consequences of an increase in unsafe sexual behaviour by men who have sex with men: how much risk behaviour occurs? What increase in HIV incidence results from relapse? Is the assumed relapse temporary or permanent? We shall develop two variants of the behavioural scenario: temporary and permanent relapse.

The assumed initial situation is as follows:
Large-scale behavioural changes take place among gay men in response to AIDS, leading to a fall in the incidence of HIV (and other STDs). The behavioural change proves not to be total, and the prevention effect is not permanent. There is an increase in unprotected intercourse and in incorrect or non-permanent use of condoms. This assumed initial situation leads to an increase in HIV incidence.

7.3.2.2 *Temporary versus permanent relapse*

Temporary relapse
The behavioural scenario for temporary relapse is based on the assumption that, in addition to a small proportion of the population which permanently displays high-risk behaviour, temporary relapse also occurs among constantly varying sections of the population.

The following factors play a role:

- Condom use is not consistent or permanent. In particular, condoms are not always used with steady partners, or partners with whom regular contact occurs;
- Young people have more unprotected contacts than older people. Unprotected contact is also a fairly regular feature of social life. Targeted information and prevention produces a rapid and adequate response to warnings of an increase in unprotected contacts;
- There are periods when anal contact takes place with more sexual partners than average. This is related to various factors such as age, being in love, periods between steady relationships and a decrease in awareness of the risks of unprotected anal contact.

This scenario has the following assumed consequences:
Due to the high seroprevalence, relapse into risk behaviour is associated with a high risk of HIV. Temporary relapse therefore leads to small outbreaks of HIV. A second wave of HIV infections does not occur in this scenario, however; the epidemic can be said to be under control.

Permanent relapse
The assumed initial situation is as follows:
The behavioural change among men with multiple male partners is not permanent. A growing proportion of men with multiple male partners relapses and virtually ceases using precautions with changing sexual contacts.

The following factors play a role:
- Awareness of the acute need for protected sexual contact declines. A sense of security and the idea that the HIV epidemic is under control as a result of the behavioural change achieved in the 1980s, combined with high resistance to condom use, play a role here.
- Safer sex does not become a social norm, and information about AIDS has less effect with the passage of time.
- The HIV/AIDS prevention programme has difficulty reaching men who are afraid to "come out" regarding homosexual contacts. The AIDS information campaign also has difficulty in achieving contact with young people, people with an active social life and travellers. With regard to the latter group, the increased number of people from countries of Central and Eastern Europe should be borne in mind; there is no informational material for this group.
- Differences between countries make HIV/AIDS prevention more difficult. Among men from countries where the HIV/AIDS prevention programme encourages monogamy and abstinence from anal contact, there are misunderstandings concerning the need for protected anal contact. The Dutch HIV/AIDS prevention programme has difficulty in reaching tourists with "the Dutch message".
- Seroprevalence among young male commercial sex workers and their clients has increased to such an extent that there is a considerable risk of HIV infection within this segment of the sex industry.

In this scenario, there is an explosive increase in HIV infection, with a large-scale spread of HIV extending beyond the large(er) cities. The increased mobility means that the course of HIV in the Netherlands becomes more dependant than previously on international developments in the HIV epidemic. From a socio-cultural point of view, this scenario has consequences for the tolerance of homosexuality and leads to an increasing association of homosexuality with AIDS.

7.3.2.3 *Simulations of different levels of unsafe behaviour*

Using the multi-group model in a number of simulations, we predict the consequences of changes in risk behaviour for the incidence of HIV. Table 7.3 shows the initial situation for the projections; Table 7.4 contains the transmission matrix.

Table 7.3 Initial situation for simulations of relapse by two groups of men with multiple partners.

Group size	
Group 1:	5,000 men with many multiple male partners
Group 2:	20,000 men with multiple male partners
Prevalence	
Total Group 1 and 2:5000 at t = 0	
Situation 1:	Group 1: 4000 HIV-infected persons
	Group 2: 1000 HIV-infected persons
Situation 2:	Group 1: 2500 HIV-infected persons
	Group 2: 2500 HIV-infected persons
Situation 3:	Group 1: 1000 HIV-infected persons
	Group 2: 4000 HIV-infected persons
Effect of behavioural change with respect to Table 7.4	
Condition 1:	A fall in YECR to 10% of the level in Table 7.4.
Condition 2:	Relapse in stages; YECR rises from 10% to 50% of the level in Table 7.4.
Condition 3:	A fall in YECR to 50% of the level in Table 7.4.

A total of 5,000 HIV-infected males is assumed at t = 0, of whom 80%, 50% and 20%, respectively, are allocated to Group 1, and the rest to Group 2. The level of behavioural change indicated in Table 7.3 applies for the transmission matrix in Table 7.4. In turn, Table 7.4 follows directly from the transmission matrix in Table 7.2. The values for the matrix elements t_{11}, t_{21}, t_{12} and t_{22} are taken from earlier model applications, in which the matrix elements t_{11} and t_{22} were validated (Van Druten and Jager, 1991). In the simulations we have separated the sub-epidemic among men with male partners from the other sub-epidemics. Table 7.4 therefore relates only to the spread of HIV between men who have sex with men. As a result of this separation, all matrix elements in Table 7.4 which are taken from Table 7.2, and which do not relate to contacts between men who have sex with men, have been given a value of zero.

Table 7.4 Transmission matrix. Transmission potential via anal contact for two groups of men with varying male partners (taken from Van Druten and Jager, 1991).

	1	2	3	4	5	6
1	1.5	0.2	0	0	-	0
2	0.05	0.5	0	0	-	0
3	0	0	0	0	0	-
4	0	0	0	0	-	0
5	-	-	0	-	-	0
6	0	0	-	0	0	-

0 = not applicable due to separation of sub-epidemics
- = not applicable in the transmission matrix

In Condition 1, a fall in the $YECR_{ij}$ (i = 1,2 and j = 1,2) has been assumed, to 90% of the level in Table 7.4 for contacts within and between the two groups. This fall is attributed to a reduction in the transmission risk and in the number of partners. A change in the level of safe behaviour is assumed compared with earlier model applications (Van Druten et al., 1991; see also Chapter 3).[8] Under Condition 2 we project a situation in which there is a relapse in three years' time from 90% to 50% of the level in Table 7.4. Under Condition 3, in contrast to Condition 1, a constant level of safe and unsafe behaviour is projected which is 50% of the level in Table 7.4. Translated into the behavioural scenarios, the simulation under Condition 1 constitutes a projection under the assumption of a permanent positive effect of behavioural change; under Condition 2 we project a gradual

[8] The Yearly Effective Contact Rate from Group 1 to Groups 1 and 2 is $YECR_{11}$ + $YECR_{12}$, ie. 1.5 + 0.2 = 1.7. The YECR from Group 2 to Groups 1 and 2 is 0.05 + 0.5 = 0.55. Under Condition 1, there is a fall in the number of new infections in Groups 1 and 2 caused by a single infected person in group 1 during one year, from 1.7 to 0.17. The annual number of infections caused by a single infected person in Group 2 falls in this condition from 0.55 to 0.055.

decrease in the effects of prevention, and the simulations under Condition 3 relates to the scenario of a permanent relapse into risk behaviour.

Figure 7.4 **HIV prevalence (*1,000) under three conditions with differing distributions of the initial prevalence: 7.4a situation 1; 7.4b situation 2 and 7.4c situation 3 (see Table 7.3 for conditions and situations).**

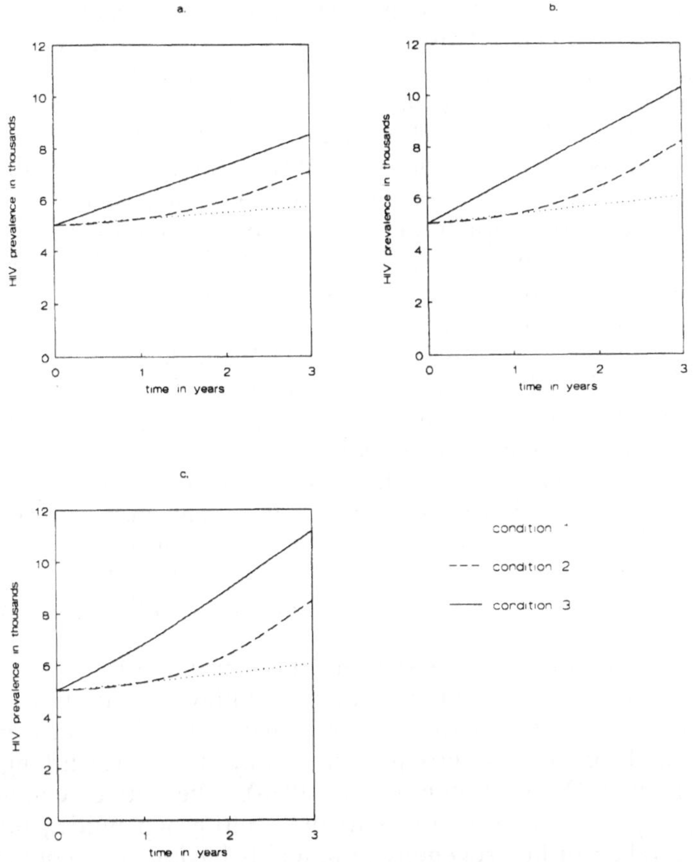

Figures 7.4abc show the results of the simulations, with each of three figures showing the HIV prevalence under the three conditions. For each situation, it can be seen that the lowest prevalence of HIV infections is found under Condition 1. This is particularly true in situation 1, with 4,000 HIV-infected persons in the group with many multiple partners (Figure 7.4a). The projection under Condition 2 shows a considerable effect on the HIV prevalence over a period of

three years. Depending on the number of HIV-infected persons in Group 2 at t = 0, the HIV prevalence can even increase to around 8,000 (Figure 7.4c). The simulations under Condition 3 lead to a seroprevalence which can increase to almost 11,000. Just as in Condition 1, the HIV prevalence rises as the number of HIV-infected persons in Group 2 increases at t = 0.

7.3.3 Commentary on Scenarios I and II

A number of simulations have been used to show the major consequences which relapse into risk behaviour can have for HIV prevalence. The simulations show that a constant high level of safe behaviour is necessary in order to permit the spread of HIV to be controlled. They also show that the effect of relapse will be greater as the virus spreads further beyond the group of men at the highest risk. Saturation effects in Group 1 also play a role here. Although HIV spreads more rapidly in Group 1, the men with many multiple partners, than among men in Group 2, the cumulative HIV incidence reaches its maximum value - infection of the whole group - more quickly than in Group 2.

How great the increase in HIV incidence due to relapse will be in practice also depends on a number of factors which are not explicitly incorporated in the simulation, such as geographical variations in seroprevalence, a difference in condom use during casual and regular/stable sexual partners, duration of the relapse and inflow and outflow to and from the core groups. The influx of young men who are becoming sexually active, the outflow from the group as a result of progression to AIDS and death, and the effects of age on sexual activity, are of particular importance for simulations covering a longer period.

Because of the danger of distortion of the results occurring through failure to take account of inflow and outflow, these simulations relate to a period of three years (see also 7.1.2). By using a so-called "open single group" model, projections over a longer period are possible (Van Druten et al., 1988). The model contains only one group so that, in contrast to the multi-group model, no account can be taken of heterogeneity in sexual behaviour and contacts with other core groups.

Figure 7.5 shows the hypothetical HIV prevalence in a homogenous group over a period of 40 years (the so-called "long-term prevalence"). The effectiveness of a prevention programme is expressed as a decrease in the YECR. The Basic Reproduction Rate (BRR) is in turn derived from the YECR and, unlike the latter, also takes account of the duration of the infectious period.[9] Changes in the infectious period or the YECR are related to the BRR. The BRR is shown on the x-axis, with the prevalence of HIV infections in per cent being shown on the y-axis.

Figure 7.5 **Hypothetical long-term effects on HIV prevalence (in per cent) with a decrease in YECR. Source: Van Druten et al., (1988).**

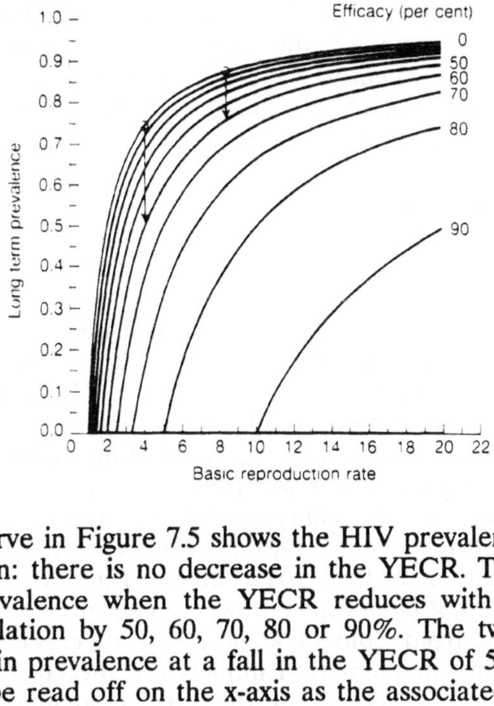

The upper curve in Figure 7.5 shows the HIV prevalence in the baseline simulation: there is no decrease in the YECR. The other curves show the prevalence when the YECR reduces with respect to the baseline simulation by 50, 60, 70, 80 or 90%. The two arrows show the decrease in prevalence at a fall in the YECR of 50%. The values 4 and 8 can be read off on the x-axis as the associated values for the BRR. These values relate to the initial situation, i.e. prior to the decrease in the YECR.

The graphs show that in the longer term, the decrease in prevalence is considerably less than the decline in the YECR: a reduction of 50% in the YECR has a relatively small effect over the long term. A BRR value of 10, for example, ultimately only produces a fall from 90% to 80% in long-term prevalence. The aim of the prevention effort must be to reduce the YECR by 90% or more (Van Druten et al., 1988; Van Druten and Jager, 1991).

---

9 For a discussion of the BRR we refer to the simulations in this chapter of the transmission of HIV via heterosexual contact.

In the Netherlands, in addition to an observed large-scale change in behaviour and a fall in the incidence of STD and HIV, there has also been an increase in relapse among visitors to STD clinics. Mooij (1990) and Van de Laar et al. (1990) refer in this connection to indications for a small group which has not changed its behaviour. A link is made between the recently observed increase in HIV in the Amsterdam cohort study and a non-permanent, inconsistently maintained change in behaviour, involving periods with an increase in unprotected anal contact and incorrect and inconsistent use of condoms (Kuiken et al., 1990; De Wit et al., 1991). Against this background, the scenario showing temporary relapse at a high level of safe behaviour would seem to the most applicable *at this moment*. An increase in sexual contact with a risk of HIV infection, possibly leading to permanent relapse, can in no way be ruled out, however.

7.4 HIV among IDUs

7.4.1 Introduction

Attempts to reconstruct the epidemic of HIV infections among IDUs using the back-calculation method have not produced satisfactory results. A combination of suggestions of a peak in HIV incidence among IDUs in Amsterdam in 1983-1984, and a seroprevalence of 30% in 1985, would require a longer incubation period among IDUs than among gay men in order to produce an epidemiological course which approximates to the reality according to the Amsterdam cohort study (Van Haastrecht et al., 1991ab; Van den Hoek, 1990). Indications for a longer incubation period among IDUs than among other core groups have not been found, however (Rezza et al., 1990).

More data from epidemiological and socio-scientific research and supplementary mathematical models are therefore needed for a reconstruction and projection of the HIV epidemic among IDUs. From an epidemiological perspective, this might mean a seroprevalence study, while in the socio-scientific field, a study of the determinants of drug use would be useful. The international literature suggests starting points for mathematical modelling of the spread of HIV among IDUs (Ahlgren et al., 1988; Kaplan, 1989c; Knox, 1988; Moss, 1987).

Two transmission routes of HIV are applicable to IDUs, namely shared use of injection equipment and the spread of HIV via sexual contact. We have drawn up two scenarios for the spread of HIV among IDUs. In line with the baseline analysis, in Scenario III we have projected a saltatory spread versus a ceiling in HIV infections. Scenario IV consists of simulations relating to the question of the spread of HIV among IDUs and from IDUs to other groups. The spread of HIV via contacts with commercial sex workers is discussed in Section 7.4.3.

7.4.2 *Scenario III: introduction and rapid spread versus a plateauing in HIV infections*

Introduction and rapid spread

The assumed initial situation for saltatory increase is that the introduction of HIV into different regions and into new "generations" of IDUs forms the starting point for a rapid increase in HIV incidence, which then rapidly reaches a maximum. Introduction into a subsequent network of IDUs produces a new wave of HIV infections in its turn. This pattern leads to a large-scale spread of HIV among IDUs.

The following assumed developments are associated with this scenario:

- The number of IDUs increases, with an increase both in the number of IDUs among young people, and in the level of intravenous use by hard-drug users who did not previously inject.
- The drug outreach and HIV/AIDS prevention programmes are unable to come into contact with new generations of users, users from ethnic minorities, and heroin-using tourists from the US and the countries of Southern, Western and Eastern Europe.
- The risk profile among IDUs, which has fallen as a result of the needle exchange schemes, increases once again. Additional prevention measures have no effect. The increasing shared use of injection equipment expresses itself in reduced use at home and less use alone, and an increase in shared use with people other than established friends and acquaintances.
- The risk profile among IDUs increases as a result of changes in the drug use itself, in particular an increase in the use of cocaine.
- The shared use of injection equipment among IDUs increases as a result of increasing mobility. This leads in a short time to an increase in the seroprevalence among IDUs in the Netherlands, to more than 30%.
- The decline in the effects of HIV/AIDS prevention is accompanied by a decrease in the use of condoms in sexual contacts, both private contacts and contacts in the sex industry. This leads to an increase in HIV incidence among non-IDUs, who in turn are responsible for a further spread of HIV through changing sexual contacts within the sex industry and the heterosexual

population in general. The increase in HIV within the sex industry subsequently contributes to yet another increase in HIV injections among drug-dependent commercial sex workers.

We assume that this variant of Scenario III leads not only to an increased HIV-related mortality and morbidity, but also to an increase in the demand for care by IDUs who until now have not made any demands on the care services in connection with AIDS or HIV-related problems. These persons often enter the health care system at the last moment, and HIV and AIDS-related problems frequently form part of a range of health problems.

Plateauing in HIV infections
The assumed initial situation in the case of a ceiling in HIV infections is a levelling off of the HIV epidemic among IDUs. There is a low annual HIV incidence, and the epidemic of HIV infections remain restricted to a few large cities. There are virtually no HIV infections in the border region. The following factors play a role here:

- There is a taboo on injecting among new, young users and users from groups and regions with which the drug-aid agencies traditionally have had little contact.
- Insofar as injecting does occur, there is virtually no shared use: equipment is used alone and at home. In addition, there are few contacts between generations of users and IDUs from different towns.
- The needle exchange programmes, supplemented by HIV/AIDS prevention campaigns, are effective. The successful HIV/AIDS prevention programme also means that contact is made with the majority of drug users. Instead of contacts with 70% of drug users as with the methadone supply programme, there is now contact with virtually all drug users in the Netherlands.
- Seropositive drug users are virtually inactive in commercial sex work. These users often withdraw voluntarily. Where clients require unprotected contacts, the self-efficacy is high.

This variant of Scenario III has the following assumed consequences: Little care is necessary for IDUs with problems related to AIDS or HIV. On the other hand, improved contacts enhance the opportunities for controlling the adverse effects of hard-drug use on the health and social functioning of hard-drug users.

7.4.3 *Scenario IV: spread via sexual contact and/or shared use of injection equipment*

We use a number of simulations to predict transmission routes of HIV among IDUs. We look at heterosexual transmission of HIV and the interaction between the spread of HIV via sexual contact and shared use of injection equipment. In heterosexual transmission the potential "bridging function" from IDUs to persons who either do not inject drugs or do not use hard drugs at all, is an important factor. We have actualized this in the simulations as "proportional mixing" or arbitrary partner selection, and "selective mixing" in which IDUs have a preference for partners from the IDU group. Table 7.5 shows the initial situation for the simulations. Groups 3 to 6 are important for these simulations, namely female IDUs (3), male IDUs (4), heterosexual men with multiple partners (5) and heterosexual women with multiple partners (6).

In determining the group sizes for (3) and (4), we have taken as a basis the estimate of 20,000 hard-drug users reported in the baseline analysis, with a male:female ratio of 3:1 and a percentage of 30% IDUs. On the basis of the Amsterdam cohort study, we have assumed a seroprevalence among IDUs of 30% at $t = 0$ (Van den Hoek, 1990); for the Netherlands as a whole, this figure may be too high. The assumptions for seroprevalence and group size in Groups 5 and 6 are based on data from sexological and socio-epidemiological research (see Chapters 3 and 4).

We identify four conditions in the simulations. Conditions 1 and 2 differ on the point of arbitrary or selective partner selection. The assumption in Condition 2 is that 50% of the partners of IDUs are also IDUs. Condition 3 is included as a control condition and relates to the transmission of HIV via heterosexual contact. Under this condition, all contacts between IDUs and non-IDUs are severed. Condition 4 sets out the initial situation for a combined projection of the HIV prevalence caused by both shared use of injection equipment and sexual transmission. On the basis of data from Dutch research on the sexual partners of hard-drug users, we have opted for selective mixing in this condition (Van den Hoek, 1990).

Table 7.5 Initial situations for simulations of the spread of HIV among IDUs.

Group size	
Group 3:	2,000 females, IDUs
Group 4:	6,000 males, IDUs
Group 5:	200,000 males, non-IDU
Group 6:	200,000 females, non-IDU
Prevalence t = 0	
Groups 3 and 4:	30%
Groups 5 and 6:	0.1%
YECR	
Sexual contact[1]:	0.050 if the woman is infected 0.098 if the man is infected
Shared use of injection equipment	0.5
Contacts between and within groups	
Condition 1:	Proportional mixing: arbitrary partner selection
Condition 2:	Selective mixing: 50% of sexual partners of IDUs are also IDUs
Condition 3:	No sexual contacts between IDUs and non-IDUs
Condition 4:	20% of the IDUs share injection equipment; selective partner choice for sexual contact

1 The YECR of 0.050 relates to a female IDU and indicates the number of infections via sexual contacts during one year in the two groups of men: $YECR_{34} + YECR_{35}$ The YECR of a non-injecting woman in the two groups of men is equivalent to the YECR of the female IDU: $YECR_{64} + YECR_{65} = YECR_{34} + YECR_{35} = 0.050$. Similarly the YECR of a non-injecting man in the two groups of women is equivalent to that of a male IDU, namely 0.098.

Due to the lack of detailed empirical data concerning the number of sexual partners of IDUs and infectiousness, we have accorded hypothetical values to the YECRs. It is assumed that the YECR for shared use of injection equipment is 10 times the YECR for vaginal intercourse with an infected woman. This assumption is based on the assumed high risk of infection where injection equipment is shared. It has also been assumed that 20% of the IDUs use shared injection equipment. On the basis of findings in the literature, the risk of infection from men to women has been assumed to be twice as great as that from women to men during vaginal contact. This leads to a higher YECR for an infected man than an infected woman. The fact that the YECR of the man is not precisely twice as great as that of the woman is due to differences in group size (206,000 men against 202,000 women). If 202,000 women have, say, five partners per year, men can have only 4.9 partners per year. The difference in group size results from the subconditions of the multi-group model (See the Appendix to Chapter 2). Table 7.6 contains the transmission matrix for Condition 1.

Table 7.6 **Transmission matrix. Transmission potential via sexual contact for 2,000 female IDUs (3), 6,000 male IDUs (4), 200,000 heterosexual men with multiple partners (5) and 200,000 heterosexual women with multiple partners (6)**

	1	2	3	4	5	6
1	0	0	0	0	-	0
2	0	0	0	0	-	0
3	0	0	0	0.0029	0.0970	-
4	0	0	0.0005	0	-	0.0485
5	-	-	0.0005	-	-	0.0485

0 = not applicable due to separation of groups
- = not applicable in the transmission matrix

Just as in Scenario II, the matrix in Table 7.6 is taken from the transmission matrix in Table 7.2. The simulations relate to four groups, and Figure 7.6 shows the results of the simulations in four smaller figures. Time is represented on the x-axis, with the cumulative HIV incidence on the y-axis. The scale on the y-axis is different in each figure, so as to express the differences between the simulations in each of the four figures as clearly as possible. For each of the four groups the cumulative HIV incidence under the four conditions is given *from* t = 0.[10]

[10] For the sake of completeness, we would point out that the HIV prevalence at t = 0 cannot be read off in Figure 7.6.

Figure 7.6 **Cumulative HIV incidence from t = 0 via sexual contact and (where applicable) shared used of injection equipment among female IDUs, male IDUs, heterosexual men with multiple partners and heterosexual women with multiple partners.**

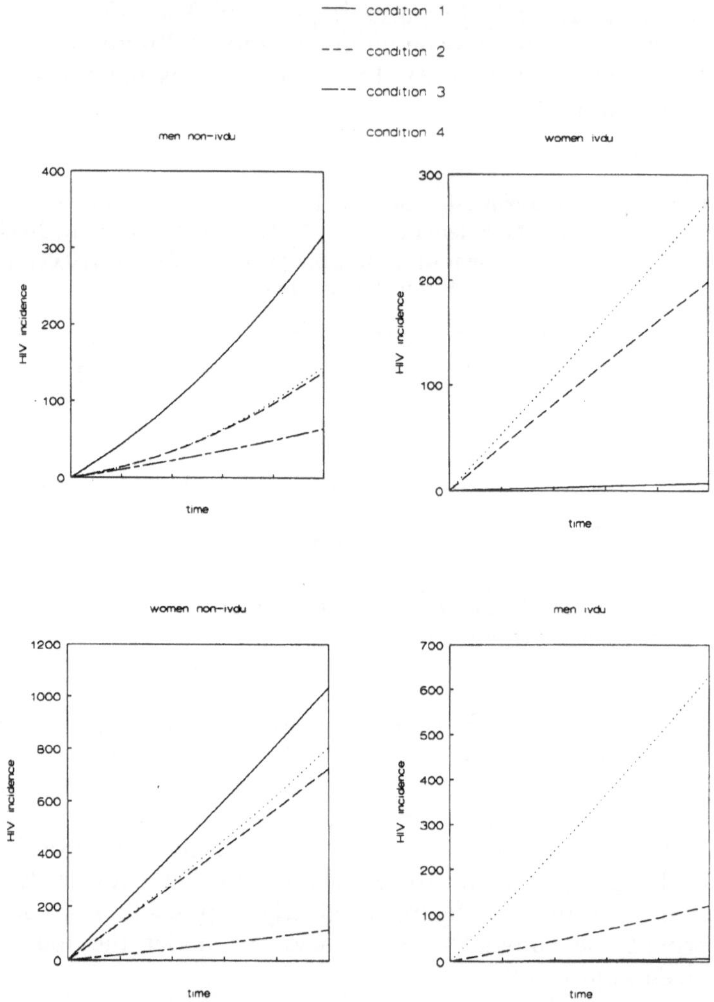

It can be seen from the figure that in the control condition (Condition 3) there is a very limited HIV incidence, irrespective of the risk of transmission via sexual contact. By contrast, Condition 1 - proportional mixing - leads to a considerable spread among non-injecting male and female drug users. In particular, the spread of HIV from the group of male IDUs to heterosexual women appears to be substantial. Condition 1 leads to virtually no infections via sexual contact among the IDUs. This is not surprising, since the assumed arbitrary partner selection means that IDUs enter into sexual contacts primarily with non-IDUs.

Selective mixing - Condition 2 - by contrast, leads to a significant cumulative HIV incidence among IDUs via sexual contact. The most striking feature however, is that, compared with proportional mixing (Condition 1), Condition 2 by no means leads to a halving of the cumulative incidence among non-injecting female drug users. Under condition 1 the cumulative incidence for all groups is considerably higher among women than among men. The assumed differences in risk of transmission by heterosexual contact play a role here.

The introduction of a second transmission route among IDUs in Condition 4 mainly effects the cumulative HIV incidence among male IDUs. In this group, the cumulative incidence is between four and six times higher than in the other conditions.

7.4.4 Commentary on scenarios III and IV

The potential cumulative HIV incidence among IDUs and among non-injecting male and female drug users was studied in a number of simulations. The simulations lead to the hypothesis that, in addition to the prevention of unsafe injection behaviour, the prevention of unsafe sexual contact is also of great importance, particularly for female injectors. For male IDUs the risk of infection via unsafe injection behaviour is of particular importance in these simulations.

The projections of the spread of HIV beyond the group of IDUs show that several hundred HIV infections are possible in the short term. The cumulative HIV incidence among women is particularly striking. In an absolute sense, this is in part related to the differences in group size as based on the literature, and to the transmission risks. The introduction of shared needle use has little effect in these simulations on the spread of HIV among men and women who do not inject drugs.

The scenarios relating to the possible spread of HIV project two potential future end-situations. The scenario of a saltatory increase in HIV infections paints a sombre picture for the future, while the scenario of a levelling off of the epidemic is optimistic. The differences between the two scenarios relate to the affects of prevention, contacts between groups of users and the potential transmission routes of HIV. It is not possible to indicate which of the two scenarios describes the most likely end-situation for the future. The scenarios reflect above all the uncertainty surrounding the course of the HIV epidemic among intravenous drug users up to the year 2000, and the effects of the AIDS prevention programme in the medium term.

7.5 *HIV among heterosexuals*

7.5.1 *Introduction*

It was concluded in the baseline analysis that there appears to be no evidence thus far of a substantial spread of HIV among the heterosexual population in general, or within the sex industry. In two independent scenarios, we briefly outline a number of possible developments in the spread of HIV infection, and carry out simulations of (1) the conditions for an independent epidemic among the heterosexual population and (2) the possible incidence of HIV within the sex industry.

7.5.2 *Scenario V: HIV among heterosexuals; independent epidemic of HIV*

The assumed development in Scenario V is that the danger of HIV infection via heterosexual transmission is being underestimated. In practice, there is evidence of a certain HIV incidence: there are men with both male and female sexual partners, clients of female IDUs, non-injecting drug using sexual partners of IDUs, travellers and "sex tourists" who lay a "bridge" between sexual networks within which multiple contacts take place. This leads to the creation of an epidemic within the population of exclusively heterosexual contacts.

7.5.2.1 *Scenario V simulations*

The simulations relate to a group of 400,000 men and women with heterosexual contact as the risk factor for HIV. This group has two partners per year in Condition 1 and five partners per year in Condition 2. This average of five partners per year is higher than the average found in a recent study of "Sexuality in the Netherlands". The heterosexual respondents in this study report approximately two partners in the last five years. Men in the age-group 18-35 and women between 18 and 25 report more than three partners per year (Van Zessen, 1991). Our simulation therefore relates to a group with a high average number of sexual partners. The assumed group size has been based on data from socio-sexological research. Our experiment is based on proportional mixing, i.e. arbitrary partner selection, and assumes a rise from 0.1% to 1% in cumulative HIV incidence over a period of five years, and examines what transmission risk per partner is needed for such an increase in HIV infections. We also determine the Basic Reproduction Rate (BRR) and on the basis of this, investigate the possibility of an independent epidemic arising. Table 7.7 sets out the initial situations of our simulations.

Table 7.7 **Initial situations for simulations of HIV among heterosexuals.**

Group size	males:	200,000
	females:	200,000
Infection risk per partner:	man - woman transmission = 2 x woman - man transmission	
Number of partners:	2 - 5 per year	
Seroprevalence		
t = 0:	males:	200
	females:	200
t = 5:	males:	2000
	females:	2000

Table 7.8 shows the transmission risks per partner, which would be required on the basis of the initial situations in the table for the epidemiological course assumed in our projection. In addition, Table 7.8 shows the Yearly Basic Reproduction Rate (YBRR) as it applies to this experiment.

In this report we define the YBRR as the number of new infections which a single infected person causes during a period of one year within his or her own group.[11] Multiplying the YBRR by the length of the infectious period produces the BRR.

On the basis of the BRR it is possible to determine whether an independent epidemic exists. It is of great importance here whether the BRR is greater or smaller than 1. If the BRR is less than 1, then the epidemic is dying out; a BRR greater than or equal to 1 indicates an independent epidemic (Kermack and McKendrick, 1927). Table 7.8 shows that in this scenario an infectious period of more than three years is needed for a BRR greater than 1.

[11] There is a fixed relationship between YECR and YBRR. These cannot be simply equated to each other, however. For the precise relationships we refer to Bailey (1957), Anderson (1982) and Conway (1984).

Table 7.8 **Transmission risk per partner, differentiated according to sex, required for an increase in seroprevalence from 0.1% to 1% over a period of five years.**

	transmission risk per partner		YBRR
	woman HIV +	man HIV +	
Number of partners per year			
2	0.113	0.226	0.32
5	0.045	0.090	0.32

In a virtually identical analysis, Bonneux and Houweling (1989) determined a BRR in the range 0.8 to 2.0. They assumed three to five partners and a risk of infection of between 10 and 15%.[12] They assume the duration of the infectious period to be 2.7 years. In common with Anderson and May (1988), they conclude that an independent epidemic among heterosexuals is unlikely in Europe or the US. Van Druten et al. (in preparation) refer in this connection to the potential effect of bridges between sub-epidemics. In an explorative scenario developed by them, they conclude that separation of the epidemic among gay men from the epidemics in the other core groups leads to a situation in which there is no longer an HIV epidemic among the heterosexual population. Scenario V appears to correspond with the above findings: only where the infectious period lasts for something over three years, or longer, and where the number of sexual partners in this group is higher than average, does an independent epidemic occur. This conclusion can be supported further by a comparison of the transmission risks. Our estimated transmission risks *per partner* in male-female transmission proved to be 50-150 times as great as the transmission risk estimated by Wiley et al. (1989) *per unprotected vaginal contact*. In other words, approximately 50-150 unprotected vaginal contacts per partner are needed to make

[12] The fact that the transmission risk per partner in heterosexual contact is greater in the simulations than the risk of transmission in unprotected anal contact among homosexual males may appear strange. It must be borne in mind that this is a *transmission risk per partner*, and not a transmission risk per contact. Estimations of the transmission risks in the literature are carried out by setting the number of infections against the number of contacts or partners. Where there is a low number of partners and many contacts per partner, this results in a high transmission risk per partner.

our transmission risk match the findings of Wiley et al. (1989).

7.5.2.2 Commentary on Scenario V

The simulation above leads to the conclusion that, under special conditions, an independent epidemic is possible within a population with only heterosexual contact as the risk factor. It is not possible to make a definitive statement, however, since simulations of this type are heavily dependent on the assumed group sizes, the number of partners and the transmission risks. In our case, the transmission risk has been estimated on the basis of assumptions of the number of partners per year and the group size, in combination with an increase in HIV incidence. The number of partners per year we have assumed appears to be on the high side. Validation of the group size is not possible, although it does seem unlikely that we have assumed the group sizes to be too low by a factor of 10. In addition, developments in the HIV incidence could also lead to completely different results. For the time being, the assumption of a seroprevalence of 0.1% does not seem to be in conflict with the findings reported in Chapter 3 from epidemiological studies among pregnant women and heterosexuals with multiple partners (Van Lith et al., 1989; Coutinho et al., 1989, 1990; Hooykaas et al., 1989; Van der Linden et al., 1990).

Our simulation is also in line with the conclusions reached in the study "Sexuality in the Netherlands", namely that a substantial spread of HIV within the heterosexual population as a whole seems unlikely in the short term. This is explained by Van Zessen and Straver (1991) on the basis of the relatively inefficient transmission via vaginal contact, the lower number of partners per year, the presence of selective partner choice, the low frequency of multiple partners as a component of a long-lasting sexual lifestyle and the present lack of any evidence for a "bridging" function to the heterosexual population from men with both male and female partners and from clients of commercial sex workers. Van Zessen and Straver reach the following conclusion with respect to heterosexual networks:

> "In heterosexual networks the necessary stability is lacking, very probably as a result of the constantly changing composition of the group exhibiting risk behaviour and the low average number of sexual partners. This means that the chains and circuits which are created..... are not stable over longer periods. Chains are created and break again, and circuits tend to fragment again relatively quickly." (p.222).

This conclusion does not rule out a certain spread of HIV among the heterosexual population, however. For example, circumstances may coincide to form chains and circuits which lead to a certain spread of

HIV, or there may be a concentration of HIV infections within sections of the heterosexual population (McClumeck et al., 1989). The developments posited in Scenario V are therefore possible. We shall return to considerations affecting HIV/AIDS prevention arising from this scenario in the general commentary.

7.5.3 Scenario VI: HIV among commercial sex workers and their clients

The development assumed in Scenario VI is that there is a spread of HIV among commercial sex workers and their clients, resulting from incorrect and inconsistent use of condoms. Commercial sex workers who inject drugs are particularly susceptible to persuasion by clients to enter into unprotected sexual contact, although non-drug-dependent sex workers also engage in unprotected sexual contact with regular clients.

7.5.3.1 Simulations in Scenario VI

Using the multi-group model, we projected the cumulative HIV incidence within the sex industry over a period of five years. The simulations relate to vaginal contact between female sex workers and male clients. Sex workers who inject drugs have been looked at separately. In the simulations we varied the seroprevalence at $t = 0$ and the level of unprotected contacts. Table 7.9 summarizes the assumed initial situations for the commercial sex work groups. We have distinguished six different conditions: in each of the Conditions 2 to 6 we have varied one parameter with respect to Condition 1. We made use of the multi-group model structure for the simulations, although the definition of the groups deviates from earlier applications of the model: in this scenario, Group 3 in the original model is taken to be the group of sex workers who inject drugs, Group 6 are sex workers who do not inject drugs, and Group 5 consists of clients of sex workers. The groups should be regarded as sub-groups of the original Groups 3, 5 and 6.

Table 7.9 **Initial situations in simulations of the spread of HIV among commercial sex workers and their clients.**

Group size	
Group 3:	2,000 sex workers who inject drugs
Group 4:	13,000 sex workers who do not inject drugs
Group 5:	125,000 clients of sex workers
Condition 1:	
Seroprevalence t = 0:	
Group 3:	30%
Group 6:	0.1%
Group 5:	0%
Number of partners:	
Clients:	12-48 sex workers per year
Transmission risk:	risk of transmission man - woman = 2 x risk of transmission woman - man
Protected contact:	
Group 1:	50% condom use
Group 2:	95% condom use
Condition 2:	95% condom use in Group 3; other variables same as Condition 1
Condition 3:	Seroprevalence in Group 6 at t = 0: 10%; other variables same as Condition 1
Condition 4:	Seroprevalence in Group 6 at t = 0: 50%; other variables same as Condition 1
Condition 5:	Seroprevalence in Group 5 at t = 0: 0.1%; other variables same as Condition 1
Condition 6:	Seroprevalence in Group 5 at t = 0: 10%; other variables same as Condition 1

The size of the groups was determined in accordance with the estimates contained in Table 3.4 in Chapter 3. For Group 3, we took as a basis an estimate for Amsterdam. In order to take into account the lack of clarity and the uncertainty regarding the frequency of visits to commercial sex workers, as well as regarding the seroprevalence and condom use, we selected a range of values for these points. We varied the frequency of visits to sex workers from once per month to once per week, and assumed that the risk of HIV infection during each contact with a sex worker is equal to the risk of infection during vaginal contact. The value for infectiousness is taken from Wiley et al. (1989) who estimate the risk of transmission of HIV from man to woman at 0.0014 during unprotected contact. The simulations are based on proportional mixing of arbitrary partner selection. The difference in the level of unprotected contacts between Group 3 and Group 6 is the result of practical observations that sex workers who inject drugs may be easy to persuade to engage in unprotected contact (Van den Hoek, 1990). The seroprevalence is based on the results given in Chapter 3 of epidemiological research among hard-drug users and heterosexuals with multiple partners.

Table 7.10 contains the transmission matrix for these simulations. As in other experiments, we have separated out a number of sub-epidemics, by allocating the value 0 in the transmission matrix to groups which are not relevant to these simulations.

Table 7.10 **Transmission matrix. Transmission potential via vaginal contact for 2,000 commercial sex workers who inject drugs (3), 13,000 sex workers who do not inject drugs (6) and 125,000 clients of commercial sex workers (6). Initial situation: Condition 1 from Table 7.9, with 24 contacts with sex workers per client per year.**

	1	**2**	**3**	**4**	**5**	**6**
1	0	0	0	0	-	0
2	0	0	0	0	-	0
3	0	0	0	0	0.07	-
4	0	0	0	0	-	0
5	-	-	0.0011	-	-	0.0007
6	0	0	-	0	0.007	-

0 = not applicable due to separation of groups
- = not applicable in the transmission matrix

The transmission matrix is based on 24 sex worker contacts per client per year. The YECR of the sex workers, calculated on the basis of Table 7.10, is 0.035 for sex workers who inject drugs, 0.0035 for non-drug- dependent sex workers and 0.0018 for the clients. The BRR has not yet been defined for a model with three groups (Heesterbeek, in preparation). Table 7.11 shows the results of simulations and gives the cumulative HIV incidence among both clients and sex workers. The figures between brackets relate to the cumulative HIV incidence in five years' time among sex workers from Groups 3 and 6.

Table 7.11 Projections of cumulative HIV incidence within the sex industry during a period of five years under six conditions at t = 0 (see Table 7.9).

Condition	**1**	**2**	**3**	**4**	**5**	**6**
Contacts by clients per year						
12	104 (0)[1]	11 (0)	126 (0)	173 (0)	106 (2)	97 (94)
24	210 (2)	22 (0)	255 (2)	348 (2)	212 (4)	212 (187)
48	422 (6)	43 (0)	513 (7)	699 (8)	426 (10)	437 (369)

* The cumulative HIV incidence between brackets relates to the HIV incidence among sex workers from Groups 3 and 6.

Table 7.11 contains the following indications for the spread of HIV among sex workers and their clients:

- Only at a constant high level of protected contact, as in Condition 2, is there a low HIV incidence during a period of five years. Under the other conditions, cumulative HIV incidence can increase to almost 700 among clients, or more than 350 among sex workers and almost 450 among clients.
- Condition 6 differs from all other conditions in that the HIV incidence among clients and sex workers is virtually identical; this contrasts to the other conditions, where few if any HIV infections are found among the sex workers. It is striking that there is no significant difference between Conditions 4 and 6 in terms of cumulative incidence, whereas there are considerable differences between the two conditions in terms of spread of HIV among sex workers and clients.
- An increase in the seroprevalence among sex workers at t = 0 (Conditions 3 and 4) has some effect when compared to Condition 1, although the difference between Conditions 1 and 3 is not particularly large. This is related to the assumed high level

of 95% for protected sexual contacts with sex workers who do not inject drugs.

7.5.3.2 *Commentary on Scenario VI*

The cumulative HIV incidence over five years was projected under six conditions within the sex industry. Our projections show that at a high level of safe behaviour within the sex industry produces only a low incidence of HIV.

There are plenty of indications that 100% condom use does not occur in the sex industry (see Chapter 3); it remains to be seen whether this will lead to dozens or hundreds of infections in the short term. The simulations show that, without a high level of condom use, hundreds of infections among both commercial sex workers and their clients are possible. The projections also show that large-scale HIV infection among sex workers only takes place once a certain HIV prevalence among clients has been reached, as in Condition 6. For the present, no indications have been found of a seroprevalence of 10% or more among clients of sex workers, which leads to the suggestion on the basis of the simulations that *at this moment* clients of sex workers, in particular, are at risk from HIV infection. For the HIV/-AIDS prevention programme, this would mean that particular attention needs to be focused on urging clients to protect themselves against HIV infection. For commercial sex workers, the message is that matters will take their own course if the demands of clients requesting unprotected contact are not resisted. If this should lead to a seroprevalence of 10% or more among clients, then the commercial sex workers' own risk of HIV infection will have increased considerably.

7.6 *General commentary*

Against the background of the reference scenario, six scenarios and a series of simulations were used to project developments which may lead to an increase in the number of HIV infections. The scenarios and simulations show above all the great importance of a permanent high level of safe behaviour, and also illustrate the need for continued HIV/AIDS prevention efforts.

This applies in any event for men who have sex with men. Within this group there is an accumulation of factors which contribute to promoting the spread of HIV: anal contact as transmission route, large number of partners per year and a significant seroprevalence. Simulations show that a permanent relapse into high-risk behaviour, or a reduction in the level of safe behaviour, could lead to hundreds of new HIV infections in the short term. The goals of the HIV/AIDS prevention programme with respect to this group seem to be clear; the main objective is the prevention of permanent relapse. Since at the moment there appears to be no evidence of a permanent relapse, or relapse on a large scale, efforts are particularly needed which are geared to the preservation of the behavioural change and to pointing out the risks of HIV infection during temporary relapse.

An important factor will be whether the large-scale behavioural change seen to date will lead to what Moerkerk (1990) calls the "prevention paradox": when effective prevention appears to bring about a fall in the impact of AIDS, there is a risk that attention for HIV/AIDS prevention will reduce, which may in turn lead to a resumption of the increase in HIV incidence. Both scenarios relate to a group whose behaviour does not change. Insofar as these are groups which have not (yet) been reached by the HIV/AIDS prevention programme, extra efforts would appear to be justified, for example via the small-scale prevention activities described in Chapters 3 and 4. It would seem to be inevitable that there will be some relapse or that there will be a small group which does not change its behaviour. However, this need not mean that the HIV/AIDS prevention programme fails. Kaplan and Abramson (1989) have shown using mathematical models that even a prevention programme that is not entirely perfect (i.e. where there is some relapse) can lead to great benefits in the long term, and they state that a prevention programme must be assessed on its long-term effects rather than what is achieved in the short term.

The same applies for IDUs as for men who have sex with men. The rapid increase in HIV through shared use of injection equipment points to the need for safe injection behaviour. In addition, our simulations show the importance of taking precautions during sexual contacts. If this is neglected, the result may be a high HIV prevalence, particularly among female IDUs.

The scenarios mapping out the spread of HIV among IDUs reflect the great uncertainty surrounding the future course of HIV infections within this group. The results of current socio-epidemiological research among hard-drug users outside Amsterdam will answer questions arising from our scenarios with respect to the seroprevalence, the extent of injection drug use outside the large cities, and the effects of the HIV/AIDS prevention programme. Moreover, the expectation would appear to be justified that the number of needles exchanged will increase during the coming years, and results may be expected from supplementary prevention activities such as bleach campaigns and individual counselling. The degree to which there will be an increase in the numbers of IDUs reached, and what permanent effects can be expected from the prevention efforts, remains uncertain.

Within the sex industry, there appears at the moment to be no evidence of a large-scale spread of HIV outside the group of commercial sex workers who are also injecting drug users. The simulations of the potential HIV incidence show that hundreds of HIV infections are possible within a relatively short time if no protective measures are used during contacts with commercial sex workers. Only when widespread condom use is predominant in the sex industry can the HIV epidemic said to be under control.

Our projections of the spread of HIV within the heterosexual population as a whole support findings that the risk of a substantial spread of HIV among this group is not high in the short term, and that the immediate risk of HIV infection is small, though not absent. As a corollary to this, we look briefly at the consequences of this for the HIV/AIDS prevention programme directed at the general population.

In the first phase of the AIDS information programme, an unsensational, factual information campaign was used with success to increase the level of knowledge concerning the transmission of HIV infection and the importance of protected sexual contact. One of the basic principles of the HIV/AIDS prevention programme is that both overestimation and underestimation of the risk of HIV infection can have adverse consequences for the results achieved by the AIDS information campaign.

The indication that unprotected heterosexual contact carries some - albeit small - risk of HIV infection, puts the taking of precautions in heterosexual contact in a different light than homosexual contact, contacts with commercial sex workers or sexual contact with an IDU. The point here, rather than an attempt to avert an acute threat, is the avoidance of potential risks. Protection during heterosexual contact therefore plays more of a role in the averting of a potential epidemic in the longer term than in combating an existing epidemic among the general population. This makes AIDS information and prevention campaigns aimed at the general population difficult, since the presentation of a detailed message amounts to a description of what is a small risk in comparison with other threats to health. It may be that an explicit link between HIV/AIDS prevention and STD prevention will provide rather more motivation: the precautionary measures taken not only give protection against HIV infection, but also against other - in view of the risk of transmission, more direct - threats from bacterial and viral STDs. For the AIDS control effort, this creates a more direct link with other, real, threats to health, while the benefit for the STD control programme lies in the expertise and experience built up in the AIDS control programme in the area of primary prevention. This can be of particular importance in combating STDs for which, just as with AIDS, no treatment is available.

7.7 *Summary*

The scenarios in this chapter are based on a group-oriented approach. The effect of behaviour and behavioural change on the incidence and prevalence of HIV is assessed in six scenarios. The choice of the scenarios is founded on the baseline analyses in Chapters 3 and 4, which set out the potentially important developments for the various core groups. The six scenarios are:

Scenario I	HIV/AIDS among men who have sex with men; scenario and subscenario;
Scenario II	HIV among men who have sex with men; temporary versus permanent relapse;
Scenario III	HIV among IDUs; introduction and rapid spread versus plateauing of HIV infections;
Scenario IV	HIV among IDUs; spread via sexual contact and/or shared use of injection equipment;
Scenario V	HIV among heterosexuals; independent epidemic of HIV infections;
Scenario VI	HIV among commercial sex workers and their clients.

In studying the above subjects within the scenarios, an approach was adopted in which qualitative data from sociological and sexological research were applied in combination with the multi-group model.

The projected incidence of HIV among men who have sex with men in the period 1989-2000, assuming continuous growth in accordance within the reference scenario, is almost 7,500. Simulations demonstrate that relapse has a major effect if the virus spreads beyond the group of males exhibiting high-risk behaviour. In addition, reference is made to the importance of a high effectiveness of the HIV/AIDS prevention programme. It is concluded that permanent relapse appears less likely at the moment than temporary relapse. As regards the spread of HIV among IDUs via the shared use of injection equipment, two entirely different scenarios appear possible: a saltatory increase, in which the introduction of HIV into a new network of IDUs leads to a new wave of HIV infections, and secondly a scenario in which there is a levelling off of the HIV epidemic among IDUs. Simulations using the multi-group model show the importance of HIV/AIDS prevention for IDUs and their sexual partners. For the female sexual partners of IDUs, in particular, prevention of unsafe sexual practice appears to be of great importance.

Simulations support the finding that a substantial spread of HIV among the heterosexual population as a whole appears unlikely in the short term, although some spread remains possible under certain circumstances. The consequences of this for HIV/AIDS prevention among the population in general is considered.

Hundreds of infections appear possible in the sex industry over the next five years. As far as the commercial sex workers are concerned, it can be said for the present that they only run a significant risk of infection when the seroprevalence among their clients approaches 10%. However, this does not alter the fact that sex workers and their clients have a common interest in preventing the transmission of HIV.

References

Ahlgren D.J., B.F. Lewis, A.C. Stein
A model of Human Immunodeficiency Virus Transmission Among Intravenous Drug Users
AIDS & Public Policy Journal, 4 (1989), 2, 83-91

Anderson, R.M. (ed.)
Population dynamics of infectious diseases; theory and applications
Chapman and Hall, London, 1982

Anderson, R.M., G.F. Medley, R.M. May, A.M. Johnson
A Preliminary Study of the Transmission Dynamics of the Human Immunodeficiency Virus (HIV), the Causative Agent of AIDS
IMA Journal of Mathematics Applied in Medicine and Biology, 3 (1986), 228-263

Anderson, R.M.
Data needs and a theoretical transmission model
In: HMSO: Her Majesty's Stationery Office, *Future trends in AIDS*; proceedings of a seminar organized by the British Department of Health & Social Security on the 23 March 1987 at the Queen Elizabeth II Conference Centre, London, 6-21

Anderson, R.M.
The epidemiology of HIV infection: variable incubation plus infectious periods and heterogeneity in sexual activity
Journal of the Royal Statistical Society; 151 (1988a), 1, 66-98, series A (Statistics in Society)

Anderson, R.M.
The Role of Mathematical Models in the Study of HIV Transmission and the Epidemiology of AIDS
Journal of Acquired Immune Deficiency Syndromes, 1 (1988b), 241-256

Anderson, R.M., R.M. May
Epidemiological parameters of HIV transmission
Nature, 333 (1988), 514-522

Anderson, R.M.
Editorial review; Mathematical and statistical studies of the epidemiology of HIV
AIDS, 1989a, 3, 333-346

Anderson, R.M.
Prospects for the UK: the AIDS epidemic in the UK; past trends and future projections
In: UK Health Departments, Health Education Authority, *HIV & AIDS:*

An assessment of current and future spread in the UK; proceedings of the Syposium held on Friday 24 November 1989b, Queen Elizabeth II Conference Centre, Westminster, London, 1990, 24-30

Aron, J.L., E.P. Wileyto
Behavioral data and models of the AIDS epidemic
In: J.C. Jager en E.J. Ruitenberg (eds.), *AIDS impact assessment; modelling and scenario analysis*, RIVM/Bilthoven, in voorbereiding

Bailey, N.T.J.
The mathematical theory of epidemics
Charles Griffin & Company limited, London, 1957

Bailey, N.T.J.
Review of available and required data for applied modelling of HIV/AIDS, with special reference to assisting public health decision-making; consultant's report to the global programme on AIDS World Health Organisation
WHO, Geneve, 1988

Bailey, N.T.J.
Operational modelling of HIV/AIDS to assist public health policy making and control
In: J.C. Jager en E.J. Ruitenberg (eds.), *AIDS impact assessment; modelling and scenario analysis*, RIVM/Bilthoven, in preparation

Bonneux, L., H. Houweling
Is een epidemie van heteroseksueel overgedragen HIV-infectie mogelijk in Europa?
Nederlands Tijdschrift voor Geneeskunde, 133 (1989), 39, 1922-1926

Castillo-Chavez, C. (ed.)
Mathematical and Statistical Approaches to AIDS Epidemiology
Springer-Verlag, Berlijn, 1989, Lecture Notes in Biomathematics

Conway, G.R. (ed.)
Pest and pathogen control; strategic, tactical, and policy models
International Institute for Applied Systems Analysis, Chichester, 1984

Coutinho, R.A., K. Boer, M.F. Schutte, W.J. van der Velde, D.K.F. Mulder, G.J.J. van Doornum
HIV-prevalentie bij zwangeren in drie poliklinieken in Amsterdam
Nederlands Tijdschrift voor Geneeskunde, 133 (1989), 19, 978-980

Coutinho, R.A., K. Boer, M.F. Schutte, W.J. van der Velde, D.K.F. Mulder-Folkerts, G.J.J. van Doornum
HIV-prevalentie bij zwangeren in en rond Amsterdam in 1989

Nederlands Tijdschrift voor Geneeskunde, 134 (1990), 26, 1264-1267

Cox, D., R.M. Anderson, A.M. Johnson, M.J.R. Healy, V. Isham, A.D. Wilkie, N.E. Day, O.N. Gill, A. McCormick
Short-term prediction of HIV Infection and AIDS in England and Wales; report of a working group
Her Majesty's Stationery Office, London, 1988

Dangerfield, B., C. Roberts
A role for system dynamics in modelling the spread of AIDS
Trans Inst MC, 11 (1989), 4, 187-195

DeGruttola, V., G.R. Seage III, K.H. Mayer, C.R. Horsburgh jr.
Infectiousness of HIV between male homosexual partners
Journal of Clinical Epidemiology, 42 (1989), 9, 849-856

Des Jarlais, D.C., A.A. Ehrhardt, M.T. Fullilove, K. Hein, J. Menken, B.S. Mensch, H.G. Miller, C.F. Turner
AIDS and adolescents
In: H.G. Miller, C.F. Turner, L.E. Moses (eds.), *AIDS: the second decade*, National Academy Press, Washington D.C., 1990, 147-252

Druten, J.A.M. van, Th. de Boo, A.G.M. Reintjes, J.C. Jager, S.H. Heisterkamp, R.A. Coutinho, J.M. Bos, E.J. Ruitenberg
Reconstruction and prediction of spread of HIV infection in populations of homosexual men
In: J.C. Jager, E.J. Ruitenberg (eds.), *Statistical Analysis and Mathematical Modelling of AIDS*, Oxford University Press, Oxford, 1988

Druten, J.A.M. van, J.C. Jager
AIDS: Statistical analysis and mathematical modelling of the acquired immunodeficiency syndrome (AIDS); with a view to scenario-analysis
Katholieke Universiteit Nijmegen (KUN) / Rijksinstituut voor Volksgezondheid en Milieuhygiëne (RIVM), RIVM, Bilthoven, 1991, report number 958501004

Van Druten, J.A.M. van, M.J.J.C. Poos, J. Hendriks, J.C. Jager
HIV epidemics in linked risk groups; a move to exploratory scenario-analysis
In: J.C Jager, E.J Ruitenberg (eds.) *AIDS impact assessment; modelling and scenario-analysis*, RIVM/Bilthoven, in preparation

Fusaro, R.E., N.P. Jewell, W.W. Hauck, D.C. Heilbron, J.D. Kalbfleisch, J.M. Neuhaus, M.A. Ashby
An Annotated Bibliography of Quantitative Methodology Relating to the AIDS Epidemic
Statistical Science, 4 (1989), 3, 264-281

Geneeskundige Hoofdinspectie van de Volksgezondheid (GHI)
anonymous records of AIDS-diagnoses
GHI, Rijswijk, continuous records

Grant, R.M., J.A. Wiley, W. Winkelstein
Infectivity of the Human Immunodeficiency virus: estimates from a prospective study of homosexual men
Journal of Infectious Diseases, 156 (1987), 189-193

Griensven G.J.P. van, E. de Vroome, P. Veugelers
Heterogeneity and fluctuations in homosexual behaviour: implications for modelling the AIDS epidemic
Presented at the *VI International Conference on AIDS*, San Francisco 1990, (Th.C.112)

Griffiths, J.D., J.E. Williams
Identification of some important factors in modelling the spread of AIDS
In: J.C. Jager and E.J. Ruitenberg (eds.), *AIDS impact assessment; modelling and scenario analysis*, RIVM/Bilthoven, in preparation

Haan, B.J. de, M.G.W. Dijkgraaf
An age structured model for HIV transmission
In: J.C Jager, E.J Ruitenberg (eds.) *AIDS impact assessment; modelling and scenario-analysis*, RIVM/Bilthoven, in preparation

Haastrecht, H.J.A. van, J.A.R. van den Hoek, C. Bardoux, A. Leentvaar-Kuypers, R.A. Coutinho
The course of the HIV epidemic among Intravenous Drug Users in Amsterdam, The Netherlands
American Journal of Public Health, 81 (1991a), 1, 59-62

Haastrecht, H.J.A. van, J.A.R. van den Hoek, G. Mientjes, R.A. Coutinho
The early course of the HIV-infection epidemic among injecting drug users in Amsterdam, The Netherlands
Poster at *VII International Conference on AIDS*, Florence, 1991b (W.C. 3288)

Heesterbeek, J.A.P.
An example of the use of the Basic Reproduction Ratio R_0 in scenario analysis
In: J.C. Jager en E.J. Ruitenberg (eds.), *AIDS impact assessment; modelling and scenario-analysis*, RIVM, Bilthoven, in voorbereiding

Heisterkamp, S.H., B.J. de Haan, J.C. Jager, J.A.M. van Druten, J.C.M. Hendriks
Short and middle term projections of the AIDS/HIV epidemic by a dynamic model with an application to the risk-group of homo/bisexual

men in Amsterdam
Statistics in Medicine, submitted

Hoek, A. van den
Epidemiology of HIV infection among drug users in Amsterdam
Rodopi, Amsterdam, 1990, academic thesis

Holmberg, S.D., C.R. Horsburgh jr., J.W. Ward, H.W. Jaffe
Biological factors in the Sexual Transmission of Human Immunodeficiency Virus
The Journal of Infectious Diseases, 160 (1989), 1, 116-125

Holmes, K.K.
HIV-infection in the context of changing epidemiological patterns of sexually transmitted disease
Presented at the *V International Conference on AIDS*, Montreal, 1989

Hooykaas, C., J. van der PLigt, G.J.J. van Doornum, M.M.D. van der Linden, R.A. Coutinho
Heterosexuals at risk for HIV: differences between private and commercial partners in sexual behavior and condom use
AIDS, 3(1989), 525-532

Jewell, N.P., S.C. Shiboski
Statistical Analysis of HIV Infectivity Based on Partner Studies
Biometrics, 46 (1990), 1133-1150

Kaplan, E.H.
What are the risks of risky sex? Modeling the AIDS epidemic
Operations Research, 37 (1989a), 2:198-209

Kaplan, E.H.
Can Bad Models Suggest Good Policies? Sexual Mixing and the AIDS Epidemic
The Journal of Sex Research, 26 (1989b), 3, 301-314

Kaplan, E.H.
Needles That Kill: Modeling Human Immunodeficiency Virus Transmission via Shared Drug Injection Equipment in Shooting Galleries
Reviews of Infectious Diseases, 11 (1989c), 2, 289-298

Kaplan, E.H., P.R. Abramson
So What if the Program ain't Perfect? A Mathematical Model of AIDS Education
Evaluation Review, 13 (1989), 2, 107-122

Kaplan, E.H.
Modeling HIV Infectivity: Must Sex Acts be Counted?

Journal of Acquired Immune Deficiency Syndromes, 3 (1990), 55-61

Kaplan, E.H., Yew Sing Lee
How Bad Can it Get? Bounding Worst Case Endemic Heterogeneous Mixing Models of HIV/AIDS
Mathematical Biosciences, 99 (1990), 157-180

Kermack, W.O., A.G. McKendrick
Contributions to the mathematical theory of epidemics
Proceedings of the Royal Society, series A, 115 (1927), 700-721

Knox, E.G.
HIV transmission in drug-injectors, and needle exchange schemes
Presented at *Second Workshop on Quantitative Analysis of AIDS*, RIVM, Bilthoven, July 1988

Kuiken, C.L., G.J.P. van Griensven, E.M.M. de Vroome, R.A. Coutinho
Risicofactoren en sexuele gedragsverandering in voor HIV-antilichamen geseroconverteerde homosexuele mannen
Tijdschrift voor Sociale Gezondheidszorg, 68 (1990), 329-334

Laar, M.J.W. van de, J.A.R. van den Hoek, J. Pickering, G.J.P. van Griensven, R.A. Coutinho, H.P.A. van de Water
Dalende trend van gonorroe in Nederland: betekenis voor de AIDS-epidemie
Nederlands Tijdschrift voor Geneeskunde, 134 (1990), 13, 647-652

Lagergren, M.
A family of models for analysis and evaluation of strategies for preventing AIDS
In: J.C. Jager en E.J. Ruitenberg (eds.), *AIDS impact assessment; modelling and scenario analysis*, RIVM/Bilthoven, in preparation

Lith, J.M.M. van, Tj. Tijmstra, G.H.A. Visser
De houding van zwangeren ten aanzien van het onderzoek op HIV-infectie
Nederlands Tijdschrift voor Geneeskunde, 133 (1989), 25, 1273-1277

McClumeck, N., H. Taelman, P. Hermans, P. Piot, M. Schoumacher, S. de Wit
A cluster of HIV-infection among heterosexual people without apparent risk factors
New England Journal of Medicine, 321 (1989), 1460-1462

Moerkerk, H.
Presentation in connection with the VI International Conference on AIDS
Utrecht, *AIDS Symposium San Francisco '90*, 1990

Mooij, A.
De ziektes van de revolutie; geslachtsziekten in Nederland vanaf de jaren zestig
In: G. Hekma, B. van Stolk, B. van Heerikhuizen, B. Kruithof (sam.), *Het verlies van de onschuld; seksualiteit in Nederland*, Amsterdams Sociologische Tijdschrift / Wolters Noordhof Groningen, 1990, 121-150

Moss, A.R.
AIDS and intravenous drug use: the real heterosexual epidemic
British Medical Journal, 294 (1987), 389-390

Rezza, G., A. Lazzarin, G. Angarano, A. Sinicco, A. Zerboni, R. Aiuiti, R. Pristerà, B. Salassa, M. Barbanera, S. Gafà, L. Ortona, P. Costigliola, U. Tirelli, P. Pezotti
AIDS free time after seroconversion in injecting drug users and other risk groups
Poster at *VI International Conference on AIDS*, San Francisco, 1990 (Th.C. 647)

Roberts, C., B. Dangerfield
Modelling the epidemiological consequences of HIV infection and AIDS: a contribution from operational research
Journal of the Operational Research Society, 41 (1990), 4, 273-289

Solomon, P.J., J.A. Donst, S.R. Wilson
Predicting the course of AIDS in Australia and evaluating the effect of AZT: a first report
National Centre for Epidemiology and Population Health, The Australian National Universtity, Canberra, 1989

Solomon, P.J., C. Fazekas de St. Groth, S.R. Wilson (eds.)
Projections of Acquired Immune Deficiency Syndrome in Australia using data to the end of September 1989
National Centre for Epidemiology and Population Health, The Australian National University, Canberra, 1990

Wiley, J.A., S.J. Herschkorn, N.S. Padian
Heterogeneity in the probability of HIV transmission per sexual contact: the case of male-to-female transmission in penile-vaginal intercourse
Statistics in Medicine, 8 (1989), 1, 93-102

Wit, J.B.F. de, E.M.M. de Vroome, T.G.M. Sandfort, G.J.P. van Griensven, R.A. Coutinho
Stijging van de incidentie van HIV-infectie, het gevolg van een toename in onveilig seksueel gedrag? Bevindingen in een cohort homoseksuele mannen in Amsterdam
Tijdschrift Sociale Gezondheidszorg, 69 (1991), 1, 26-30

Withers, C.S.
AIDS: References on modelling -with comments-; update: september 22, 1989
Applied Mathematics Division, department of Scientific and Industrial Research, Wellington, New Zealand, 1989

Zessen, G.J. van
Seks en Levensloop
In: G.J. van Zessen en Th. Sandfort (red.), *Seksualiteit in Nederland; seksueel gedrag, risico en preventie van AIDS*, Swets & Zeitlinger, Amsterdam/Lisse, 1991, 35-58

Zessen, G.J. van, C. Straver
De mogelijke verspreiding van HIV onder de Nederlandse bevolking
In: G.J. van Zessen en Th. Sandfort (red.), *Seksualiteit in Nederland; seksueel gedrag, risico en preventie van AIDS*, Swets & Zeitlinger, Amsterdam/Lisse, 1991, 205-224

8 Health care and medical technology

8.1 Introduction

The reference scenario indicates that on a national level AIDS will lead to a considerable, though manageable, burden on health care facilities over the next decade. The situation is different at the level of care provision and the relationship between care-provider and patient. The care and treatment of people with an HIV or AIDS demands a great deal of time and involves high (additional) costs for the often very intensive medical, nursing and psychosocial help and the expensive medication (Dutch Lower House, 1987, 1989; NCAB, 1988; KPMG, 1989; Postma et al., 1991).

The rapid pace of medical developments demands a high level of specialized expertise. In order to maximize this know-how and the quality of care, 11 hospitals were nominated in 1990 to act as regional centres for the treatment, care and study of AIDS patients, with the AMC functioning as a national reference centre (Dutch Lower House, 1989). One of the tasks of these regional hospital centres is to pass on knowledge to other institutions, so that adequate care can continue to be provided to the increasing number of patients (Health Council, 1987; NCAB, 1991). Early intervention and prophylactic treatment of infections can enable the diagnosis of AIDS to be delayed and opportunistic infections to be prevented (Volberding et al., 1990; Health Council, 1990; Langer and Goudsmit, 1989; Biglioni et al., 1991). The advancing developments in diagnostics and treatment methods have a favourable effect on the welfare of people with AIDS. Although many HIV-infected persons face serious psychosocial and psychiatric problems, the demand for assistance has been below expectations. Intensive counselling and initiatives in social support may have played a role here (King, 1990; Van Beuzekom et al., 1991; Van den Boom et al., 1991a). The fear of infection among care-providers, and the unfamiliarity and discomfiture felt with gay or drug using patients, or patients who are commercial sex workers have not led to large-scale discrimination. In addition to the setting up of regional hospital centres, a number of initiatives in care, which are to some extent innovative, have been started in response to AIDS, such as the stimulation of patient-oriented nursing, the recruitment of AIDS consultants, involvement of the patient in the care and treatment provided, experiments with intensive home care, the starting of volunteer projects and the carrying out of clinical trials among healthy asymptomatic HIV-infected persons. These developments give rise to a number of questions for scenario analysis.

Figure 8.1 shows the most important elements and relationships, taken from the conceptual model in Chapter 1, for scenarios in the area of care and medical technology. Both the AIDS incidence and the HIV/AIDS prevalence, as well as the care provided, are influenced by medical technology. As far as care is concerned, this influence is a two-way process: the demand and need for care among people with HIV and AIDS influences the supply of care; in turn, the supply of care influences the demand for that care. Medical technology is also influenced by the care: the increasing experience and expertise within the care sector lead to improvements in the diagnostic techniques and treatment methods.

Figure 8.1 Relations between medical technology, care, HIV and AIDS.

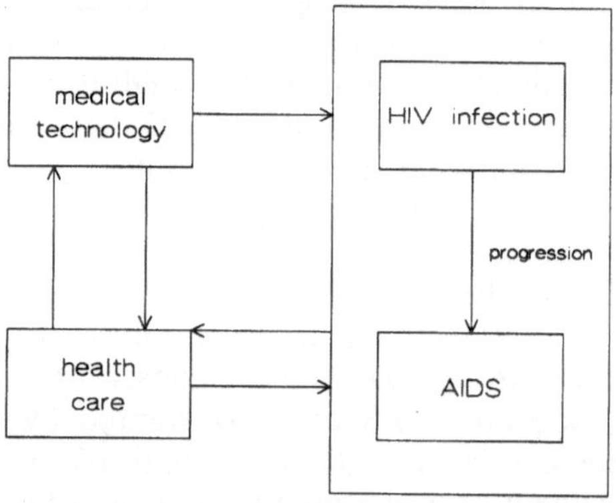

The central questions for scenarios relate to the influence of developments in the care sector, medical technology and the treatment of AIDS on the supply, matching and coordination of the care. What is the influence of developments in medical technology on incidence and prevalence, and on the demand for care? What are the costs for the health care sector of the various developments in treatment possibilities? What are the consequences for health care if AIDS increasingly becomes a chronic disease which requires (life)long treatment, but which is no longer acutely life-threatening?

Three scenarios are used to develop projections relating to the above questions. These scenarios are as follows:

Scenario I Extension of the survival time after diagnosis of AIDS.

Scenario II	Early intervention; delaying progression to AIDS
Scenario III	AIDS as a chronic disease[1]

The first two scenarios relate to the short and medium term, while the third scenario is a long-term projection. Scenarios I and II are developed quantitatively, while Scenario III is reflective in nature. Table 8.1 shows the parameters which are varied with respect to the reference scenario and the indicators used to express the impact of the changes.

Table 8.1 Parameters and indicators of scenarios relating to care and medical technology.

Parameters		**Indicators**	
	Scenario I survival period	Scenario II early intervention	Scenario III chronic disorder
Epidemiology:			
survival period incubation period	AIDS prevalence	AIDS prevalence AIDS incidence HIV prevalence	AIDS/HIV incidence -prevalence
Economy:			
Inpatient	bed need and hospital/nursing home costs	bed need and hospital/nursing home costs	bed need hospital/ nursing home
Outpatient	hours and costs of regular and intensive home care GP consultations	outpatient care at trial centres costs of AZT GP consultations	hours of regular and intensive home care general practitioner trial centres
Volunteers	hours and requests buddy help informal network		requests for buddy help other volunteers informal network
Programme costs	tests	number and costs of tests	test policy
Organization of care:	regional centres substitution volunteers	regional centres trial/treatment centres pre & post-test counselling	category-specific vs non-category-specific care

[1] The possibility of a vaccine is not explored in this scenario. It is not possible to predict when a vaccine might become available, what its effects would be and who would be eligible for vaccination. It is also not known what consequences this might have for the HIV and AIDS epidemic (Koff and Fauci, 1991; Bolognesi and Schild, 1990; Redfield, 1991; Goldsmith, 1991).

The left-hand column of the table shows the epidemiological, economic and sociocultural parameters. The indicators are listed under each of the scenarios. Thus, for example, the effect of the parameter "extension of the survival period" is studied on the basis of the AIDS prevalence, the need for care and the organization of that care.

8.2 Methods and underlying principles

We have assumed in the scenarios that all people with AIDS will make use of the health care facilities sooner or later. The main questions in the health care scenarios are as follows:

- What is the effect of an increase in the survival period on the demand for care and the composition of the care package. What are the implications of meeting a proportion of the need for in-hospital care with 24-hour intensive home care?
- What are the consequences for care of an increase in the length of the pre-AIDS stage as a result of early intervention and symptom control?
- What are the consequences for the organization and provision of care if AIDS becomes a chronic disease?

The projections in this chapter are carried out using the coherent system of assumptions from the reference scenario. The methods, data and assumptions on which the epidemiological developments and the economic evaluation are based are discussed in Chapter 2, while the classification of the costs is set out in Chapter 5. As can be seen from Table 8.1, although the epidemiological parameters are varied in the scenarios, the emphasis in this chapter is on changes in the need for care and the duration of care. In common with the working method adopted in the reference scenario, we also indicate the change in impact with respect to the subscenario, which is based on estimated developments in the HIV epidemic up to 1.1.1989.

The scenarios are largely reflective. We look at changes in the care package, (financial) limiting conditions for the care-provision services, changes in the relationship between care-provider and patient, quality of care, and the consequences of developments in medical technology for the testing policy. We also look at the question of whether the present facilities will be able to meet the expected future need for care. The chapter concludes with a commentary in which the variants referred to are discussed.

We have assumed in the scenarios that neither a curative therapy nor a vaccine are yet available. We have also assumed that all people with AIDS have a need for care, that a demand for care is always met, and that the care provided is of good quality. We set the scenarios against the background of current developments in health care, such as the aim of reducing the length of hospital stays, substitution by out-of-hospital facilities, and the promotion of home care (Ministry of Welfare, Health and Cultural Affairs, 1989; Dutch Lower House, 1987). It is assumed that these developments will continue unchanged in the future.

8.3 Scenario I: Increase in the survival time after diagnosis of AIDS

Assumptions

In Scenario I we assume that there will be an increase during the period 1990-2000 in the survival period after diagnosis of AIDS, from two to three years. This is related to improved diagnosis and developments in treatment methods. Depending on the severity of the pathological process, this will lead to a change in the demand for care and the duration of that care. In addition, substitution will lead to a change in the supply of care.

AIDS prevalence

In Scenario I we select three variants of an increase in the survival period from two to three years, achieved in four years' time. Figure 8.2 shows the corresponding AIDS prevalence in the period 1990-2000. From 1992 onwards, the effect of the increasing survival period with respect to the reference scenario (and the subscenario) becomes apparent. After four years it is clear that there is a higher AIDS prevalence than that observed in the reference scenario. The HIV prevalence/incidence and the AIDS incidence do not change with respect to the reference scenario and subscenario, because the assumed change only takes place after diagnosis of AIDS.

Figure 8.2 **AIDS prevalence (at 31.12) for a survival period after the diagnosis of AIDS of two (reference scenario) and three years (scenario I), including respective subscenarios.**

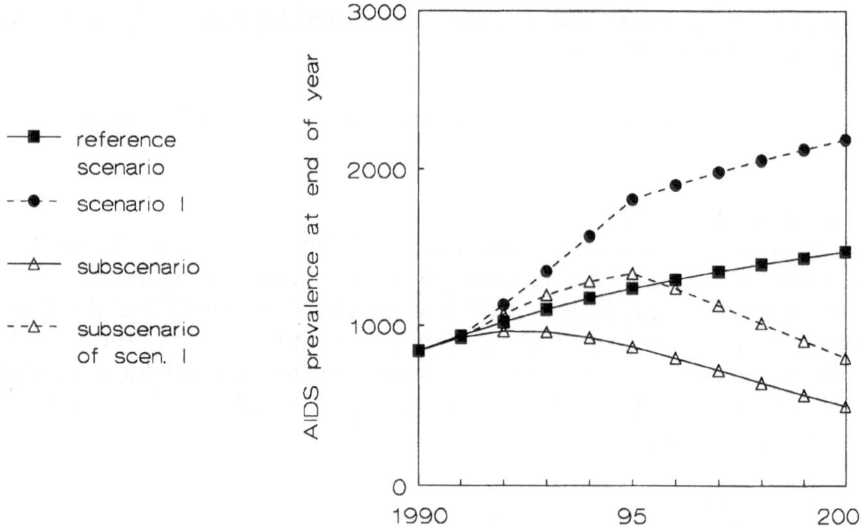

8.3.1 *Variant A: Unchanging intensity of care with a survival period of three years*

In Variant A we assume the same need for care *per person-year* as in the reference scenario; this means that people with AIDS have the same need for care in the third year of survival as in the foregoing two years.

Use of care
As a result of the higher AIDS prevalence, the need for care increases. Demand for both in-hospital and out-of-hospital care rises in proportion to the increase in the survival period to three years. Table 8.2 summarizes the demand for care for HIV or AIDS. Our estimates for hospital beds are based on the most recent information on bed requirements. (Dijkgraaf et al., 1991).

Figure 8.3 and Table 8.2 show that the number of hospital beds halfway the year in Variant A is almost one-and-a-half times as great as in the reference scenario or the subscenario. With a three-year survival period, the number of hospital beds required is 177 in 1995 and 224 in 2000; the number of nursing home beds is 14 and 18, respectively. In common with the working method used in the reference scenario, calculations have also been carried out for the subscenario. Lengthening the survival period by one year amounts to increasing the bed requirement from 95 to 137 in 1995 and from 57 to 89 in the year 2000. The demand for home nursing, home help, intensive home care and general practitioners is also one-and-a-half times the figure in the reference scenario.

Figure 8.3 **The need for hospital beds (on 30.6): comparison of reference scenario with Variant A (constant level of care) from Scenario I, including respective subscenarios.**

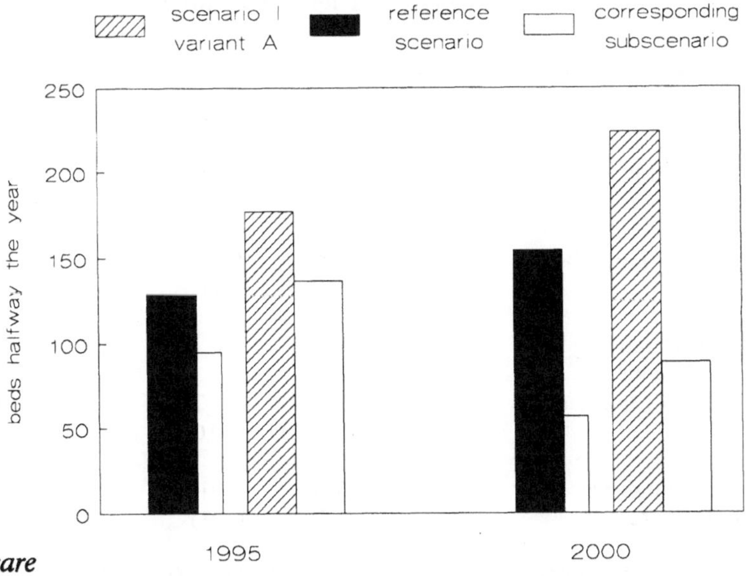

Costs of care

It was stated in the reference scenario that the cost implications of a reduction in the average length of hospital stay from 51-53 to 27 days per person year are still unclear. In the calculations, we have taken the cost studies based on 53 days as a yardstick. For out-of-hospital care we estimate the costs for a survival period of three years at NLG 14 million for 1995, and NLG 18 million for the year 2000.

The total of direct patient-related costs in the year 2000 is NLG 39 million higher than the costs in the reference scenario, if the survival period is extended to three years. For the subscenario, an extension of the survival period produces an increase in the patient-related costs of NLG 24 million in 1995.

The costs can be compared with the estimate produced by the Financial Statement on Health Care 1991 (FOZ, 1991). For a survival period of three years, the costs in 1995 amount to 0.39% of the total costs of the care categories studied. The calculation for the sub-scenario shows that, with an increased survival period, these costs take up over 0.30% of the total. For the year 2000 these percentages are 0.48% and over 0.19%, respectively.[2] Just as in the reference scenario, therefore, there is a considerable though manageable burden on the total health care costs. The calculations for the subscenario make clear that averting HIV infections can result in a considerable reduction in the patient-related costs.

Table 8.2 **Reference scenario compared with Variant A, including respective subscenarios: patient-related economic impact of AIDS in 1995 and 2000 with a survival time of two and three years.**

	Survival time	1995		2000	
Hospital beds[2]	2 years	128	(95)	154	(57)
	3 years	177	(137)	224	(89)
Nursing home beds	2 years	10	(7)	12	(4)
	3 years	14	(11)	18	(7)
District nursing and home help: Hours of home care	2 years	37,500	(27,700)	45,200	(16,400)
	3 years	52,500	(40,600)	66,700	(26,300)
Days' intensive home care	2 years	664	(491)	801	(290)
	3 years	932	(721)	1,184	(466)
General practitioner consultations	2 years	24,000	(17,900)	27,900	(11,500)
	3 years	28,900	(22,100)	34,900	(14,700)
Outpatient costs[1] x NLG 1,000,000	2 years	10.1	(7.5)	12.2	(4.5)
	3 years	14.0	(10.9)	17.8	(7.0)
Total costs[1] x NLG 1,000,000	2 years	77.6	(57.4)	92.6	(34.8)
	3 years	104.8	(80.9)	131.8	(52.6)

1 Costs converted to 1988 levels
2 Based on Dijkgraaf et al. (1991)

2 As in the reference scenario, a nominal growth of 2% in the costs of AIDS has been assumed.

8.3.2 *Variant B: Intensification of home care*

Assumptions
In this projection, people with AIDS require an ever-increasing amount of care. Following diagnosis of AIDS, the steadily deteriorating immune system allows more and more frequent occurrence of complex infections. Combating these requires specialized treatments, leading to an increase in hospital admissions, although improved treatment methods mean that the duration of each admission is shorter. In Variant B, we assume that the shortening of the length of hospital stay, together with a simultaneous increase in the number of admissions, result in a bed requirement of 27 days, the same as that in the reference scenario and in Variant A of Scenario I.

As well as inpatient help, people with AIDS also need additional care. This cannot be provided by the informal support network alone, which means that investment in home care is required. In order to continue providing the progressively deteriorating AIDS patient with adequate, high quality care, the out-of-hospital help given per observation year must be twice as high as in the reference scenario.

Use of care
For an impression of the total length of stay and the total costs, we refer to the data relating to a three-year survival period in Table 8.2. Variations from the reference scenario arise in a number of areas, including in the district nursing service and in the number of consultations with general practitioners. Table 8.3 reflects the need for home care and number of general practitioner consultations for Variant B.

Table 8.3 **Variant B: Out-of-hospital help needed in the case of an increase in survival period to three years: 1995 and 2000, based on the AIDS prevalence in the reference scenario (and subscenario).**

	1995		2000	
District nursing and home help:				
- Hours of home care	105,000	(81,300)	133,500	(52,500)
- Days of intensive home care	1,900	(1,400)	2,400	(900)
GP consultations	45,800	(35,200)	56,400	(23,200)

The increased need for home care in Variant B is a result of the assumptions made in this variant. The increase is therefore unrelated to substitution of in-hospital care by out-of-hospital care.

It would seem reasonable to assume that the increase in the need for general practitioner consultations and home care in this variant will become particularly noticeable in the final stages of the disease. Apart from an increase in actual care and assistance, the attention given to matching and coordinating of the care also increases. The help-providers here are AIDS consultants, social workers, the general practitioner, home helps and district nurses. The demand and pressure on the social network will also increase. The informal network has for some time supplemented the (more intensive) care provided for those closest to the patient with voluntary help, district nursing and home help.

Costs of care
The costs of inpatient and outpatient hospital care are the same as in Variant A, i.e. NLG 91 million and NLG 114 million in 1995 and 2000 respectively. The costs of out-of-hospital care double, amounting to NLG 18.5 million in 1995 and NLG 23.4 million in the year 2000. Comparison with the Financial Statement on Health Care (FOZ, 1991) shows that the costs of AIDS and HIV in the year 2000 in Variant B account for 0.50% of the total costs of the care categories studied. Figure 8.4 shows a comparison for the outpatient costs of Variants A and B.

It is apparent from Figure 8.4 that the difference between the variants is fairly small. This is because a proportion of the costs of out-of-hospital care, namely the consultations with general practitioners, occur in the pre-AIDS stage, whereas these variants relate to patients already diagnosed with AIDS. It has also been assumed that the annual use of AZT, both at home and in hospital, is the same as in the reference scenario. The increased costs of the out-of-hospital help in Variant B do not therefore lead to significant differences with respect to Variant A.

Figure 8.4 **Outpatient patient-related costs (in millions NLG, cost level 1988) for an increase in survival time to three years: comparison of variant A (constant level of care) and B (increased level of home care), including respective subscenarios. Hospital outpatient costs excluded.**

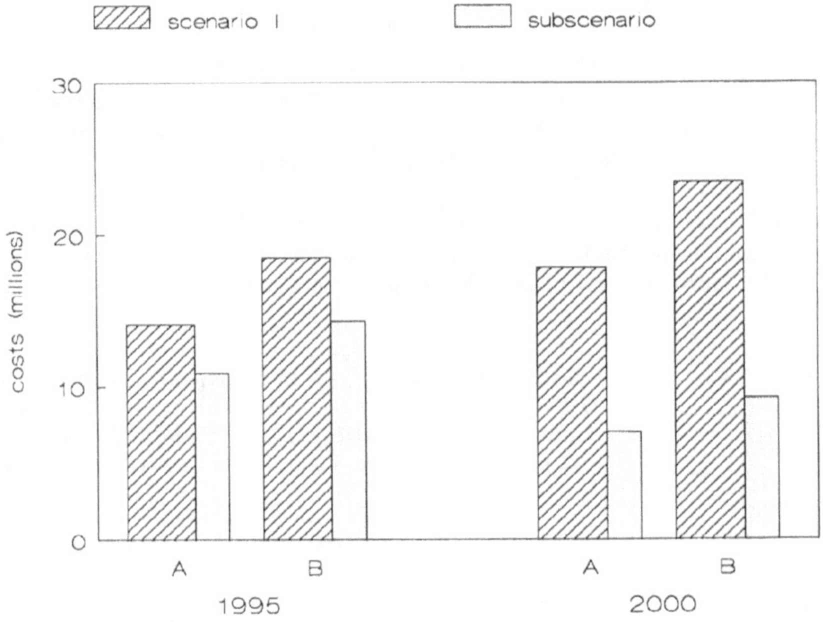

8.3.3 *Variant C: Substitution*

Assumptions

In this variant we assume that the need for care per observation year is the same as in the reference scenario (and the subscenario). We also assume developments in the possibilities for treating people with AIDS which allow a proportion of the inpatient care to be replaced by intensive home care. This substitution is made possible by medico-technological developments in home care, and is encouraged by the government through the provision of adequate funding. The need for inpatient care remains the same as in the reference scenario during the three-year survival period, i.e. 27 days per observation year.

We project a situation in which a maximum of seven inpatient days are replaced by seven days of 24-hour intensive home care, thus leading to a reduction in the number of hospitalization days from 27 to 20 days per observation year. The intensive home care is supplemented by regular home care, volunteers and the informal support network.

Use of care

Table 8.4 shows the bed requirement for a substitution from inpatient to outpatient care from 27.3 hospitalization days per observation year, as in the reference scenario and the subscenario, to 20 hospitalization days. In Variant C of this scenario, a survival period of three years leads to a need for 132 beds in 1995, against 166 in the year 2000. This represents a reduction in the hospital bed requirement compared to Variant A (Table 8.2). This is offset by a clear increase in demand for home care, volunteer help and the services of the informal support network. The latter is provided by the partner, family and/or friends, with additional support from volunteers. This scenario leads to an increase in the demand for buddies. The matching and coordination of inpatient care and home care demands a good deal of attention from AIDS consultants, specialists, general practitioners, the district nursing service and the home help service.

Table 8.4 **Substitution from inpatient to outpatient care of 7 out of 27 hospitalization days per observation year. Costs (in million NLG; cost level 1988) in 1995 and 2000 compared with reference scenario, including respective subscenarios.**

		1995	2000
Beds:	reference scenario	96 (71)	115 (43)
	variant C	132 (102)	166 (66)
Outpatient costs: (x NLG 1 million)	reference scenario	11.8 (8.7)	14.2 (5.2)
	variant C	20.1 (15.6)	25.5 (10.1)

The possibilities and conditions which form the basis of the care model described are an important aspect of this scenario. Intensive home care is only possible if an intensive support network is in place or can be organized (Tjadens et al., 1991), and there must be an adequate supply of buddies to provide the volunteer assistance required.

Costs of care

Substitution from inpatient to outpatient care will take place for the so- called "low-care" days, with the least intensive level of care. The AZU has calculated the marginal costs per low-care hospitalization day at NLG 332. The Dutch Health Service funds intensive home care up to NLG 200 per day; on the basis of this maximum amount, the saving per AIDS patient comes to 7.3 x NLG 132, i.e. approximately NLG 1000.

The costs of outpatient care are higher than in the reference scenario, where in the year 2000 the total patient-related costs for a survival period of two years amounts to NLG 93 million; in the event of substitution this total drops to NLG 91 million for the same survival period. The move towards substitution boils down in this projection almost entirely to a commitment to improving the quality of life, by allowing the patient to remain in the home situation for as long as possible. This projection leads only to a slight cost saving.

8.3.4 Commentary on Scenario I

An increase in the survival period following diagnosis of AIDS has many consequences for the direct care of people with AIDS. Figure 8.5 reflects the consequences for patient-related costs, which will increase significantly if the survival period is extended to three years. Variant B, intensification of home care, brings the highest costs. The differences between Variants A and C, however, are not especially large.

The number of hospital and nursing home beds needed for people with AIDS as a result of an increased survival period will not create any capacity problems at a national level. Set against the anticipated increase in the need for (intensive) home care for the elderly, the chronically sick, patients prematurely discharged from hospital and terminal patients, the absolute bed requirement of AIDS patients will also not be particularly large, although a necessary condition here is that home care is sufficiently well organized to be able to absorb the expected increase in demand in the future.

It was concluded in the reference scenario that, particularly in the health care sector, the impact of AIDS would only become fully apparent in the 1990s. An extension of the survival period, and the resultant higher patient-related costs compared with the reference scenario, serve only to reinforce this conclusion. Such an increase in the survival period would also have consequences beyond the year 2000, since a proportion of the care per patient would be displaced to the period after that year.

Figure 8.5 **Patient-related costs (in million NLG; cost level 1988) for both inpatient and outpatient care, for an increasing survival time: comparison with the reference scenario. A: constant level of care, B: increasing level of home care, and C: substitution of home care for care. Including respective subscenarios.**

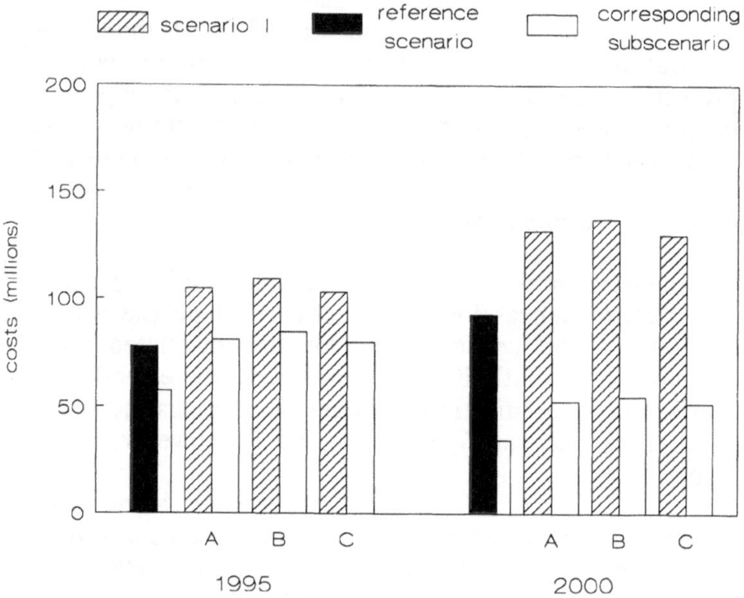

As regards the level at which care is actually provided, this scenario leads to conclusions which are unchanged from the baseline analysis: fear of infection or ignorance concerning the living situation of the person can still hinder a proper care-provider relationship and thus create problems (Dutch Lower House, 1987). In addition, the anticipated number of people with AIDS will be at least double that in the preceding decade. More people with AIDS will find themselves in the care system for a longer period as a result of the extended survival period and increasing treatment possibilities. For the regional centres this will mean an increase in the pressure on special AIDS units and nursing staff. A shorter stay per hospital admission does not imply cheaper care per se: often, extremely specialized treatments are needed which require intensive, complex and expensive care, in order to combat the AIDS-related complaints. In connection with developments such as the lengthening of the duration of care and intensification of home care, we would also point out the increasingly important part played by AIDS consultants and AIDS internists in the regional centres. Adequate coordination between the various care-providers is necessary, and the allocation to one of the care-providers of a case-management or coordinating role would seem to be a useful step in organizing the home care for and with the patient. This role is often assumed by the AIDS internist or AIDS consultant, but it could also be carried out by the general practitioner, the professional home care provider or another care-provider. It is important that this is taken into account when looking at questions of capacity.

A growing need for care, and the substitution of care, will lead to an increase in the pressure placed on the social network as compared to the reference scenario. The partner, family or friends will have to provide care for a longer period for a patient whose condition is steadily worsening. Gay men generally have a fairly well-functioning social network, which provides the necessary informal support (Arno, 1986; De Rijk et al., 1991; Van den Boom et al., 1991a). The question for this group is what effect an increase in the survival period and substitution will have on the ability of the informal support network to cope. In the case of IDUs, on the other hand, a different situation reigns, since the social network of this group is limited in size and offers little in the way of support (Driessen et al., 1991). An extended period of care is likely to bring more problems for this group than for gay men.

It would seem reasonable to expect that this scenario will lead to an increasing demand for supplementary support from the buddy care system. On a national level, this may not create capacity problems, since the present demand for buddies outside the large towns is lower than the supply. However, increasing demand could well lead to shortages of buddies in towns with a high concentration of people with AIDS.

8.4 Scenario II: Early intervention; delaying progression to AIDS

Assumptions

Research into therapies for HIV infections and AIDS is producing an ever-increasing flow of results. AIDS-inhibiting agents are becoming more effective, and by 1995 a therapy is applied to all HIV infected persons capable of delaying progression to AIDS. The effect of the therapy is that the immune system remains intact for longer.

There is an extension of the asymptomatic stage and consequently of the incubation period, and a shift takes place from in-hospital to out-of-hospital care with treatment being largely on an outpatient basis. The number of studies in the trial/treatment centres increases. The effects of the AIDS-inhibitors is such that HIV-tests are considered useful for everybody, which in turn leads to an increase in the demand for psychosocial care and counselling. All HIV-infected persons take advantage of the possibilities of early intervention.

Incidence and prevalence of HIV and AIDS
The HIV prevalence, and the AIDS incidence/prevalence, will change as a result of successful early intervention. We have projected the consequences for the care sector in two variants: (1) a one-year extension of the incubation period from 1995 onwards for all HIV-infected persons in CDC group II, (2) ditto with a three-year extension. Due to the uncertainty of the effect of early intervention on the survival period of people with AIDS, we have allowed for both a two-year and a three-year survival period. The projected impact of AIDS is compared with the reference scenario.

Figures 8.6 a to d show the AIDS incidence and AIDS/HIV prevalence in this scenario, based on the HIV incidence in the reference scenario. Extension of the incubation period has a direct effect on HIV prevalence and AIDS incidence, while the increase in the survival period affects the AIDS prevalence. The impact of the extension of the infectious period on HIV incidence has been left out of consideration here.

Use of care

Figures 8.6a to d show that an extension of the asymptomatic period leads to a decrease in the incidence and prevalence of AIDS, accompanied by an increase in the prevalence of HIV. This applies both to a two-year and a three-year survival time. This scenario leads to a decrease in the time spent in hospital, but an increase in outpatient care. The therapy means that the immune system remains intact for longer and that hospital admissions are delayed. An extension of one year in the incubation time and two years in the survival time leads to an expected bed requirement of 141 in the year 2000; if the survival period is three years, the number of beds required increases to 203.

Figure 8.6 **Effect of early intervention: extension of incubation time by one year and three years. Comparison with the reference scenario;**
8.6a: prevalence in the pre-AIDS stage; 8.6b: AIDS incidence; 8.6c: AIDS prevalence with a two-year survival time; 8.6d: AIDS prevalence with a three-year survival time. Including respective subscenarios.

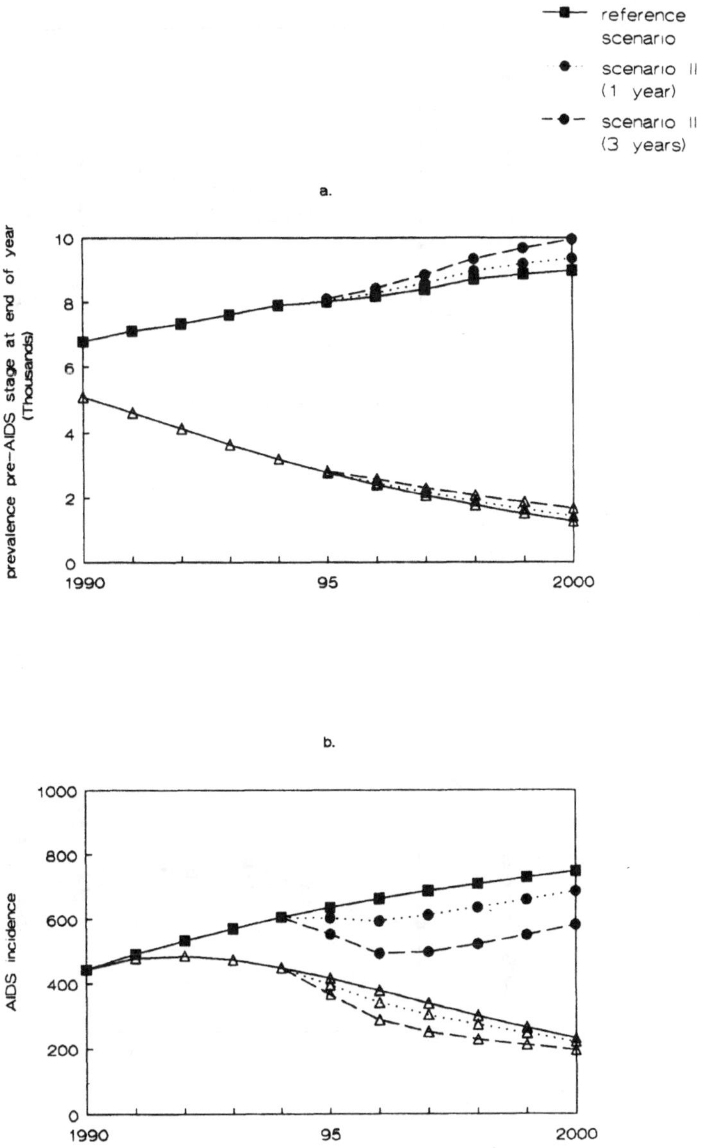

- vervolg Table 8.6 -

—△— subscenario

··△·· subscen. II (1 year)

–△– subscen. II (3 years)

c.

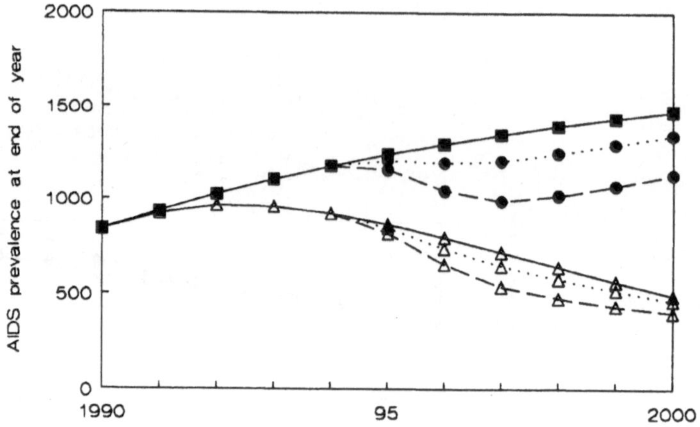

d.

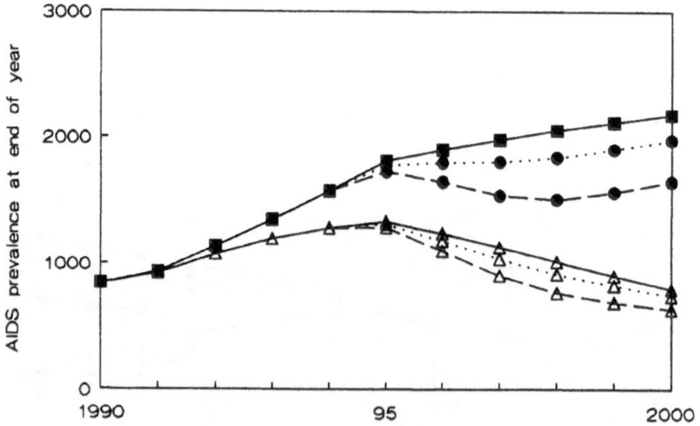

If the incubation period increases by three years and if the survival period is *two* years, the bed requirement falls to 120 in the year 2000. A three-year increase in the incubation period combined with a survival period of *three* years creates a bed requirement of 120 in 1995 and 170 in the year 2000. This figure is lower than the 224 beds required for an increase in the survival period in Variant A of Scenario I (Table 8.2). In looking at this fall in bed requirement in the year 2000, however, it should be borne in mind that this scenario involves a delay in the occupancy of hospital beds, with the consequences of AIDS being spread out over a longer period.[1]

The favourable results of early treatment mean that, in this scenario, a large number of (potentially) HIV-infected persons requests a test. The general practitioner is a key figure in the pre and post-test counselling of persons who have requested a test. Despite the positive results of early treatment, the future for HIV-infected persons remains extremely uncertain: AIDS remains a fatal disease. Now that more people are aware of their serostatus, there is increasing demand for psychosocial help, a demand which is being met by general practitioners, social workers and the RIAGGs. In the period between the test results and the onset of treatment, the general practitioner assists and monitors the patient.

The developments in early intervention mean that HIV-infected persons enter the health care system earlier than in the reference scenario, even where no symptoms of disease are present. Judging when early intervention should begin and deciding on the treatment itself, are the tasks of the AIDS internists in the regional centres or hospitals where relatively high numbers of people with HIV are seen. The outpatient clinic would seem to be the logical place for treatment, although it may be increasingly possible to provide treatment at home. Developments in medical technology lead to an increase in the number of clinical trials, which take place chiefly in the regional hospitals centres. These trials are coordinated by the National AIDS Therapy and Evaluation Centre (NATEC).

Costs of care

Putting off the progression to AIDS leads to a noticeable fall in the costs of inpatient care for AIDS patients. However, since there is no question of eradication of AIDS, this scenario shows only a temporary fall in the burden on the care system and the costs of inpatient care.

---

[1] Obviously, the consequences of early intervention can also be determined on the basis of the course of events as portrayed in the subscenario. For the sake of clarity we have not presented these results here. In general, the findings from calculations based on the subscenario tend to be similar to the results given in the text.

Unless early interventions before the year 2000 are followed by an effective therapy for people with AIDS, the developments emerging from this scenario will lead to a large increase in the costs of in-patient care after the year 2000.

It is unclear what the costs of early intervention will be. In addition to the costs of AZT, PCP prophylaxes and other drugs, this scenario will also lead to an increase in costs for medical resources, space and staff, as well as an increase in psychosocial care. The lack of sufficient data precludes the presentation of actual costs or figures, though it would seem reasonable to assume that considerable cost items are involved.

No more than an indication can be given of the costs of monitoring and early intervention. If the incubation period increases by one year or three years after 1995, monitoring and early intervention will increase the costs of the reference scenario by NLG 18 million in 1995 and NLG 28 million in the year 2000. The patient-related costs in the reference scenario amount to NLG 124 million in 1995 and NLG 139 million in the year 2000, so that early intervention leads to a significant increase in these costs. A decrease in the costs as compared to the reference scenario on certain aspects is not addressed to here.

The costs of testing for HIV-antibodies can be estimated at a minimum of NLG 4.3 million, the seroprevalence in the pre-AIDS stage of 7,900 for the year 1995 as set out in the reference scenario. These are the costs of the test, consultations and pre and post-counselling. The calculation shown in Appendix B is based on the NCAB assumptions (1990).

8.4.1 Commentary on Scenario II

It is difficult to give an indication of which consequences of early intervention have the greatest effect on the care for people with HIV and AIDS (GR, 1990; NCAB, 1990). Since people with HIV remain asymptomatic for longer, demand for inpatient care declines. On the other hand, they become eligible for prophylactic treatments in a stage which there are still no symptoms, and become "patients" earlier, with a resultant load on the general practitioner, the specialist, psychosocial help and outpatient care. The regional hospital centres play an important role in the early treatment; in addition to the treatment of the HIV-infected persons, they have a task in research and clinical trials. The costs of early intervention such as prophylaxes, AZT and other AIDS-inhibitors, and the number of diagnostic procedures such as counting the number of T-cells, rise sharply in comparison with the reference scenario due to the increase in the number of people who are covered by these treatments.

In spite of the extensive therapeutic possibilities presented in this scenario, the psychosocial drawbacks of tests remain. It is important that the government takes steps to safeguard the rights of people with HIV and to prevent the accessibility of health care and certain social facilities becoming restricted, including where an ever-growing number of people have themselves tested. We have not looked in this scenario at the social consequences of an increase in the number of test requests. In accordance with the baseline analysis, it has been tacitly assumed that no tests take place *except* at the request of the person undergoing the test. Similarly it has been tacitly assumed that the present problems surrounding access to social facilities for HIV-infected persons, such as life insurance, will have been solved.

8.5 Scenario III: AIDS as a chronic disease

Introduction

There is no uniform definition of the concept "chronic disease". However, there is a general description which can also be applied to AIDS (Van den Bos, 1989; Dutch Lower House, 1991): An illness is chronic if there is a demonstrative progressive deterioration; if the illness is long-lasting; if the seriousness of the illness is such that it hampers the general daily functions. The illness implies a certain burden on the care system.

It would be premature at this stage to discuss chronicity in any detail, given that the life-expectancy of people with AIDS is still extremely limited. A frequently voiced opinion, however, is that AIDS is increasingly taking on the form of a chronic disease with manifestations of acute illness (Bilheimer, 1989).

In Scenario III we explore the impact of AIDS as a chronic disease for the demand, organization and costs of care, and also look at the consequences for society of such a development. The underlying principle in this scenario is the need for care and support for the physical and psychological problems faced by people with AIDS. This contrasts with the reference scenario and the other care scenarios, in which the acute care provided was the main focus.

Assumptions

As a result of the successes achieved in the treatment and care of AIDS, the disease loses its acute life-threatening character and becomes a serious, progressively deteriorating chronic illness, ultimately leading to death following a protracted period of illness.

It is assumed that developments in the biomedical field have advanced to such an extent that the survival period of people with

AIDS increases to around 15 years. This is made possible by developments in medication. In this scenario, people with AIDS have a continuous need for drugs in order to maintain the immune system, and as a result they are under constant supervision by the general practitioner and the AIDS internist. No cure is possible, the disease is irreversible, and progressive deterioration leads to a gradual decline in the physical and mental faculties. This leads to increasing demand by AIDS patients for health care facilities.

Use of care

The care and support needed can be provided to a large extent by the general practitioner, supplemented by outpatient checks by the AIDS specialist. As the patient's health deteriorates, the regular and intensive home care system is called on to an increasing extent, assisted by the informal support network. The progressive deterioration caused by the disease means that psychosocial problems account for a major proportion of the demand for care. The general practitioner, RIAGGs and social work service (AMW) are the main care-providers in this area. Acute infections require short-term hospital admission. In the event of a serious deterioration of physical and mental functions, AIDS patients can be placed in a nursing home. Supplementary home care is required in the case of terminal patients.

Costs of care

The costs of providing care and treatment to people with AIDS relate chiefly to the costs of drugs, general practitioner costs and the costs of professional home care. The long-term use of medication, in particular, means that the total costs in this scenario are considerably higher than in the reference scenario, though it is not possible to give an indication of the actual costs of Scenario III. Compared to the foregoing scenarios, the need for nursing home beds and, to a lesser extent, hospital beds will be greater. Scenario III leads to a clear increase in the demand for general practitioner help and psychosocial care as compared with the reference scenario. A wider-ranging and longer-lasting burden placed on the support provided by the social network and volunteers, as a supplement to and support for the professional and intensive home care.

Organization of care

The care available must be matched to the individual needs of the chronic AIDS patient. The need for care is variable and depends partly on the availability of an informal support network. More attention than at present needs to be focused on proper organization and coordination of inpatient and outpatient care and the availability of resources for expanding home care. Case managers will be needed to ensure this proper coordination. This case manager may be the patient him or herself, someone from their immediate circle, or a care-provider. The psychosocial assistance forms part of the integrated provision of care. Regional hospital centres play a key role in the diagnosis, care, treatment and guidance of persons with AIDS. The specific nature of AIDS and the limited number of persons with the disease, means that not every care-provider will be able to respond adequately to the demand for care. This creates a need for a pooling of knowledge in regional AIDS centres. In addition, information will have to be provided on a national scale to general practitioners, district nursing services, home help services, and other relevant care-providers and professional groups.

8.5.1 Commentary

Those suffering from chronic disorders face, in addition to the physical trials, many adverse social and financial consequences of their illness. Access to the labour market is limited and as a result of a lack of concessions in the work situation, participation in the work process is for many not (or no longer) possible (Dutch Lower House, 1991). Problems can also arise concerning access to insurance and social facilities and, as a result of their physical restrictions, people may face a lack of understanding from those around them, as well as problems in general daily life. The decreased participation in social life increases the risk of social isolation.

To some extent, these problems are already a reality for people with AIDS; a much longer survival period will only reinforce them. Policy measures such as those proposed in the Policy Document on Chronic Disorders (Dutch Lower House, 1991), should also apply to people with AIDS on these points. Special attention also needs to be given to the availability and support of the informal network and volunteers, whose help is required to a varying degree over a long period. A further problem is the assumed lifelong infectiousness: if people with AIDS live with their disease for 15 years or more, this means an infectious period of more than 25 years, if the incubation period is also taken into account. This in turn has consequences for prevention and public information, which will have to focus attention for a considerable period on the need for safe sexual and injection behaviour.

Special attention will also be needed for women with AIDS who have become infected during their fertile years (Coates et al., 1991). Problems associated with the desire for children, pregnancy and fear of infection of the child will increase. Women are also often responsible for bringing up children, something which will become a steadily more difficult task in view of their decreasing ability to carry out daily tasks.

8.6 General commentary

In this chapter the consequences of varying developments in the care, medical technology and treatment of AIDS were explored in three scenarios. Scenarios I and II have a quantitative basis; Scenario I looks at an extension of the survival period following diagnosis of AIDS, while Scenario II deals with early intervention and the delay of progression to AIDS. Scenario III, AIDS as a chronic disorder, is reflective in nature; this scenario can be considered to be a variant of Scenario I. By reinforcing the developments in the extension of the survival period, Scenario III gives an indication of what consequences an extremely long survival period following diagnosis of AIDS can have for the care system. This scenario may be applicable to the long term, while Scenarios I and II explore situations in the short and medium term.

The care scenarios support and reinforce the conclusion drawn from the reference scenario, that the impact of AIDS will only become fully apparent in the health care sector in the second decade of the AIDS epidemic.

The scenarios relate to the delay of illness, suffering and death for the patient and to the possible spread of, or shifts within the same or a larger care package. For the person with AIDS this means no change in the sombre perspective; for the health care system it means that the total demand for health care facilities per patient will increase rather than decrease. In this way the care scenarios, more emphatically than the reference scenario, presage the period beyond the year 2000; extending the survival period and delaying progression to AIDS means that more people with AIDS than in the reference scenario will only begin to need inpatient care after the year 2000.

Scenarios I and II explore different projected end-situations independently of each other, but can also be seen in relation to each other: Scenario II, just as Scenario I, deals with an increase in the survival period following the diagnosis of AIDS, from two to three years. It is also possible that other developments in Scenario I and II may take place simultaneously, for example a simultaneous increase in the number of HIV-infected persons needing outpatient care facilities, and substitution of the care for AIDS patients. The demand for and costs of the care for HIV-infected persons and AIDS patients will prove higher in such a case than is projected in this chapter.

Apart from developments in care, the epidemiological course

also has an effect on the scale of the costs of care. This chapter uses the data emerging from the reference scenario with respect to the scale and spread of the epidemic. If there were a relapse into unsafe behaviour or a spread of HIV beyond the core groups, this would in time lead to a greater demand for care facilities. Conversely, developments which lead to an HIV/AIDS incidence which corresponds more closely to the non-preventable developments outlined in the subscenario, would result in a lower demand for care.

Besides changes in the epidemiological course, other intervening developments are also possible, for example the disappearance of the support provided by the informal network and volunteers, leading to more frequent and earlier need for professional health care. The availability of an effective therapy or vaccine is another factor which would lead to totally different situations than those projected in the scenarios.

Scenarios I and II show that an increase in the survival period, intensification of home care, substitution of care and early intervention will lead to an increase in the patient-related costs of AIDS as set out in the reference scenarios. In some scenarios this increase in costs is of the order of tens of millions of guilders - a significant increase compared with the reference scenario. On the other hand, the variants do not lead to a doubling or tripling of the patient-related costs. The finding in the reference scenario that AIDS will lead to a considerable but manageable burden on the total health care budget would therefore seem to apply also to Scenarios I and II.

An indication is given for each scenario and each variant within those scenarios of what shifts they will produce in the care sectors. As far as inpatient care is concerned, Scenarios I and II appear not to lead to any problems. Just as in the reference scenario, it seems possible, given present capacity, to meet the bed requirement of AIDS patients within the existing facilities. This conclusion also applies to the bed requirement in the event that Scenarios I and II occur simultaneously, i.e. in the event of an extension of the survival period following diagnosis of AIDS and a simultaneous delay of the progression to AIDS. Such a development could, however, lead to problems in the outpatient care sector.

These health care scenarios make it clear that the care of people with AIDS and HIV continue to demand attention. AIDS remains an incurable disease which requires specialized, sometimes extremely intensive care, support and guidance. In addition, there is no reason to assume that the psychosocial consequences of AIDS for the care-provider and those close to the person will decrease in the future. The rapid developments in treatment and research will continue to demand attention for proper organization, matching, coordination and content of the care. In other words, the budgetary consequences of the AIDS epidemic appear to be manageable, while the impact of AIDS for the content and organization of the care will continue to demand undiminished attention.

The care provided to people with AIDS and HIV has until now been organized within the normal health care system, if necessary supplemented and supported by category-specific facilities. In the area of inpatient care, the knowledge and experience of treatment is pooled in regional centres (regional hospitals). The setting up of these specialized centres is justified by the seriousness and specificity of the AIDS problem. An important question for the future is how long this special attention will be necessary and what need exists for regional hospitals. To date, the basic aim has been that in time all general hospitals will be able to care for people with AIDS: however, a development is also possible in which the number of patients and the complexity of the treatment provided lead precisely to the desirability of a concentration of care facilities. In such a case, the goal would change and would be replaced by a commitment to designating one or more hospitals with a special, permanent AIDS department.

As far as outpatient care is concerned, the increasing demand on the health-care system may lead to capacity problems in the future. Where substitution takes place, intensive home care will often become the "hospital at home", performing complex and labour-intensive nursing tasks, and thus exerting additional pressure on these facilities. The need for home care is currently already greater than the supply, and this development will continue, partly as a result of the increasing ageing of the population and the shortening of the length of stay in hospitals. In conjunction with this development, the need for support by volunteers and the informal support network will also increase, whereas the supply of "traditional volunteers" is not expected to grow (SCP, 1990). This means that, irrespective of developments in the AIDS epidemic, home care and informal care for people with AIDS and HIV may come under pressure (Tjadens et al., 1990; Schrijvers and Van Londen, 1990abc).

A separate area of concern is the spread of care facilities. In anticipation of a heavy burden on the health care system, a range of measures have been taken throughout the Netherlands. At the moment, however, there is a concentration of people with AIDS in the large cities, particularly Amsterdam. One of the results of this is that Amsterdam is facing a shortage of buddies, whereas in other parts of the Netherlands a large number of buddies are still awaiting their first client (De Rijk et al., 1991). There are also large regional differences in the number of inpatient beds occupied at regional hospitals centres. It is not certain whether the concentration of the

AIDS epidemic in the large cities will be a permanent feature, and there is currently no obvious solution to this problem. Only when the margins of uncertainty on the future incidence of AIDS are smaller, and when regional estimates of the expected number of people with AIDS become possible, will it be possible for planners of health care facilities to solve this dilemma. In any event, a shortage of facilities appears undesirable.

Up to now, only the location of the care of people with AIDS and HIV in the care system has been considered. In addition, however, AIDS also has an effect on general health care in the Netherlands. We examine the initiatives in connection with AIDS, as well as the problems surrounding clinical trials of drugs. Initiatives in the care of people with AIDS may also be applicable to other illnesses besides AIDS; examples of such initiatives might include the buddy care system, contact with fellow patients, the use of a care file, as well as the experiences of the AIDS consultants and the experiments with intensive home care.

In the area of clinical trials there may be increasing issues in the near future. It is expected that an increasing number of HIV-infected persons will be considered for clinical trials, and that more new drugs will become available; in addition, pressure from patient organizations will increase for the lowering of the entry requirements for participation in a trial, as well as for more research and a speeding up of the registration process for new drugs (Byar et al., 1990; Danner, 1990; Hellman and Hellman, 1991; Passamani, 1991). Dissatisfaction regarding the lengthy approval procedures for new drugs which appear on the market led to initiatives by the pressure group "Fight for Life" which resulted in the setting up in 1991 of the organization's own trial centre in Amsterdam. It is possible that in the future the role of the patient will increase in other illnesses as well. This too can be regarded as a social development which has come about partly as a result of AIDS (Van den Boom et al., 1991b).

8.7 Summary

In this chapter the effect of developments in health care, medical technology and the treatment of people with HIV and AIDS on the demand, supply, costs, coordination and matching of the care is considered in three scenarios. In the first scenario, an increase in the survival period to three years following diagnosis of AIDS, three variants are developed: (A) unchanged intensity of care, (B) intensification of home care and (C) substitution. The second scenario explores the consequences of early intervention for the care system, while the third scenario looks at the consequences for care if

AIDS can be considered as a chronic disorder. All three scenarios lead to an increase in the patient-related impact of AIDS when compared with the reference scenario. The burden on health care facilities remains considerable though manageable.

In these care scenarios, AIDS remains a serious, complicated illness which demands intensive, specialized treatment and care. Problems may be expected particularly at the level of care provision, and in the organization, matching and coordination of the care. The organization and availability of professional home care, volunteers and the informal support network also demands special attention, in order to be able to provide adequate care and support for the increasing number of people who will require outpatient facilities.

References

Arno, P.
The nonprofit sectors' response to the AIDS-epidemic: community based services in San Francisco
American Journal of Public Health, 76 (1986), 11, 1325-1330

Beuzekom, M. van, F. van den Boom, H. Kroon, J.G. Storosum, H.N. Sno, H. van Dis
Psychisch dysfunctioneren (SCL-90) bij symptomatische HIV-infectie en AIDS-patiënten
Tijdschrift voor Psychiatrie, 33 (1991), 5, 331-343

Biglino, A., A. Pugliese, B. Forno, A.M Pollono, M. Busso, P. Gioannini
Effects of Long-Term Zidovudine Treatment on Cell-Mediated Immune Response and Lymphokine Production
Journal of Acquired Immune Deficiency Syndromes, 4 (1991), 3, 261-266

Bilheimer, L.
Data gaps in modeling AIDS Service Utilization and Costs
Presented at *V International Conference on AIDS*, Montreal, June 8, 1989

Bolognesi, D.P., G.C. Schild
Vaccines and immunology: overview
AIDS, 1990, 4, S127-S128

Boom, F. van den, T. Gremmen, H. Roozenburg
Leven rond de dood; nabestaanden over ziekte, dood en rouw
NcGv, Utrecht, 1991a, NcGv-reeks 91-16

Boom, F. van den, D. Reinking, P. Schnabel
AIDS als bedreiging en uitdaging voor de homobeweging
Tijdschrift voor Gezondheid en Politiek, september 1991b, 2-5

Bos, G.A.M. van den
Zorgen van en voor chronisch zieken
Bohn, Scheltema & Holkema, Utrecht, 1989, academisch proefschrift

Byar, D.P., Schoenfeld, S.B. Green, D.A. Amato, R. Davis, V. De Gruttola, D.M. Finkelstein, C. Gastonis, R.D. Gelber, S. Lagakos, M. Lefkopoulou, A.A. Tsiatis, J. Peto, L.S. Freedman, M. Gail, R. Simon, S.S. Ellenberg, J.R. Anderson, R.R. Collins, R. Peto, T. Peto
Design considerations for AIDS trials
New England Journal of Medicine, 232 (1990), 19, 1343-1348

Coates, T.J., D.C. Des Jarlais, H.G. Miller, L.E. Moses, C.F. Turner, D. Worth
The AIDS epidemic in the second decade

In: H.G. Miller, C.F. Turner, L.E. Moses (eds.), *AIDS: the second decade*, National Academy Press, Washington D.C., 1990, 38-80

Danner, S.A.
AIDS, interventiestudies en patiëntendruk
Nederlands Tijdschrift voor Geneeskunde, 134 (1990), 38, 1835-1836

Dijkgraaf, M.G.W., J.J.C. Borleffs, M.J.J.C. Poos, J.C. Jager, A.J.P. Schrijvers
Monitoring hospital resource use and cost: a three-and-a-half year follow up
Presented at *VII International Conference on AIDS*, Florence, 1991 (MD 112)

Driessen, A., L.van de Velden, F. van den Boom, J. Derks
Steun van de Regenboog; vrijwillige hulpverlening aan verslaafde AIDS-patiënten
NcGv, Utrecht, 1991, NcGv reeks 91/12

Goldsmith, M.F.
AIDS vaccines, inch closer to useful existence
JAMA, 265 (1991), 11, 1356-1357

Health Council (GR)
De zorg voor patiënten met AIDS en andere ziekteverschijnselen als gevolg van infectie met het humaan-immunodeficiëntievirus
GR, The Hague, 1987, no. 26

Health Council (GR)
Vroege medische interventies bij personen die met AIDS-virus zijn geïnfecteerd
GR, The Hague, 1990, no. 16

Hellman, S., D.S. Hellman
Of mice but not men; Problems of the Randomized Clinical Trial
New England Journal of Medicine, 324 (1991), 22, 1585-1589

King, M.B.
Psychological aspects of HIV infection and AIDS. "What have we learned?"
British Journal of Psychiatry, 156 (1990), 151-156

Koff, W.C., S. Fauci
Human trials of AIDS vaccines: current status and future directions
AIDS, 1989, supplement, S125-129

KPMG Klynveld Bosboom Hegener, Organisatie-adviseurs
Kosten en meerkosten van ziekenhuiszorg voor HIV-geïnfecteerden
KPMG, Utrecht, 1989

Lange, J.M.A., J. Goudsmit
Vroege behandeling met zidovudine; een keerpunt in de strijd tegen AIDS?
Nederlands Tijdschrift voor Geneeskunde, 133 (1989), 2599-2601

Lower House of the Dutch States General (TK)
- Policy document on AIDS policy
Lower House of the States General, session 1986-1987, 19218, nos. 8-9 (TK, 1987)
- Letter from the State Secretary for Welfare, Health and Cultural Affairs
Lower House of the States General, session 1988-1989, 19219, no. 30 (TK, 1988)
- Letter from the State Secretary for Welfare, Health and Cultural Affairs
Lower House of the States General, session 1989-1990, 19218, no. 38 (1989)
- Chronisch-Ziekenbeleid, chronische patiënten niet buiten spel
Lower House of the States General, session 1990-1991, 22025, no. 1. (1991)
- Financieel Overzicht Gezondheidszorg (Financial Statement on Health Care) 1991
Lower House of the States General, session 1990-1991, 21 812, no. 1-2 (FOZ, 1991)

Miltenburg, T.
Experimenten thuisverpleging; een tussentijdse evaluatie
Instituut voor Toegepaste Sociale Wetenschappen, Nijmegen, 1989

Ministry of Welfare, Health and Cultural Affairs (WVC)
Doelgericht veranderen, Ontwerp-Kerndocument Gezondheidsbeleid voor de jaren 1990-1995
WVC, Rijswijk, 1989

Nationale Commissie AIDS Bestrijding (NCAB)
- *Raamplan AIDS en de psychosociale zorg*
NCAB, Amsterdam, 1988
- *Vroegtijdige interventie bij personen met een HIV-infectie*
NCAB, Amsterdam, 1990
- *Een kader voor de invulling van de centrumfunctie voor AIDS bij ziekenhuizen*
NCAB, Amsterdam, 1991

Passamani, E.
Clinical Trials - Are They Ethical?
New England Journal of Medicine, 324 (1991), 22, 1589-1591

Postma, M.J., M.G.W. Dijkgraaf, J.C.C. Borleffs, D.P.Reinking, F.M.L.G. van den Boom, J.C. Jager
Omvang en kosten van ziekenhuiszorg voor HIV-geïnfecteerden; een vergelijking en integratie van Nederlandse studies
Tijdschrift voor Sociale Gezondheidszorg, 1991, geaccepteerd

Redfield, R.R.
A phase I evaluation of the safety and immunogenicity of vaccination with recombinant gp 160 in patients with early HIV-infections
The New England Journal of Medicine, 324 (1991), 24, 1677-1684

Rijk, K. de, J. Drent, F.van den Boom
Buddy-zorg in perspectief; vrijwilligershulpverlening voor mensen met AIDS: meerwaarde en grenzen
NcGv, Utrecht, 1991, in preparation

Social and Cultural Planning Office (SCP)
Sociaal and Cultural Report 1990
Rijswijk/Alphen a/d Rijn, SCP/Samsom, 1990

Schrijvers, A.J.P., J. van Londen
Ontwikkelingen in de thuiszorg, 1: Begripsomschrijvingen
Medisch Contact, 45 (1990a), 22, 707-712

Schrijvers, A.J.P., J. van Londen
Ontwikkelingen in de thuiszorg, 2: Vraag en aanbod
Medisch Contact, 45 (1990b), 23, 745-747

Schrijvers, A.J.P., J. van Londen
Ontwikkelingen in de thuiszorg, Slot: De toekomst
Medisch Contact, 45 (1990c), 24, 768-772

Tjadens, F., N. Welling, C. Tunissen
Experimentele thuisverpleging (1), Achtergronden van intensieve thuiszorg
Medisch Contact, 46 (1990) 4, 107-108

Volberding, P.A., S.W. Lagakos, M.A. Koch
Zidovidine in asymptomatic human immunodeficiency virus infection: a controlled trial in persons with fewer than 500 CD-4 positive per cubic milimeter
New England Journal of Medicine, 322 (1990), 941-949

Appendix A

Assumptions and calculations for Scenario I: extension of the survival period after diagnosis of AIDS

The step-by-step increase in the survival period was calculated as follows.

In 1990 25% of diagnosed people with AIDS have an average survival period of three years, with two years for the remaining 75%. This gradually changes over a period of four years until in 1994 all people with AIDS have an average survival period of three years.

In the reference scenario, the consequences of AIDS were calculated on the basis of a length of nursing care of both 53 and 27 days per observation year; in Scenario I we explore only the consequences of an average length of nursing care of 27 days per observation year.

Assumptions concerning the increase in survival period are based on present medical developments, literature studies and consultation. The estimated need for intensive home care is based on an experiment in three Dutch Health Service regions and has been set at 0.55 days per observation year per AIDS patient (Miltenburg, 1989).

For all three variants of Scenario I the costs, bed use, hours of care, consultations and days of care are derived from the AIDS prevalence halfway through a year, multiplied by the estimated costs per observation year.

With regard to use of medication at home, only the use of AZT was considered in the reference scenario (and its subscenario); no data are available on other agents. In projections based on a survival period of three years, it would be necessary to take account of a potential resistance to AZT and a resultant decline in AZT use per observation year. In these projections we have assumed that in such cases AZT-replacement drugs are used, whose costs compare with those of AZT. This leads to the assumption that the home use of AIDS-inhibitors per observation year remains constant.

Appendix B

Assumptions and calculations for Scenario II: early intervention

The costs of the number of tests carried out in 1995 are based on the data relating to HIV prevalence as at 31.12.1994. The number of HIV-infected persons on 31.12.1979 is 7,900 in the reference scenario. The calculation is as follows. In line with the reference scenario, it has been assumed that 25% of the HIV-infected persons are aware of their seropositivity. This results in the following calculations on the costs of tests, consultations and pre and post-test counselling (Table B1). The cost calculation method for early intervention devised by the NCAB (1990) has been used:

Table B.1 **Number and costs of tests and consultations, including pre and post-test counselling in Scenario II: early intervention** (derived directly from the reference scenario, using the NCAB calculation method (1990))

Tests:			
new HIV +:			
ELISA test	5,925 x fl. 25	=	fl. 148,125
repeat of ELISA:			
all HIV +	7,900 x fl. 25	=	fl. 197,500
2 x Western Blot:			
new HIV +;			
1 x Western Blot:			
aware HIV +	13.825 x fl. 200	=	fl. 2,765,000
Total tests:			fl. 3,110,625
Consultations:			
General practitioner:			
3/5 Health Service:	11.850 x fl. 24.50	=	fl. 290,325
2/5 private:	4,740 x fl. 30.20	=	fl. 143,148
Municipal Medical & Health Authority/no-threshold clinic:			
10% physician:	1,185 x fl. 25	=	fl. 29,625
90% nursing:	10,665 x fl. 17	=	fl. 181,305
Pre and post-test counselling:			
average 1 hour @ NLG 75			
all tests			fl. 592,500
Total consultations:			fl. 1,236,903
Total tests/consultations:			fl. 4,347,528

Table B.2 shows the same calculations applied to the subscenario. Based on the assumptions in the subscenario, 50% of patients are aware of their seropositivity.

Table B.2 **Number and costs of tests and consultation, including pre and post-test counselling in Scenario II: early intervention** (derived directly from the subscenario, using the NCAB calculation method (1990))

Tests:			
new HIV +:			
ELISA test	1,600 x fl. 25	=	fl. 40,000
repeat of ELISA:			
all HIV +	3,200 x fl. 25	=	fl. 80,000
2 x Western Blot:			
new HIV +;			
1 x Western Blot:			
aware HIV +	4,800 x fl. 200	=	fl. 960,000
Total tests:			fl. 1,080,000
Consultations:			
General practitioner:			
3/5 Health Service:	2,880 x fl. 24.50	=	fl. 70,560
2/5 private:	1,920 x fl. 30.20	=	fl. 57,984
Municipal Medical & Health Authority/no-threshold clinic:			
10% physician:	480 x fl. 25	=	fl. 12,000
90% nursing:	4,320 x fl. 17	=	fl. 73,440
Pre and post-test counselling:			
average 1 hour @ NLG 75			
all tests			fl. 240,000
Total consultations:			fl. 453,984
Total tests/consultations:			fl. 1,533,984

Both tables are based on the assumption that all HIV-infected persons are tested at the start of a programme of early intervention; in practice it may not be possible to achieve this. On the other hand, the option of early intervention may lead to test requests from a large number of persons who prove not to be infected with HIV. No basis has been found for correct assumptions about this.

Costs of early intervention and monitoring

For the distribution of HIV-infected persons over the various CDC groups we refer to Figure 2.3 in Chapter 2, in which HIV-infected persons are divided into (1) acute infection, (2) asymptomatic stage, (3) symptomatic stage (pre-AIDS). Group (2) consists of persons eligible for early intervention. In our calculations we have assumed that transition from Group (2) to Group (3) is delayed by early intervention. It is assumed that, at 1.1.1995, early intervention leads to an increase in the incubation period of between one and three years for all members of Group (2) who are liable to move on to Group (3). This assumption implies that everyone who is eligible takes part in early intervention programmes.

Monitoring applies to HIV-infected persons in Groups (1) and (2). For the calculations relating to monitoring it has been assumed that everyone in Groups (1) and (2) who does not take part in an early intervention programme participates in a monitoring programme. The assumed 100% participation results in a maximum estimate of the number of participants in the monitoring programmes. In practice, not every HIV-infected person will be eligible for monitoring. However, a situation other than this hypothetical one did not seem appropriate given the state of present knowledge.

On the basis of the NCAB estimate (1990), costs of early intervention have been assumed to be NLG 15,000 per year, while the costs of monitoring have been put at NLG 1,400. This results in two summaries of the costs of early intervention and monitoring in the year 2000. Table B.3 shows the summary based on the reference scenario, while Table B.4 relates to the subscenario. As can be seen from Table B.3, the costs of early intervention and monitoring range from just under NLG 18 million to more than NLG 27.5 million, depending on the extension of the incubation period. In the subscenario (Table B.4) the cost estimates, again depending on the extension of the incubation period, range from NLG 4 million to almost NLG 8 million. The difference in costs is caused by the number of participants in early intervention programmes.

Table B.3 Number of persons eligible for early intervention and monitoring in the year 2000 (epidemiological basis: reference scenario)

	Increase in incubation period	
	1 year	**3 years**
Number and costs		
Participants in early intervention:	429	1,074
Costs:	fl. 6,435,000	fl. 16,110,000
Participants in monitoring:	8,162	8,162
Costs:	fl. 11,426,800	fl. 11,426,800
Total costs:	fl. 17,862,000	fl. 27.539,000

Table B.4 Number of persons eligible for early intervention and monitoring in the year 2000 (epidemiological basis: subscenario)

	Increase in incubation period 1 year	3 years
Number and costs		
Participants in early intervention:	165	422
Costs:	fl. 2,475,000	fl. 6,330,000
Participants in monitoring:	1,150	1,152
Costs:	fl. 4,085,000	fl. 7,940,000
Total costs:	fl. 6,550,000	fl. 14,270,000

9 The response to AIDS: strategies for AIDS control and care

9.1 Introduction

The response to AIDS throughout the Western world shows both a number of similarities and several - rather more significant - differences. The similarity lies in the fact that all countries take seriously the threat posed by AIDS to public health and that in response to this, public information about AIDS, epidemiological surveys of the number of HIV-infected persons and biomedical research into developing treatments have all been started. Initiatives have also been taken in every country in the area of care for people with HIV and AIDS.

There are great differences in the scale on which the fight against AIDS has been tackled and the choices which have been made between the available intervention strategies. Moerkerk (1990) has reflected on the divergent HIV/AIDS prevention strategies in Europe. He observes large differences in the involvement of pressure groups in the prevention policy, the degree of attention given to the social impact of AIDS, the tone and content of the message conveyed by the public information programme and the making available of resources for large-scale information programmes about AIDS. As a corollary to this, reference can also be made to the wide international differences in testing policy and the legal framework within which AIDS is situated.

There are obvious differences here between the Netherlands and Sweden. In the Netherlands, AIDS is not approached from a basis of existing legislation relating to the combating of infectious diseases; further, a restrained testing policy has been adopted, and an HIV-test carried out other than at the request of the person involved is considered to be in conflict with individual civil liberties with respect to privacy and the protection of the integrity of the body. In Sweden, by contrast, AIDS has been incorporated into the Swedish law on the combating of infectious diseases and detection of the cause of disease, and a test-promoting policy is pursued. In extreme cases, the AIDS control programme has legal powers to impose short periods of enforced isolation, in which patients work under supervision towards reintegration in society (Karamoustafa, 1990).

The above, sometimes diametrically opposed, choices in the AIDS control effort are no doubt related to expectations concerning the course of the HIV/AIDS epidemic, but there is also a very strong link with wide-ranging factors such as the way health problems are tackled, the influence which those directly involved have on policy, the legal/ethical choices where there are conflicting interests between the individual and those involved in care provision, institutions with financial interests and the interests of public health, and the importance which is attached to countering the negative social impact of AIDS. For each country, this results in an AIDS control scenario which can only be described in close relation to the social context which forms the basis of the response to AIDS.

In this chapter we use two strategic scenarios to explore alternative paths by which AIDS control targets can be achieved. These two scenarios, which are described against the background of the response to AIDS to date, are referred to as the Self-regulation strategy (I) and the Detection Strategy (II).

The care provided for people with AIDS and HIV can also be expressed in strategic scenarios. In the Netherlands, a choice has been made for an integrated approach to the biomedical and social problems, and the care provided has been linked to the existing system of health care facilities. In addition to this it was felt that extra attention should be given to care for people with AIDS, and this led among other things to concrete initiatives such as the setting up of regional hospital centres, the subsidising the ancillary costs of AIDS, the dissemination of experience and expertise and infection control measures for care-providers. and the making available of additional resources for initiatives in the area of psychosocial support. The aim of this strategy is to provide high-quality support to people with AIDS. We examine alternatives for the organization of the care provided to AIDS patients in two strategic care scenarios: a Regular care strategy (I) and an AIDS-specific care strategy (II).

9.2 *Development and background*

The AIDS control scenarios consist of an action plan relating to epidemiological monitoring, HIV/AIDS prevention, testing policy and access to social facilities; the strategies relating to care concern the organization of the support provided. In the commentary we consider the changes in the two scenarios with respect to the present approach to AIDS control and care. We also examine the potential social impact of the two scenarios. The strategies are developed and discussed against the background of the baseline analyses and, in particular, those sections of these which relate to the Dutch policy on AIDS.

The goal of the AIDS control programme is the same in the Self-regulation and the Detection strategy, namely to prevent HIV infections as far as possible. There are, however, radical differences on some aspects of the development of the scenarios. The Self-regulation strategy is linked to the present AIDS control strategy, while the Detection strategy, by contrast, is based on the assumption of a radical deviation from the present AIDS control programme.

The Self-regulation strategy contains the additional assumption that the approach to AIDS is regarded as an example for the control of all threats to health, and to sexually transmitted diseases in particular. The Detection strategy is based on the contrasting assumption that a reappraisal of the underlying principles of AIDS control is necessary. In this scenario there is a shift in the approach both to the policy on testing and HIV/AIDS prevention.

The two strategic care scenarios have the same objective: "to offer high-quality psychosocial and somatic care to people with HIV and AIDS". We assume in the care strategies that there are differences of insight regarding the degree of integration of the help offered to people with AIDS in the existing system of health care facilities. In the regular care strategy, we assume that the special attention given to the care of people with AIDS is run down. In the AIDS-specific care strategy, we examine what plan of action is needed for the specialized care of people with AIDS.

With regard to HIV/AIDS incidence and the care provided, we have assumed that the strategies are founded on future expectations derived from the reference scenario. In other words, an explosive increase in HIV is not expected within the next ten years. As far as care is concerned, we have assumed the availability of care as set out in the reference scenario. Table 9.1 contains the key parameters and indicators which are considered in the scenarios.

For the sake of completeness we would emphasize right at the start that the scenarios do no more than *project* in general terms a number of divergent strategies for AIDS control and the organization of care. The scenarios have been constructed in order to throw light on a number of alternative paths, and are not intended as alternatives to the present AIDS policy.

Table 9.1 **Strategic scenarios relating to AIDS control and the organization of the care of people with AIDS.**

	AIDS control		Organization of care	
	Strategy I Self-regulation	Strategy II Detection	Strategy I Regular care	Strategy II AIDS-specific care
AIDS/HIV inc./prev	ref.	ref.	ref.	ref.
Epidemiological monitoring	bas.	early detection	n/a	n/a
HIV/AIDS prevention	non-AIDS-specific	AIDS-specific incl. additional measures	n/a	n/a
Testing policy	voluntary testing	test-promoting policy, compulsory test if necessary	n/a	n/a
Priority: individual liberties	+	-		
public health interest	bas.	+		
third-party interest	bas.	+		
Organization of care	n/a	n/a	within existing system of health care	special facilities/ measures

ref. = in accordance with reference scenario
bas. = baseline analysis
\- = less than described in baseline analysis
\+ = more than described in baseline analysis

9.3 Strategies for AIDS control

9.3.1 Strategy I: Self-regulation

Topology

In this strategy great importance is attached to safeguarding the right to privacy, the right to self-determination and the individual responsibility of the citizen. The testing policy formulated in connection with AIDS remains unchanged. Access to social facilities is guaranteed in this scenario by extra protection of the legal position of the individual with respect to medical examinations.

The compilers of this strategy consider that the approach towards HIV and AIDS may serve as an exemple for STD control in general. While it is true that HIV differs from a number of other STDs as a result of its long incubation period, in a prevention policy based on the personal responsibility of the individual this is not a decisive argument for a different approach. The benefit gained from a period of public information directed specifically at AIDS is translated into changes in the STD control programme, in which the emphasis is shifted towards primary prevention.

9.3.1.1 Development of Self-regulation strategy

Monitoring and AIDS prevention
The Self-regulation strategy is based on the view that it is known which groups face an increased risk of HIV infection. The results of epidemiological monitoring of a small number of groups are sufficient for the production of estimates of the seroprevalence. Participation in epidemiological surveys is voluntary.

The main element of the control strategy is a sober, factual information programme which relies on the personal responsibility of the individual. The view here is that the increased attention being given within the health care sector and within society as a whole to health, a healthy lifestyle and prevention of disease, the growth in public health information and education, and the experience and expertise gained in the context of AIDS control with respect to public information, in principle offer sufficient guarantees for effective HIV/AIDS prevention. It is also considered essential that the expertise built up in AIDS control should be more widely applied. As far as HIV/AIDS prevention is concerned, this means that the information must relate to all sexually transmitted diseases; for the STD control programmes, it means that information will to a large extent take the place of early detection and curative treatment.

The objectives for prevention are derived directly from the objectives of the former HIV/AIDS prevention programme, namely a high level of knowledge about STDs, including HIV, safe sex as a social norm, and the presence of the necessary social interactive skills (assertiveness) to enable the use of condoms to be openly discussed where necessary. There is a realization that providing information is a continuous activity. As with other forms of behaviour which carry a health risk, such as smoking, alcohol and drug use and driving habits, the level of knowledge must be kept up. Young people and people who are hard to reach through general public information campaigns form a special group. Young people are reached through education, with health education in the broad sense becoming a compulsory subject and including information about STDs HIV/AIDS. Information activities among groups which are hard to reach take place on the basis of small-scale campaigns. Special training schemes and courses are also provided, designed to preserve changes in behaviour and to prevent relapse.

Hard-drug users form a special group, if only because in this group communicable diseases are also spread via the shared used of injection equipment. In conjunction with drug aid programmes and via a combined approach of needle- and syringe exchange schemes, cleaning of needles and, if necessary, individual counselling, the aim is to keep the risk profile among injecting drug users at a permanently low level. This approach fits into a wider strategy whose main aims are to combat deterioration in the health of hard-drug users and to promote their social integration.

Separate attention is also devoted to the transmission of STDs in the sex industry. A distinction is made in the prevention campaigns between drug-dependent commercial sex workers, foreign sex workers and other sex workers, and information campaigns geared to each of these sectors are started, aimed at the clients, the sex workers themselves and those who manage the sex workers. The attention devoted to the health of sex workers forms part of a wider strategy geared to the integration of sex workers into society. One component of this strategy is the recognition of sex work as a profession.

Testing policy/access to social facilities

The right to privacy and self-determination are the key points of this strategy. This translates into a firm intention to adhere to a restrained test policy, even where changes take place in the treatment available. No circumstances are imaginable which would justify infringement of individual liberties through legislative rules. The importance attached to individual liberties is also expressed in measures which give extra protection to the individual in medical examinations. It is forbidden to perform an HIV-test during a medical examination for a job application. The guiding principle for such examinations, and for life assurance, is that an HIV-test is only permitted in cases where a sum insured is requested which, in the opinion of a forum of experts, is considered to be at odds with the real level of need of the applicant given his or her social circumstances. In order to combat adverse financial consequences for life insurance companies, a guarantee fund is set up. These measures also apply to tests for hereditary disorders when a proposer applies for insurance.

The testing policy for HIV is held up as an example for the testing policy with respect to other STDs. Testing without consent cannot be permitted. A test also carries an information obligation. Pre and post-test counselling are a permanent feature in requests for tests for STDs or HIV.

9.3.2 *Strategy II: Detection*

Topology
The compilers of this strategy posit that there is every reason for a reappraisal of the underlying principles of the AIDS control programme. The need to counter a large-scale spread of HIV, the long incubation period of HIV and the incurability of AIDS demand a special effort. Public information and the promotion of behavioural change are insufficient on their own. Its long incubation period means that the virus can spread unnoticed, possibly leading in the long term to a large-scale spread of HIV. A system of source and contact detection is adopted, in which an HIV-test can be administered without the consent of the person directly concerned in which restrictive measures can also be applied if necessary in the case of persons who prove reluctant to change their behaviour. The lack of an available treatment makes AIDS sufficiently different from many other STDs that there can be no question of integrating the AIDS and STD control programmes. A special approach is need for the primary prevention of HIV.

The reappraisal of the underlying principles of the AIDS control programme results in a completely different vision of the legal/ethical aspects of the AIDS situation. The right to privacy and self-determination is recognized within the limits created by the needs of the AIDS control programme. It is also intended that control of the disease should as far as possible be based on the individual responsibility of the citizen. A test-promoting policy is adopted.

9.3.2.1 *Development of Detection strategy*

Monitoring and AIDS prevention
According to the Detection strategy, the fact a large-scale epidemic has so far not developed offers no guarantee whatsoever for the course of the HIV epidemic in the medium term, something which in the long term could potentially lead to a slow but substantial spread of HIV among the entire population. The approach adopted is based on the conviction that a sober, factual information campaign is feasible for the majority of the population, but not for everyone. Some groups exist are difficult to reach, making it necessary to combine targetted information programmes with a system of intensive contact tracing, partner notification and compulsory reporting of HIV infection. The system of early detection is targeted in particular at groups in which there is an existing HIV epidemic, i.e. men who have sex with men and IDUs. Special attention is also focused on the sex

industry and the sexual contacts of HIV-infected persons. In addition, some people remain indifferent to the prevention message, and extra prevention efforts are needed if it is apparent from the behaviour of these persons that appealing to individual responsibility has no effect. In extreme cases legal powers may be sought to administer compulsory treatment in the context of a reintegration programme.

Participation in epidemiological studies is encouraged and in some cases compulsory. For example, HIV-testing is compulsory for travellers to and from the US, Central Africa and other countries where a large-scale epidemic exists. HIV-infected persons without Dutch nationality are refused entry to the Netherlands.

Integration of the AIDS control programme and the STD control programme is rejected. The STD control programme can benefit from the experience and expertise gained in the area of public information and the promotion of behavioural change, while the AIDS control effort can learn from the experiences of the STD control programme in the area of early detection. As long as there is no adequate treatment for HIV infection, and HIV infection persists for life, a stricter detection policy is needed for HIV/AIDS than for STDs where curative medical intervention is possible.

Testing policy and access to social facilities

The development of this control strategy requires legislation to establish in which cases and under what conditions an HIV-test can be carried out without consent. This legislation would also stipulate that the medical information so obtained must not be used for any purpose other than combating AIDS. The legislation would also establish the procedure to be followed when a decision is taken to apply restrictive measures to persons who fail to change their behaviour. A guarantee fund would be set up to compensate for the adverse negative consequences of HIV for the individual. HIV-infected persons who are able to demonstrate that they have become infected through no fault of their own would be eligible to receive monies from this fund. A decision would also be taken to extend the psychosocial support system in order to relieve the adverse psychological consequences of HIV for the individual. Provision would be made for sanctions to combat discrimination and ostracism as a result of AIDS or HIV.

The underlying principle is that all measures are specifically geared to AIDS. It is the express intention that this approach must not set a precedent for the approach to other communicable diseases.

9.3.3 Commentary on AIDS control strategies

In a commentary on Strategies I and II it is useful to draw a distinction between (1) the need and the return in an epidemiological and preventive sense, and (2) the consequences, desirability and permissibility from a social and legal point of view. We shall compare the two strategies on the basis of this distinction.

9.3.3.1 Epidemiology and prevention

Both strategies are based on the epidemiological course outlined in the reference scenario, and both assume that it is possible to arrive at a situation in which there is no longer any significant incidence of HIV. The usefulness of and need for epidemiological research and HIV/AIDS prevention are not disputed here.

The Self-regulation strategy will have achieved its aims if it becomes apparent that the present HIV/AIDS prevention programme is largely effective, and is thus able to demonstrate that a control strategy based on personal responsibility of the individual is possible. The AIDS control programme will then act as an example for the approach to sexually transmitted diseases in general.

For the moment, it is not possible to make any definite statements on these matters, since the effects of a prevention strategy are difficult to determine. Moreover, few effect-evaluations are known which allow a comparison between different prevention strategies, and it is only recently that the first publications have appeared detailing the development of a methodology focused on programme evaluation in HIV/AIDS prevention (Coyle, et al., 1991; Kaemingk and Sechrest (eds.), 1990; Levington et al., (eds), 1990.

The elements of the control strategies which cover HIV/AIDS prevention differ as regards integration with and linking to the public information campaigns on STDs and other health hazards. Where choices have to be made, the arguments put forward in Chapter 7 may play a role: it was stated there that a direct link between information activities can contribute to the control of STDs and HIV/-AIDS.

An integral element of Strategy II is a compulsory HIV-test in certain, well-defined situations. Set against the goal envisaged by such a compulsory HIV-test, however, there are many indications that this is a counter-productive strategy. The history of STD control can be held up as an example; this shows that compulsory measures, even where antibiotics are available, have made no positive contribution to the control of venereal diseases (Brandt, 1987; Paalman, 1986). In the case of AIDS, too, only contra-indications are available regarding compulsory testing. Thus, for example, an experiment in Illinois involving a compulsory premarital HIV test failed, while the test-promoting policy pursued in Sweden appears not to produce a reliable picture of the seroprevalence, particularly among gay men, who in general are strongly opposed to the test-promoting policy. The main consequence of a compulsory test appears to be that there is a large-scale attempt to avoid examination (Kelly and Turnock, 1989; Henrikson, 1988; Bottinger, 1989). As regards the use of the HIV-test on travellers, Canadian research points to low cost-effectiveness of a mandatory test for HIV among immigrants (Gilmore, 1991, personal communication). The Detection strategy, therefore, can be evaluated as ineffective.

The present AIDS control programme in the Netherlands is based on the Self-regulation strategy. A choice has been made for "epidemiological research on a voluntary basis" in "frontline groups situations" such as STD-outpatient clinics, for socio-sexological research into risk behaviour, sociopsychological research into behavioural changes and evaluations of the effects of public information (Dutch Lower House, 1990). It is not possible to make a definitive statement about the productivity of a strategy in which the testing policy is based entirely on a voluntary response; an important factor here will be the degree to which there is a refusal to participate in research, and what distortion of the course of HIV results from this. In the case of the Self-regulation strategy, then, it may be that the AIDS control programme fails to obtain an up-to-date picture of the course of HIV. In this connection, epidemiologists consider that the lack of a rational basis based on epidemiological data is undesirable and has a highly detrimental effect on the AIDS control effort (Coutinho, 1989; Huisman, 1989; Lumeij, 1989; Valkenburg, 1990). They refer here among other things to the results of anonymous unlinked research into HIV infections carried out in the United States and the United Kingdom (Coutinho, 1990; Ades et al., 1991; Tappin et al., 1991).

9.3.3.2 AIDS and the Dutch context

Kapilla (1990) and Moerkerk (1990) characterize the Dutch prevention strategy in an international context as rational and pragmatic, with a great deal of attention for the potential social impact of the strategy selected, and the high degree of involvement and influence of pressure groups, who determine an AIDS strategy jointly with the government and others concerned. Schnabel (1989) characterizes the Dutch policy on AIDS as "first and foremost Dutch in character, whilst also being applicable to AIDS". This "Dutch character" can be seen in the great reticence of the government to involve itself in the private lives of citizens, the commitment to achieving a jointly-formulated AIDS control strategy and the choice of a strategy which as far as possible rules out compulsion, ostracism and social isolation. With respect to AIDS, this is expressed in a high priority being given to individual liberties and the reflection of this priority in the testing policy, the efforts of the AIDS information campaign, which are geared to the creation and maintenance of public acceptance of the AIDS epidemic, and the attention given to safeguarding access for people with AIDS to social facilities. The Detection strategy is diametrically opposed to this socio-cultural framework of the AIDS control programme.

9.3.3.3 Testing policy/access to social facilities

There is a world of difference between the two strategies with respect to the testing policy and the measures relating to access to social facilities. If the two strategies are weighed against what is considered desirable, feasible and permissible from a social and legal/ethical point of view, then it becomes apparent that a good deal of the Detection strategy is diametrically opposed to the response to AIDS to date, the key elements of which, as described in some detail in Chapter 4, are the importance of the right to privacy and self-determination. Deviation from this approach is only possible in exceptional circumstances and on the basis of legislative rules. This means, for example, that an HIV-test is only possible during the course of epidemiological research if the consent requirement and the information obligation are met, and if the right to protection of the integrity of the individual is taken into account. A weighing-up process which leads to the establishment of a Detection strategy would therefore imply that there had to be decisive reasons for such a change in strategy. The fact that HIV is not transmissible through normal social contact, the great psychological burden for the individual of a positive HIV-test, the potential consequences of HIV infection for access to social facilities and the suspicion that HIV has not spread to any large extent amongst the Dutch population, all weigh against the introduction of a Detection strategy. The possibility of such a strategy being chosen can therefore be regarded as ruled out, given the Dutch legal/ethical viewpoint and the lack of decisive reasons for deviating from this view.

The Self-regulation strategy is in line with the present legal/-ethical framework of the Dutch AIDS control programme. In contrast to the present situation, it has been assumed that the insurance problem has been solved, and that self-regulation is not sufficient in the case of medicals for applying employees. As far as insurance is concerned, this means that agreement must be reached as to what should be understood to be a "realistic level of need, matching the social circumstances". With respect to medicals for applying employees this would mean that the guidelines for such medicals have in practice not led to a change in the practice of such medicals as described in Chapter 4, i.e. not meeting official guidelines.

9.4 Strategies related to the organization of care

9.4.1 Strategy I: Regular care

Topology
The underlying principle in this scenario is to reduce the extra attention given to support in cases of AIDS, to abolish special measures, and to make the initiatives geared specifically to AIDS support more general in nature. General infection control is considered sufficient in this scenario to combat the transmission of HIV in a professional care situation.

9.4.1.1 Development of Regular care strategy

The underlying principle is that the care and support of people with AIDS and HIV should take place entirely within the existing system of health care facilities. This would mean that assistance and service is available to people with HIV and AIDS in every hospital, from every general practitioner, in every district nursing and home help organization, at every RIAGG and in every social services institution. Additionally, the care and assistance offered to hard-drug users could be linked to organizations dealing with drug dependency.

This approach is based in part on the expectation that developments in biomedical research and the treatment of people with HIV and AIDS will progress less rapidly than in the past. There is also a conviction that systematic, planned dissemination of expertise and experience has led to a high level of knowledge concerning the treatment, support and relief of people with HIV and AIDS. A number of initiatives in the care and support of these persons will become a permanent feature of the regular health care sector. The range of care facilities will be expanded by the addition of emotional and practical peer support. The buddy projects broaden out to become support projects in a more general sense, being directed not only at people with AIDS, but at all persons with chronic diseases.

As far as the care provision itself is concerned, it is felt that the care of people with AIDS does not have to be seen as a special issue. The infection control measures taken to avoid transmission of HIV in a professional situation are considered adequate, and will in time reassure care-providers. The special attention given to the psychosocial burden of caring for people with AIDS would in this scenario also need to shift to attention for the burden presented by caring for terminally-ill young people. There is a recognition of the fact that prejudices about homosexuality, drug-use and prostitution can play a role in the provision of care. Initiatives designed to avoid the adverse effects of such prejudices, however, are seen as separate from initiatives in the care of people with AIDS.

9.4.2 Strategy II: AIDS-specific care

Topology
In the care of people with HIV and AIDS, the care of the latter is found to be so complex that a separate system of care facilities is considered necessary. Specially trained and selected personnel work within this AIDS-specific system providing relief, care and support to AIDS patients. The establishment of this AIDS-specific system is also seen as a way of countering the worries concerning the transmission of HIV in a professional situation.

9.4.2.1 Development of AIDS-specific care strategy

The underlying principle of the care is that the problems of caring for people with HIV and AIDS justify the creation of a specific organization. The effective, cost-efficient treatment of the disease symptoms of AIDS demand great experience and expertise, and the regional hospital centres are therefore given a permanent rather than a temporary status. In addition, the combination of drug-dependency treatment and the care and support of HIV-infected IDUs justify special care arrangements. There is also a feeling that a special approach is indicated for gay men. The support offered by RIAGGs does not match the needs of gay men who are infected with HIV.

In order to combat the fear of infection and burn-out among personnel providing treatment, it has been decided that the care for people with AIDS and HIV should be provided by specially trained personnel in both inpatient and outpatient care situations. For outpatient care, this leads to the emergence of general practitioners, district nursing staff and home help staff specializing in AIDS. The buddy help and support projects for IDUs continue to be geared specifically to the support of people with AIDS. There is a new initiative in the form of so-called Integrated AIDS Centres, where knowledge and expertise on AIDS-related care and information are pooled. These centres also have a function in the psychosocial support of AIDS care-providers, and each centre has an AIDS information line open to the general public.

9.4.3 Commentary on care strategies

The need for high quality care and support of people with HIV and AIDS in the Netherlands, with every demand for care being met, is not questioned, and we have assumed that this will continue to be the case in the future.

To date, the care and support have been provided as far as possible within the existing circuit of health care facilities. The setting up on an AIDS-specific system or special AIDS hospitals has never been considered. Many elements of an AIDS-specific care-provision strategy deviate from this underlying principle as regards the organization of care. The Regular care strategy fits in with the present strategy, and carries forward a number of developments.

There is no question of opting for one of the two strategies. Chapter 8 characterized the care of people with HIV and AIDS as unchangingly complex, and pointed to the need for specialist treatment of people with AIDS. Moreover, the lack of clarity concerning the possibilities and effects of early treatment lead to the assumption that there can be no question of reduced attention or spreading of the inpatient care of people with HIV and AIDS. Instead, we shall conclude by listing a few points for consideration in a reappraisal of the present strategy:

- At present, the recent emergence of AIDS, the seriousness of the disease, the burden for the patient, his or her environment and the care providers, and the rapid development and changes in care and research, are all reasons for devoting extra attention to AIDS (NCAB, 1991). How, and on what basis, is it possible to establish that the extra attention for AIDS can be reduced?
- The extra attention for AIDS may be significant for the health care sector as a whole. It is important in this respect to determine how positive experiences in the area of national and regional collaboration, continuity of care, and the linking of voluntary work and professional care, can be applied within the health care sector in general (NCAB, 1991). Possibilities for new care initiatives in connection with AIDS, and in accordance with the Regular care strategy, may include a broadening of the concept of buddy support. The question to be answered is for what other diseases and disorders practical and emotional support by volunteers is desirable and feasible.

- The Regular care strategy makes no statement about psychosocial support geared specifically to gay men, or a number of initiatives for IDUs with HIV infection, such as a support project. A relevant consideration in this strategy appears to be whether, and if so in what way, regular organizations are able to provide high quality psychosocial care and support to gay men, hard-drug users and those close to them (De Rijk and Van den Boom, 1989).
- Apart from developments in care itself, expectations with regard to epidemiology naturally influence the planning of care facilities. A great many care initiatives in the past have been inspired by expectations of an explosive increase in the number of people with AIDS. The fact that prognoses of the *growth* in the number of people with AIDS are less sombre than five years ago may lead to changes in the planning and organization of care.
- It is relevant to ask how necessary it is to disseminate the knowledge and experience gained in the care and support of AIDS throughout all health care organizations if expansion, modification and support of the present, concentrated care facilities mean that it is also possible to meet the demand for care. In other words, what role can Integrated AIDS Centres play within a strategy which on the one hand acknowledges the complexity of AIDS care and on the other hand seeks to organize the direct care provision as far as possible within a non-specialized system of health care facilities?

9.5 General commentary

Chapter 2 makes a broad distinction between three control strategies: (1) a "laissez-faire" strategy, (2) a provision strategy and (3) an integral AIDS-specific control strategy. The policy in a laissez-faire strategy is to take measures only in crisis situations. This must be based on the expectation that AIDS is not a problem in an epidemiological, economic or social sense. The policy in a provision strategy is to take measures in the area of controlling transmission, care and research. The underlying principle of Strategy 2 is that there is no need for special AIDS-specific efforts. This contrasts with Strategy 3, where a need is perceived for specific efforts aimed at the control and care of AIDS. This strategy also includes measures geared specifically to the social impact of AIDS.

The Policy Document on AIDS published by State Secretary Dees in 1987 can be seen as a strategic scenario, in which a choice has been made for an integral, AIDS-specific control strategy which is geared towards normalization and social integration. The justification for this policy is the potential threat of AIDS to public health, the specific nature of AIDS, specific problems of care and support, and concern regarding the reaction of society. The start of 1992 sees the establishment of the AIDS policy for the coming years. The new Policy Document on AIDS published by State Secretary Simons contains a reappraisal or evaluation of the 1987 Policy Document on AIDS.

Applied to our division into three strategic scenarios, one consideration here is whether the present integral AIDS-specific control strategy should be continued, or whether a shift in strategy or some parts of it in the direction of a provision strategy seems appropriate. The Self-regulation and Regular care provision strategies examine the choices which may then have to be made. Both scenarios give an impression of a situation in which AIDS continues to be a serious problem. Efforts in epidemiological research, public information, the promotion of behavioural change, the care given to people with AIDS, and access to social facilities, continue to be necessary. Given the seriousness, extent and uncertainty of the problem, there is no question of a shift in the direction of a laissez-faire strategy. The question here is whether an AIDS-specific strategy is necessary and, as a corollary to this question, in what respects the AIDS strategy sets an example for the approach to comparable problems. This is elaborated in the Self-regulation strategy by combining the abolition of information geared specifically to AIDS with changes in the information provided on STDs. In the Regular provision strategy, buddy projects geared to people with AIDS disappear and are replaced by general support projects. Both strategies, then, contain a double turning point; the question is whether this is possible and desirable.

This chapter describes with a good deal of certainty the social context which underlies the formulation of the AIDS control strategy applied in the Netherlands. An AIDS control strategy which fits in with the Dutch socio-cultural traditions and which takes account of the high regard for the right to privacy and self-determination, will be based on the personal responsibility of the individual, and will seek to maintain contact with HIV-infected persons and core groups. In this connection, it is important with regard to the transmission of HIV to determine to what extent the personal responsibility of the individual is also a societal responsibility. For the individual, conversely - be it gay man, hard-drug user or sex worker - it is important that he or she is approached as a responsible individual, not only in the context of AIDS control, but also within the framework of society in general. In the case of gay men, the Dutch approach has worked: in a short space of time a large-scale change in behaviour has taken place, partly through the initiatives and activities of pressure organizations set up by and on behalf of gay men. Whether the Dutch approach is equally successful for groups which are less integrated into and accepted by society, such as drug-users and commercial sex workers, appears at first sight to be less self-evident.

9.6 Summary

Four strategic scenarios have been developed in this chapter against the background of the response to AIDS thus far. Two scenario relate to diverging paths aimed at achieving particular goals in terms of AIDS control: a Self-regulation strategy and a contrasting Detection strategy. The other two scenarios relate to the organization of high quality care, and consist of a Regular care strategy and an AIDS-specific care strategy.

The AIDS control scenarios consist of strategies for epidemiological monitoring, HIV/AIDS prevention, testing policy and access to social facilities. The social context and legal framework of the AIDS control programme is emphatically linked with the development of AIDS control strategies. The Self-regulation strategy fits in with the present AIDS control programme, and contains the added assumption that the approach to AIDS can also be applied to the fight against other sexually transmitted diseases. The underlying principles of the AIDS control programme are changed in the Detection strategy. In addition to group-oriented information programmes, this strategy also entails intensive contact tracting and partner notification, a test-promoting policy and, where necessary, compulsory measures. In the commentaries on the control strategies, the Detection strategy is not considered either possible or desirable as an option for AIDS control in the Netherlands.

Strategies for the organization of care provision are developed in the care scenarios. The underlying principle in the Regular care strategy is that extra attention for the care of people with HIV and AIDS is no longer necessary, and that the care should be provided entirely within the existing system of health care facilities. In the AIDS-specific scenario, by contrast, the care is considered to be sufficiently complex to require separate facilities and care-providers specially trained in AIDS care. It is observed in the commentary that there is at this moment no question of a choice having to be made for one of the two strategies.

References

Ades, A.E., S. Parker, T. Berry, F.J. Holland, C.F. Davidson, D. Cubitt, M. Hjelm, A.H. Wilzox, C.N. Hudson, M. Briggs, R.S. Tedder, C.S. Peckham
Prevalence of maternal HIV-1 infection in Thames Regions: results from anoymous unlinked neonatal testing
Lancet, 337 (1991), 1562 - 1656

Bayer, R.
Public Health Policy and the AIDS epidemic; an end to HIV Exceptionalism?
New England Journal of Medicine, 324 (1991), 21, 1500-1504

Böttinger, M.
HIV epidemiology in Sweden
Presented at *V International Conference on AIDS*, Montreal, June 7, 1989

Brandt, A.M.
No Magic Bullet: a social history of venereal diseases in the United States since 1880
Oxford University Press, New York/Oxford, 1987

Coyle, S.L., R.F. Boruch, C.F. Turner (eds.)
Evaluating AIDS prevention programs; expanded edition
Washington DC, National Academy Press, 1991

Coutinho, R.A.,
Van pokken, syfilis en AIDS; geschiedenis van de infectieziektenbestrijding door de eeuwen heen
Drukkerij Bij, Amsterdam, 1989, inaugurele rede

Coutinho, R.A.,
Eerste resultaten van anonieme HIV-screening in de Verenigde Staten.
Nederlands Tijdschrift voor Geneeskunde, 134 (1990), 45, 2173 - 2175.

Gilmore, N.
personal communication, 1991

Henriksson, B.
Social Democracy or Societal Control; a critical analysis of the Swedish AIDS Policy
Glacio Bokförlag, Stockholm, 1988

Huisman, J.
Anoniem serologisch bevolkingsonderzoek op het vóórkomen van HIV-infektie: een noodzaak!
Tijdschrift voor Sociale Gezondheidszorg, 66 (1988), 301-302

Kaemingk, K., L. Sechrest (eds.)
Evaluation of AIDS-prevention and education programs
Evaluation and Program Planning, 13 (1990), 1, 1-107

Kapila, M.
The prevention of AIDS and other STDs: issues for policy makers
In: M. Paalman (ed.), *Promoting Safer Sex; prevention of sexual transmission of AIDS and other STD*, Swets & Zeitlinger, Amsterdam/Lisse, 1990, 233-244

Karamoustafa, A.
Sweden
In: S. Wayling (ed.), *Current status of HIV/AIDS Prevention and Control Policies in the European Region: 1990 update*, WHO, regional Office for Europe / Global Program on AIDS, Copenhagen, 1990, 145-155

Kelly, C.J, B. Turnock
Mandatory premarital HIV-antibody testing: a twelve month experience
Presented at *V International Conference on AIDS*, Montreal, June 7, 1989

Levington, L.C., A.M. Hegedus, A. Kubrin (eds.)
Evaluating AIDS Prevention: Contributions of Multiple Disciplines
New Directions for Program Evaluation, 1990, 46, 1-106

Lower House of the States General
- Nota inzake het AIDS-beleid
  Lower House of the States General, session 1987-1988, 19218, no. 8 (1987)
- Regeringsstandpunt inzake onderzoek naar de verspreiding van HIV-infectie in Nederland
  Lower House of the States General, session 1989-1990, 19218, no. 39

Lumey, L.H., H. Houweling, J.C. Jager
Noodzaak en mogelijkheden van prevalentie-onderzoek naar HIV-infectie in Nederland
Nederlands Tijdschrift voor Geneeskunde, 133 (1989), 923 - 927

Moerkerk, H.
AIDS prevention strategies in European Countries
In: M. Paalman (ed.), *Promoting Safer Sex; prevention of sexual transmission of AIDS and other STD*, May 1989 in The Netherlands, Swets & Zeitlinger, Amsterdam/Lisse, 1990, 61-75

Paalman, M.
AIDS: Welke lessen kunnen uit de SOA-bestrijding getrokken worden?.
SOA-bulletin 7 (1986), 1, 4-6

Schnabel, P.
De diepten van een epidemie: over de maatschappelijke gevolgen van AIDS
In: A. Noordhof-de Vries (red.). *AIDS; Een nieuwe verantwoordelijkheid voor gezondheidszorg en onderwijs*, Swets & Zeitlinger, Amsterdam/Lisse, 1989, 15-33

Tappin, D.M., R.W.A. Girdwood, E.A.C. Follett, R. Kennedy, A.J. Brown, F. Cockburn
Prevalence of maternal HIV infection in Scotland based on unlinked anonymous testing of newborn babies
Lancet, 337 (1991), 1565-1567

Valkenburg, H.A.
Epidemiologische aspecten
Lecture during the symposium *'Anonieme aspecten in verband met AIDS'*, Erasmus Universiteit, Rotterdam, 25-1-1990

10 Concluding remarks

10.1 Introduction

Chapters 6 to 9 explore the socio-cultural and economic impact of AIDS. In Chapter 6 the reference scenario plays a key role in these projections. Chapters 7, 8 and 9, against the background of the reference scenario, explore intervening developments in the areas of risk behaviour and the effects of prevention, the care and the choices to be made in the control and care strategies.

This concluding chapter reflects on a number of important findings from the various scenarios. We shall be guided by the following questions, which lie at the basis of this scenario project:

- What future course of the epidemic of the HIV and AIDS epidemic can be expected, what are the uncertainties and what implications does this have for the AIDS control programme?
- What burden will AIDS place on health care facilities, and what problems may be expected in the provision of care to people with HIV and AIDS?
- What social changes has AIDS brought about and, conversely, what will be the social context on which the response to AIDS will be based?

10.2 The epidemic of HIV infections and AIDS

In this scenario project, projections of developments in the epidemic form the starting point for the analysis of the impact of AIDS. Both a reference scenario and a subscenario were constructed; in the reference scenario we project the impact of AIDS if current developments remain unchanged, while the subscenario gives an impression of the consequences of HIV/AIDS which could be averted through preventive efforts. An important conclusion from the reference scenario is that the effects of AIDS will only become fully apparent in the second decade of the epidemic. This finding is drawn from the AIDS incidence figures, the patient-related costs and the mortality figures. The subscenario, in combination with the reference scenario, shows that a considerable proportion of the consequences of AIDS can still be averted through prevention and public information. Successful intervention would enable the growth in the incidence of AIDS in the medium term to be diverted in the direction of the subscenario. If the AIDS control programme fails in this attempt and developments take place as suggested by the epidemiological course emerging from the reference scenario, then the impact of the HIV/AIDS epidemic will remain considerable and their effect will continue to increase until well after the year 2000.

In addition, a comparison of the reference scenario with the subscenario shows that an equally sizeable proportion of the impact of AIDS is unavoidable given the present availability of treatment. Up to 1998, for example, the impact of AIDS for the care sector in the subscenario is larger than in 1990. The AIDS incidence figures from the subscenario are also illustrative in this connection, with an AIDS incidence being projected for 1995 which is of the same order as that in 1990, while in the year 2000 the incidence of AIDS will still be at the 1987 level. It can be concluded that control of the HIV epidemic at the start of the 1990s will not lead to a lessening of the extent of the impact of AIDS until the end of this decade. In this connection the reference scenario, which is based on the assumption of an HIV incidence of between 750 and 1000 per year, gives an impression of how far the AIDS control programme in the Netherlands has to go before achieving its goal of controlling the HIV/AIDS epidemic.

Together, the reference scenario and subscenario are a cause for sober reflection and lead us to underscore the following quotation from State Secretary Dees in the Policy Document on AIDS: "the fact that the AIDS prevention programmes will be a long-term endeavour is for me beyond doubt."
(p.8).

The commentary on the reference scenario also examines the assumed increase in growth in the incidence of AIDS and the developments in the HIV epidemic which form the basis of this growth. The possibility is considered that the reference scenario, in common with short-term predictions from the recent past, sketches a predominately sombre future projected end-situation, which in practice should be adjusted downwards. Such an experience-based fact could lead to an expected epidemiological course in which there is a greater levelling off of the HIV/AIDS epidemic than at present. In doing so more justice could be done to the successes achieved to date in HIV/AIDS prevention. After all, this has led in a short time to a high level of knowledge about AIDS and to a large-scale change in behaviour among the most seriously affected group, namely men who have sex with male partners. In expressing an expectation of a levelling off of the AIDS epidemic, however, we are primarily defining a situation which is desirable for the future. Although the baseline analysis and the reconstruction of the AID/HIV epidemic contain indications that a first step has been taken on the path to control of the AIDS epidemic, they also show the points on which AIDS remains an undiminished problem and the conditions which must be met in order to be able to speak of successes in AIDS control. This led us to construct a restrained reference scenario, in which we have incorporated the uncertainty concerning developments in the epidemic.

Part of this uncertainty results from a lack of key data, which meant that assumptions had to be made in the reference scenario regarding essential matters such as seroprevalence, infectiousness and the incubation period. By consulting with experts we have attempted as far as possible to remove the existing uncertainties, but we are aware that we have only partially succeeded in this endeavour. In this sense, the reference scenario also forms a plea for further research into the epidemiological course of HIV, infectiousness and the factors which influence progression to AIDS.

Other causes of uncertainty are related to the dynamics of a communicable disease, with behaviour as the key determinant. We have shown in the behavioural scenarios what effect changes in risk behaviour or in the effectiveness of prevention can have for the prevalence of HIV. We have opted for an approach based on a differentiation into groups: men with multiple male partners, injecting drug users (IDUs), males and females with multiple heterosexual partners, commercial sex workers and their clients. As well as developments in the HIV epidemic within risk groups which are unpredictable in the sense that they cannot be localized precisely in time, and yet which cannot be ruled out, attention has also been focused on the spread of HIV between core groups. Among other things we have given attention to the transmission of HIV to the non-injecting drug using sexual partners of IDUs and the transmission of HIV within the sex industry.

To some extent, the behavioural scenarios represent a *refining* of the reference scenario since, in contrast to the reference scenario, the behaviour which forms the basis of HIV transmission is the key factor. The consequences of *intervening* developments have also been explored to some extent, including a relapse into risk behaviour by men who have sex with men or a substantial spread of HIV among the general heterosexual population.

The most important indication from the behavioural scenarios is that there is *no reason for optimism* concerning the future spread of HIV. A large number of new HIV infections is possible in a relatively short time-frame. As a result, the behavioural scenarios are first and foremost a plea for *continued efforts* in the AIDS information campaign and the promotion of behavioural change. With respect to men who have sex with men, IDUs and the sex industry, the scenarios show that there is an *acute need* for protective measures during high-risk contacts in order to achieve control of the spread of HIV. A choice for the heterosexual population as a whole is whether to link the warnings about the risk of HIV infection to the provision of information about other sexually transmitted diseases (STDs). The recently observed increase in STDs among the heterosexual population demonstrates that continued attention for the primary prevention of sexually transmitted diseases is called for.

In this way the behavioural scenarios underpin the cautiously formulated reference scenario, since developments which cannot be ruled out, such as a mass relapse into risk behaviour or the spread of HIV to groups which have as yet not been affected on a large scale, could lead to an epidemiological course which exceeds the incidence of HIV/AIDS described in the reference scenario.

This clear, if somewhat cautiously formulated conclusion, is inspired partly by the potential extent of the HIV epidemic, and the awareness of the large number of transmission routes, which we have explored only partially in a large number of projections. Reference has been made at various points in the baseline analysis to the wide range of factors affecting the incidence of HIV, such as the introduction of HIV-2 in the Netherlands, the large-scale introduction of HIV among ethnic minorities, or the influence of "Europe 1992" and developments in countries of Central and Eastern Europe which may lead to an increase in mobility. The lack of research data, the need to make a selection from possible topics for scenario analysis, and the time we had at our disposal for the scenario projects are the reasons that these important effects are not incorporated in the scenario analysis.

A second reason for these conclusions which, despite these reservations, should be taken seriously, is also apparent in the reference scenario, namely the lack of information about the current situation in the HIV epidemic, the underlying risk behaviour and the effectiveness of prevention, all of which are essential for scenario analysis. At the moment there is insufficient knowledge in the Netherlands regarding seroprevalence outside a number of selected groups. Moreover, the data on the effectiveness of the HIV/AIDS prevention programme are inadequate and there is still insufficient understanding of the prevention of risk behaviour and of the networks within which HIV can spread. In the elaboration of the behavioural scenarios, the lack of empirical data for scenario analysis was most apparent in the future projections in the spread of HIV among IDUs. For other groups too, however, a high level of simulation was sometimes necessary, because the group size, seroprevalence, risk behaviour and effectiveness of prevention could not be established with certainty. It remains to be seen what deviations from the reference scenario and the behavioural scenarios will result from this lack of insight into the (determinants of) HIV infection. A higher incidence than that portrayed in the reference scenario may result from the projected intervening developments. Conversely, various developments are possible which could lead to a lower HIV incidence, such as increased effectiveness of prevention, the elimination of behavioural relapse, or the incorporation of the need for protection against HIV infection (and STDs) during sexual contact. Only in a situation where "a natural levelling off and dying out of the HIV/AIDS epidemic" can be expected, can the AIDS control programme be considered to be relieved of the obligation of mounting continued efforts in HIV/AIDS prevention in an attempt to keep the spread of HIV/AIDS to a minimum.

10.3 Care of people with AIDS and HIV

An essential element in the scenario analysis was the linking of the various projected epidemiological courses to the burden on health care facilities and the costs of providing those facilities. One of the most important conclusions emerging from the reference scenario was that the impact of HIV/AIDS will only become fully apparent within the health care sector in the second decade of the epidemic. In fact, the reference scenario suggests that the demand for care and the patient-related costs of AIDS in the second decade may rise to five times their level in 1988. Moreover, the subscenario shows that the developments in the HIV epidemic up to 1.1.1989 mean that the costs of AIDS up to the year 2000 will turn out to be higher than in 1988. The cost increase in the reference scenario is due entirely to developments in patient-related costs, which increase from NLG 18 million in 1988 to NLG 93 million in the year 2000. This delayed action or, to put it another way, medium-term effect, is caused by the long incubation period of HIV.

The true burden on health care facilities will depend to a great extent on developments in the incidence of AIDS/HIV. Calculations in the context of the reference scenario, for example, show that the avoidance of or failure to develop, HIV infection could lead to a reduction in the patient-related costs to 60% of NLG 93 million. In addition, advances in the diagnosis and treatment of HIV and AIDS-related complaints will also have an effect on the consequences for the health care sector. Changes in patterns up to the year 2000, which to some extent have already begun, could lead to an increase in the survival period of people with AIDS, the substitution of care, or the intensification of home care. Summarized briefly, this scenario amounts to the projection of a situation where the emphasis lies on shifts in the care package. An increased proportion of care will be provided outside hospitals, although the burden on in-hospital facilities will also increase as a result of the extended survival period. A reduction in the burden on in-hospital care will only take place in the event of a future development in which the effects of early intervention postpone the diagnosis of AIDS. However, this effect, which we project in the scenario on the impact of early intervention, is somewhat artificial in the sense that the consequences of AIDS for in-hospital care are simply postponed until after the year 2000. Equally, there is no question of a reduction in the burden on the care system, since early intervention leads to an increase in the burden on out-patient care.

One thing which all care scenarios have in common as regards health care, is that the increased life-expectancy and the delay of the onset of illness will entail an increase in costs. Set against existing capacity and current budgets for health care facilities, the reference scenario suggests a considerable (and increasing) but manageable burden on facilities. The care scenarios do not affect the essence of the conclusions drawn in the reference scenario. Although there is a suggestion of significant developments up to the year 2000, seen from the perspective of gains in terms of health and life, as well as from an economic standpoint, there will be only *relatively modest changes* with respect to the reference scenario.

The above conclusion is supported by conclusions and considerations arising from the care scenarios. Thus, for example, the care scenarios highlight the problems which may arise as a result of the expected increase in demand for out-of-hospital care and volunteers, the extra pressure on the informal support network and the matching of the care to need through substitution and increasing the length of care. As regards the content of the care, the assumption must be that the present situation will continue unchanged in the coming decades, namely expensive and complex care for people with AIDS which, just as at present, justifies additional concern and resources. At most, as suggested in the strategic care scenario, we can say that considerations may arise which will play a role if a different organization or set-up of the care appears appropriate in the medium or long term.

As a corollary to this, reference must also be made to the unchanging problem in the relationship between care-provider and HIV-infected persons, and the emotional burden placed on care-providers and those close to them, coupled with the care and support of young people suffering from a terminal illness. These matters, which were areas of concern in the 1980s, apply equally for the 1990s.

In any discussion of care, the person with AIDS him or herself naturally demands the greatest attention. A deliberate choice was made not to develop vaccine or therapy scenarios. An increase in the average survival period after diagnosis of AIDS to three years appears to be most in line with current expectations. For the person with AIDS, however, this means an unchangingly bleak future prospect: an expected increase of one year in the survival period is after all no more than a drop in the ocean.

AIDS has been approached in this report as an incurable disease, which even in our most positive scenario can only lead to a situation in which AIDS becomes a chronic disorder with an average survival period after diagnosis of AIDS of fifteen years. Insofar as this scenario is applicable, however, it relates to the period after the year 2000. Until that time, the quality of life for the person with AIDS will continue to be linked to the quality of the care for a terminally ill person.

10.4 The social context of AIDS

The fear of an uncontrollable spread of AIDS among the Dutch population appears to have ebbed away in the Netherlands. In contrast to the situation ten years ago, no-one at the start of the second decade of the epidemic takes a doomsday scenario seriously, while developments in the incidence of AIDS are leading to speculations of a levelling off of the AIDS epidemic. The failure to materialize (for the present) of a substantial spread of HIV among the heterosexual population in general may also have contributed to a lessening of the fear of AIDS. There have also been successes in HIV/AIDS prevention, which has meant that the possibility of HIV infection has lost some of its surprise element.

The behavioural scenarios shows that AIDS continues to present a serious and undiminished threat to public health. As long as there is no incorporation of the need for protection against communicable diseases during multiple sexual contacts, there remains a certain risk of HIV infection. Reference must be made in this connection to the present-day core groups and to young people, who form the potential core groups of the future.

The reference scenario is based on the implicit assumption that the HIV/AIDS prevention programme will be increasingly effective through the 1990s. This may lead in the year 2000 to a reappraisal of sexual behaviour through the linking of HIV, sexual contact and health care protection. However, this suggests an end-situation which will not develop as a matter of course. In the commentary on the reference scenario we expressed doubts as to whether it would be possible to attain such an end-situation without an intensification of prevention efforts. In line with this, the behavioural scenario points out the need for continuing research into the effectiveness of the

AIDS-information programme.

The fear that AIDS would lead to negative reactions to or discrimination against *groups* which are socially vulnerable or not widely accepted has not been borne out in the Netherlands. Such a reaction would in fact amount to a socio-cultural revolution in a Dutch climate which is strongly oriented towards integration and which in an international context is characterized by tolerance. On the contrary, the baseline analysis has shown that *the avoidance of what are considered undesirable social consequences* of AIDS have been an important area of concern in the Netherlands. The HIV/AIDS prevention policy, which also had an explicit social goal, and the testing of the AIDS policy against the individual liberties which are so highly valued in the Netherlands bear witness to this. As a corollary to this, the discussion of the strategic scenarios makes it abundantly clear that radical changes in the social sphere are unlikely and are diametrically opposed to the present legal framework of the AIDS control programme in the Netherlands.

In spite of this, however, it is still possible that AIDS could lead to situations which are considered socially undesirable, and it should be remembered that access to social facilities such as insurance are still under pressure. Equally, it is by no means certain what the consequences will be of a situation - which is feasible on the basis of the reference scenario - in which the perception of AIDS shifts from that of an unknown disease which poses a threat to public health, to become "a" communicable disease which is concentrated within a small section of society.

10.5 Conclusion

AIDS will undoubtedly continue to be a problem for the HIV/AIDS prevention programme, public health and society in general right up to the year 2000, and possibly for a long time thereafter. As a result, it may be that this report covers only the start of the period in which the consequences of AIDS will be apparent. From the reconstruction of the first decade and the projection of the second, it is above all apparent that the problems posed by AIDS remain largely unchanged and are likely to remain so until the year 2000. Infection with HIV is and for the present continues to be preventable only through protection or abstinence from high-risk contacts; AIDS itself continues for the present to be a incurable, fatal illness. However, changes are also taking place in the approach to the AIDS situation and expectations concerning the impact of AIDS. The first decade was initially characterized by questions about and confusion over the potential scale of the AIDS crisis, resulting in the setting up of the AIDS control programme and first attempts to curb the impact of AIDS. Building on this, the second decade will undoubtedly see moves towards the identification of strategies designed to lead to control of the impact of AIDS. This second phase in the AIDS control programme is likely to be characterized by efforts which ultimately lead to consolidation and extension of the successes achieved to date in HIV/AIDS prevention and the care and support of people with AIDS and HIV. In epidemiological terms, this could lead to a situation typified by small-scale outbreaks of HIV, which do not lead to a substantial spread of HIV. From a societal perspective, a natural solidarity with people with AIDS and HIV could arise, alongside a reaction to AIDS which is indistinguishable from the reaction to other communicable and/or incurable diseases.

In giving this outline of the contours of a projected end-situation, we are doing no more than identifying what for the moment appear to be the most important challenges for AIDS control up to the year 2000. Underlying the scenarios in this report is the view that there is a need for continued efforts in AIDS control. As long as AIDS continues to be a life-threatening disease and a potential threat to public health, this underlying principle would appear to be self-evident.

APPENDIX I

List of abbreviations

AIDS	Acquired Immune Deficiency Syndrome
AMC	Academic Medical Centre
AMW	Social Work
APHA	Department of Psychosocial Support for AIDS, J.A. Schorer Foundation
AZT	Azidothymidine Retrovir
AZU	University Hospital Utrecht
AZUA	University Hospital Amsterdam
BRR	Basic Reproduction Rate
CAD	Alcohol and Drugs Advisory Bureau
CaDH	Homosexuality Anti-Discrimination Centre
CBS	Central Bureau of Statistics
CDC	Centers for Disease Control
CD4+-cel	T-lymphocyte, T-helper cell
COTG	Central Council on Health Care Charges
CRM	Ministry of Culture, Recreation and Social Work
EC	European Community
EEC	European Economic Community
ELISA	Enzyme Linked Immunosorbent Assay
EUR	Erasmus University Rotterdam
FNJB	Netherlands Federation of Junkie Unions
FOZ	Financial Statement on Health Care
GGD	Municipal Medical Department
GG & GD	Municipal Medical & Health Department
GGZ	Mental Health Care
GHI	Chief Medical Officier of Health
GHW	Health Care Workers
GR	Health Council
GVO	Health Information and Education on Health
GW	Constitution
HIV	Human Immunodeficiency Virus
ICD	International Classification of Diseases
IOM/NAS	Institute of Medicine/National Academy of Sciences
IDU	Injecting Drug User
KPMG	Klynveld, Bosboom and Hegener Management Consultants
KNMG	Royal Dutch Medical Association
LADIS	National Alcohol and Drugs Information System
LAS	Lymphadenopathy Syndrome
LCA	National AIDS Coordination Team
LRC	London Rubber Company
MDHG	Medical Social Services for Heroin users
MIDAS	Modelling Incidence and Reporting Delay Adjustment Simultaneously

NATEC	National AIDS Therapy and Evaluation Centre
NCAB	National Commission for AIDS Control
NcGv	Netherlands Institute of Mental Health
NIAD	Netherlands Institute for Alcohol and Drugs
NIPG/TNO	Netherlands Institute for Preventive Health Care/Netherlands Organisation for Applied Scientific Research (TNO)
NISSO	Netherlands Institute of Sexological Health
NIVH-COC	Netherlands Association for the Integration of Homosexuality
NKV	National Home Nursing Association
NVC	Netherlands Association of Alcohol and Drug Consultation Bureaux
NVHP	Netherlands Association of Haemophilia Patients
NVSH	Netherlands Association for Sexual Reform
NZI	National Hospitals Institute
NZR	National Hospitals Council
PccAo	AIDS Research Programme Coordination Committee of the Health Research Council
PCP	Pneumociystis Carinii Pneumonia
PGL	Generalised Lymphadenopathy
PIGG	In-Hospital Mental Health Care Patient Register
PPTC	Pre and Post-Test Counselling
PYLL	Potential Years of Life Lost
RIAGG	Regional Institute for Ambulant Mental Health Care
RGO	Health Research Council
RIVM	National Institute of Public Health and Environmental Protection
RUG	State University of Groningen
RUL	State University of Leiden
RUU	State University of Utrecht
SAD	Ancillary Services Foundation
SCP	Social and Cultural Planning Office
SIG	Health Care Information Centre
SOA	Sexually Transmitted Disease(s) (STD)
SOA-stichting	Foundation for the Control of Sexually Transmitted Diseases
STG	Steering Committee on Future Health Scenarios
SZ	Slotervaart Hospital
TK	Lower House of the Dutch States General
UvA	University of Amsterdam
UN	United Nations
US	United States
VU	Free University of Amsterdam
WGBO	Medical Treatment Agreement Act
WHO	World Health Organisation
WPR	Data Protection Act
WVC	Ministry of Welfare, Health and Cultural Affairs

WvS	Criminal Code
YBRR	Yearly Basic Reproduction Rate
YECR	Yearly Effective Contact Rate

APPENDIX II

Experts consulted

P. Ansems	KPMG
E.W. Bergsma	NIPG/TNO
S. Biersteker	Foundation for the Control of STD
P.J.E. Bindels	GG & GD Amsterdam
C.A. Blom	SAD
Dr. J.C.C. Borleffs	AZU
Mrs. M. Bot	NIAD
Prof. R.A. Coutinho	GG & GD Amsterdam
Dr. J.T.M. Derks	NcGv
Dr. J.A.M. van Druten	Catholic University Nijmegen
M.G.M. Dijkgraaf	RIVM
C.J.M. van Eijk	NCAB
B.D.P. Eijrond, doctor	NCAB
R. de Graaf	NISSO
G.J.P. can Griensven	GG & GD Amsterdam
C. Hartgers	GG & GD Amsterdam
S.H. Heisterkamp	RIVM
H. Houweling	RIVM
W.M. de Jong	NCAB
L.C. de Kam	SAD
H. Laverman	NKV
R. Leidl	University of Maastricht
L.H. Lumey	RIVM
H.M. Mannaerts	National Home Nursing Association
Mrs. M.E.M. Paalman	STD Foundation
Th. Paulussen	National GVO Centre
M.J.J.C. Poos	RIVM
C.A. Postema	GHI
D.P. van Rooyen	Schorer Foundation
Dr. Th.G.M. Sandfort	State University of Utrecht
C. Smit	NVHP
Dr. C.J. Straver	NISSO
G.J. Tillemans	NCAB
Mrs. J. Vanwesenbeeck	NISSO
Mrs. A. Verster	GG & GD Amsterdam
C.C.M.C. Wiggers	NIPG/TNO
G.J. van Zessen	NISSO